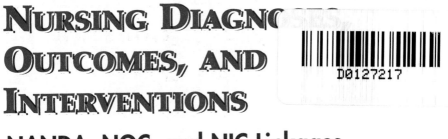

NURSING DIAGNOSES, OUTCOMES, AND INTERVENTIONS

NANDA, NOC, and NIC Linkages

Nursing Diagnoses, Outcomes, and Interventions

NANDA, NOC, and NIC Linkages

Editors

Marion Johnson, RN, PhD
Gloria Bulechek, RN, PhD, FAAN
Joanne McCloskey Dochterman, RN, PhD, FAAN
Meridean Maas, RN, PhD, FAAN
Sue Moorhead, RN, PhD

Center for Nursing Classification
University of Iowa
College of Nursing

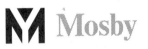

A Harcourt Health Sciences Company

St. Louis   London   Philadelphia   Sydney   Toronto

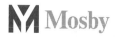

A Harcourt Health Sciences Company

Vice President/Nursing Editorial Director: *Sally Schrefer*
Executive Editor: *Barbara Nelson Cullen*
Associate Developmental Editor: *Stacy Welsh*
Project Manager: *John Rogers*
Project Specialist: *Betty Hazelwood*
Designer: *Kathi Gosche*

Mosby, Inc.
A Harcourt Health Sciences Company
11830 Westline Industrial Drive
St. Louis, MO 63146

Printed in the United States of America

International Standard Book Number 0-323-01212-4

00 01 02 03 04 GW/FF 9 8 7 6 5 4 3 2 1

PREFACE

This first edition of *Nursing Diagnoses, Outcomes, and Interventions: NANDA, NOC, and NIC Linkages* illustrates links among three of the standardized languages recognized by the American Nurses Association. These languages are the diagnoses developed by the North American Nursing Diagnosis Association (NANDA), the outcomes of the Nursing Outcomes Classification (NOC), and the interventions of the Nursing Interventions Classification (NIC). The provision of links among these classifications will facilitate the use of each of the languages in clinical practice and documentation systems as well as in education. The links also provide excellent opportunities for nurse researchers to explore the associations among diagnoses, outcomes, and interventions in conjunction with patient and organizational characteristics that might influence outcome achievement.

The first part of the book provides an introduction to the NANDA, NOC, NIC links that are presented in Part II. A brief description of the three languages, including their development and current status, is provided. This orients users who are unfamiliar with one or more of the languages to the structure of each of the languages and provides references for learning more about each of the languages. The method used to develop the linkages is described, and issues relevant to the use of the linkage work are identified. The linkages were developed at the University of Iowa by the researchers who developed the NIC and NOC classifications. The links are based on expert opinion and in some instances nursing literature. Because the links are not drawn from clinical practice or research, they are not presented as prescriptive and must be tested in the clinical setting. The last chapter in Part I describes the use of the links in care planning, electronic information systems, nursing education, and nursing research. A number of case studies are provided to illustrate the use of the links. The authors thank the students in the RN-BSN program whose case studies are presented here.

The major portion of the book is devoted to the links among the three languages. Entry to the links is through the NANDA diagnoses. The diagnoses are listed alphabetically with two exceptions: (1) all of the risk diagnoses appear in one section at the end of the linkages; and (2) the major concept, for example *thermoregulation,* has been used in the alphabetical listing rather than the modifier *ineffective.* Suggested NOC outcomes are linked to each of the diagnoses, and NIC interventions are linked to each of the NOC outcomes. Definitions are provided for each of the NANDA diagnoses in the linkage work, and definitions for the NOC outcomes and the NIC interventions are found in the appendixes.

This linkage work does not attempt to link the taxonomic structures of each of the languages. However, the links will provide language developers and users the opportunity to evaluate the similarities and dissimilarities among the languages, to suggest modifications in the links, and to evaluate the work put forth in this book. The authors appreciate all feedback from users concerning missing elements or links that are not used in the practice situation.

Marion Johnson

CONTENTS

PART I

Languages and Applications

CHAPTER 1

The Languages

For several years, the need for uniform or standardized nursing languages (SNL) has been discussed in nursing literature (Jones, 1997; Keenan & Aquilino, 1998; Maas, 1985; McCloskey & Bulechek, 1994; McCormick, 1991; and Zielstorff, 1994). A uniform nursing language serves several purposes, including the following:

- Provides a language for nurses to communicate what they do among themselves, with other health care professionals, and with the public
- Allows the collection and analysis of information documenting nursing's contribution to patient care
- Facilitates the evaluation and improvement of nursing care
- Fosters the development of nursing knowledge
- Allows for the development of electronic clinical information systems and the electronic patient record
- Provides information for the formulation of organizational and public policy concerning health and nursing care
- Facilitates teaching clinical decision making to nursing students

The contribution of standardized languages to the practice and development of nursing has been described in detail in the articles cited above as well as in the books describing the Nursing Interventions Classification (McCloskey & Bulechek, 1992, 1996, 2000) and the Nursing Outcomes Classification (Johnson & Maas, 1997; Johnson, Maas, & Moorhead, 2000).

This book illustrates linkages between three of the standardized languages recognized by the American Nurses Association (ANA): the diagnoses developed by the North American Nursing Diagnosis Association (NANDA), the interventions of the Nursing Interventions Classification (NIC), and the outcomes of the Nursing Outcomes Classification (NOC). The provision of links between these classifications is a major step forward in facilitating the use of these languages in practice, education, and research. For those unfamiliar with the languages, a brief overview of each classification follows.

NANDA

The use of standardized nursing language began in the 1970s with the development of NANDA's diagnostic classification. Professional recognition of nursing diagnoses came in 1980 when the ANA published *Nursing: A Social Policy Statement*, which stated that "nursing is the diagnosis and treatment of human

3

responses to actual or potential health problems" (American Nurses Association, 1980, p. 9). The 1995 update retains this statement and further elaborates that "Diagnoses facilitate communication among health care providers and the recipients of care and provide for initial direction in the choice of treatments and subsequent evaluation of the outcomes of care" (American Nurses Association, 1995, p. 9).

A nursing diagnosis is "a clinical judgment about individual, family or community responses to actual or potential health problems/life processes. Nursing diagnoses provide the basis for selection of nursing interventions to achieve outcomes for which the nurse is accountable" (North American Nursing Diagnosis Association, 1999, p. 149). Nursing diagnoses in NANDA are consistent with the above definition, being both actual and potential (is at risk for development). The elements of an actual NANDA diagnosis are the label, the definition of the diagnosis, the defining characteristics (signs and symptoms), and related factors (causative or associated factors), as illustrated in Table 1-1. The elements of a potential diagnosis as defined by NANDA are the label, the definition, and associated risk factors.

NANDA was formed in 1973 when a group of nurses met in St. Louis, Missouri, and organized the first National Conference Group for the Classification of Nursing Diagnoses (North American Nursing Diagnosis Association, 1999). The first conferences were invitational and included work sessions where the participants developed, reviewed, and grouped diagnoses based on their expertise and experience. By 1982 an alphabetical list of 50 nursing diagnoses had been developed and accepted for clinical testing, and the conferences were opened to the nursing community. Taxonomy development began at the third conference, and the first taxonomy was accepted at the seventh conference. Taxonomy I includes the following nine patterns that comprise the domains: Exchanging, Communicating, Relating, Valuing, Choosing, Moving, Perceiving, Knowing, and Feeling. Currently, a revised taxonomy with a multiaxial framework, Taxonomy II, has been proposed, but not approved, by the NANDA board. The work of NANDA is published every other year; the 1999-2000 edition of the NANDA classification includes 140 nursing diagnoses (North American Nursing Diagnosis Association, 1999). Methods for validation of diagnoses have been developed (Fehring, 1986; Parker & Lunney, 1998; Hoskins, 1997; and Whitley, 1999), and validation studies have become a major part of the biannual conferences. Research studies and application articles also appear in the NANDA journal *Nursing Diagnosis*, which was renamed *Nursing Diagnosis: The Journal of Nursing Language and Classification* in 1999.

A collaborative agreement for a joint venture between a research team at the University of Iowa College of Nursing and NANDA was reached to extend the NANDA work. The goal is to improve the comprehensiveness, scope, and clinical usefulness of the NANDA classification (Craft-Rosenberg & Delaney, 1997). This team submitted a number of refined diagnoses and new diagnoses for discussion at the 1998 NANDA conference. The 1999-2000 edition of the NANDA classification (North American Nursing Diagnosis Association, 1999) includes a portion of these updates and the conference proceedings describe the Nursing Diagnosis Extension and Classification (NDEC) work in full.

NANDA terminology has been translated into nine languages and is used in more than 20 countries throughout the world. NANDA celebrated its 25th anniversary in 1998. The organization that began with the varied oral and written speech of nurses in 1973 has evolved to develop a formalized, coded nursing

TABLE 1-1 ONE EXAMPLE OF A **NANDA** DIAGNOSIS

Anxiety

Definition: A vague uneasy feeling of discomfort or dread accompanied by an autonomic response; the source is often nonspecific or unknown to the individual; a feeling of apprehension caused by anticipation of danger. It is an altering signal that warns of impending danger and enables the individual to take measures to deal with threat.

DEFINING CHARACTERISTICS

Behavioral	Diminished productivity; scanning and vigilance; poor eye contact; restlessness; glancing about; extraneous movement (e.g., foot shuffling, hand/arm movements); expressed concerns due to change in life events; insomnia; fidgeting
Affective	Regretful; irritability; anguish; scared; jittery; overexcited; painful and persistent increased helplessness; rattled; uncertainty; increased wariness; focus on self; feelings of inadequacy; fearful; distressed; apprehension; anxious
Physiological	Voice quivering **Objective:** Trembling/hand tremors; insomnia **Subjective:** Shakiness; worried; regretful **Physiological:** Increased respiration (sympathetic); urinary urgency (parasympathetic); increased pulse (sympathetic); pulse dilation (sympathetic); increased reflexes (sympathetic); abdominal pain (parasympathetic); sleep disturbance (parasympathetic); tingling in extremities (parasympathetic); increased tension; cardiovascular excitation (sympathetic); increased perspiration; facial tension; anorexia (sympathetic); heart pounding (sympathetic); diarrhea (parasympathetic); urinary hesitancy (parasympathetic); fatigue (parasympathetic); dry mouth (sympathetic); weakness (sympathetic); decreased pulse (parasympathetic); facial flushing (sympathetic); superficial vasoconstriction (sympathetic); twitching (sympathetic); decreased blood pressure (parasympathetic); nausea (parasympathetic); urinary frequency (parasympathetic); faintness (parasympathetic); respiratory difficulties (sympathetic); increased blood pressure (sympathetic)
Cognitive	Blocking of thought; confusion; preoccupation; forgetfulness; rumination; impaired attention; decreased perceptual field; fear of unspecific consequences; tendency to blame others; difficulty concentrating; diminished ability to problem solve; diminished learning ability; awareness of physiological symptoms

RELATED FACTORS

Exposure to toxins; threat to or change in role status; related to unconscious conflict about essential goals and values of life; familial association/heredity; unmet needs; interpersonal transmission/contagion; situational/maturational crises; threat of death; threat to or change in health status; threat to or change in interaction patterns; threat to or change in role function; threat to self-concept; unconscious conflict about essential values/goals of life; threat to or change in environment; stress; threat to change in economic status; substance abuse

From North American Nursing Diagnosis Association. (1999). *Nursing diagnoses: Definitions & classification 1999-2000.* Philadelphia: Author.

diagnosis vocabulary; to verify the vocabulary with research; and to ensure that the language is ready for inclusion in the computerized patient record of the future. The NANDA Taxonomy I has been mapped into the World Health Organization (WHO) International Classification of Diseases, Injuries, and Causes of Death (ICD) code (Fitzpatrick, 1998).

NIC

Research to develop a vocabulary and classification of nursing interventions began in 1987 with the formation of a research team led by Joanne McCloskey and Gloria Bulechek at the University of Iowa. The team developed the Nursing Interventions Classification (NIC), a comprehensive, standardized classification of interventions that nurses perform. Unlike a nursing diagnosis or patient outcome where the focus of concern is the patient, the focus of concern with nursing interventions is nurse behavior; those things that nurses do to assist the patient to move toward a desired outcome.

The NIC language includes all interventions performed by nurses, both independent and collaborative interventions, as well as direct and indirect care interventions. An intervention is defined as "any treatment, based upon clinical judgment and knowledge, that a nurse performs to enhance patient/client outcomes" (McCloskey & Bulechek, 2000, p. *xix*). This definition was incorporated into the 1995 revision of *Nursing's Social Policy Statement* by the ANA (American Nurses Association, 1995).

Each NIC intervention consists of a label name, a definition, a set of activities that indicate the actions and thinking that go into the delivery of the intervention, and a short list of background readings as illustrated in Table 1-2. The intervention label name and the definition are the content of the intervention that is standardized and should not be changed when NIC is used to document care. Care can be individualized, however, through the choice of activities. From a list of approximately 10 to 30 activities per intervention, the nurse selects the activities most appropriate for the specific individual or family. The nurse can add new activities if needed; however, all modifications and additions should be congruent with the definition of the intervention. The classification is continually updated and has been published in three editions of the *Nursing Interventions Classification (NIC)* text. The first edition, published in 1992, contained 336 interventions (McCloskey & Bulechek, 1992); the second edition, published in 1996, contained 433 interventions (McCloskey & Bulechek, 1996); and the third edition, published in 2000, contains 486 interventions (McCloskey & Bulechek, 2000).

The 486 interventions in the third edition are grouped into 30 classes and 7 domains for ease of use. The 7 domains are (1) Physiological: Basic, (2) Physiological: Complex, (3) Behavioral, (4) Safety, (5) Family, (6) Health System, and (7) Community. A few interventions are located in more than one class, but each intervention has a unique number (code) that identifies the primary class in the taxonomy.

Whereas an individual nurse will have expertise in only a limited number of interventions reflecting his or her specialty, the entire classification captures the expertise of all nurses. NIC can be used in all settings (from acute care intensive care units to home care, hospice care, and primary care settings) and in all specialties (from pediatrics and obstetrics to cardiology and gerontology). Although the entire classification describes the domain of nursing, some of

TABLE 1-2 ONE EXAMPLE OF A NIC INTERVENTION

Anxiety Reduction

Definition: Minimizing apprehension, dread, foreboding, or uneasiness related to an unidentified source of anticipated danger

Activities

Use a calm, reassuring approach

Clearly state expectations for patient's behavior

Explain all procedures, including sensations likely to be experienced during the procedure

Seek to understand the patient's perspective of a stressful situation

Provide factual information concerning diagnosis, treatment, and prognosis

Stay with patient to promote safety and reduce fear

Encourage patients to stay with child, as appropriate

Provide objects that symbolize safeness

Administer back rub/neck rub, as appropriate

Encourage noncompetitive activities, as appropriate

Keep treatment equipment out of sight

Listen attentively

Reinforce behavior, as appropriate

Create an atmosphere to facilitate trust

Encourage verbalization of feelings, perceptions, and fears

Identify when level of anxiety changes

Provide diversional activities geared toward the reduction of tension

Help patient identify situations that precipitate anxiety

Control stimuli, as appropriate, for patient needs

Support the use of appropriate defense mechanisms

Assist patient to articulate a realistic description of an upcoming event

Determine patient's decision-making ability

Instruct patient on the use of relaxation techniques

Administer medications to reduce anxiety, as appropriate

From J.C. McCloskey & G.M. Bulechek (Eds.). (2000). *Nursing interventions classification (NIC)* (3rd ed.). St. Louis: Mosby.

the interventions can be provided by other disciplines. Health care providers other than nurses are welcome to use NIC to describe their treatments.

Multiple research methods were used in the development of NIC. An inductive approach was used to build the classification based on existing practice. Original sources included current textbooks, care planning guides, and nursing information systems. Content analysis, focus group review, and questionnaires completed by nurse experts in specialty areas of practice were used to augment the clinical practice expertise of team members (McCloskey & Bulechek, 1992). Methods used to construct the taxonomy included similarity analysis, hierarchical clustering, and multidimensional scaling (McCloskey & Bulechek, 1996). Over time, more than 1000 nurses have completed questionnaires, and approximately 50 professional associations have provided input about the classification. Through clinical field testing, steps for implementation were developed and tested, and the need for linkages between NANDA, NOC, and NIC was identified. The NIC books and numerous other publications provide more information about the research used to construct and validate NIC. A video made by the National League of Nursing describes the early work and is now available for rent from the Center for Nursing Classification at the University of Iowa.

NIC interventions have been linked with NANDA diagnoses, Omaha System problems, and NOC outcomes. The NIC classification has been translated in five languages; five additional translations are now in progress. Use of NIC to document the practice of nursing is expanding rapidly, both nationally and internationally. The classification is continually updated through an ongoing process of feedback and review. Instructions for how users can submit suggestions for modifications to existing interventions or propose a new intervention can be found in the back of the NIC book. Work that is done between editions of the NIC book and other relevant publications that enhance the use of the classification are available from the Center for Nursing Classification at The University of Iowa, College of Nursing, Iowa City, IA 52242. Current information is available on the Center for Nursing Classification web page: http:// www.nursing.uiowa.edu/cnc.

NOC

Since the 1960s, considerable effort has been expended on developing outcome measures useful for evaluating nursing practice (Horn & Swain, 1978; Marek, 1989; Martin & Scheet, 1992; McCormick, 1991; Waltz & Strickland, 1988). In 1991 a research team, led by Marion Johnson and Meridean Maas, was formed at the University of Iowa to develop a classification of patient outcomes correlated with nursing care. The work of the research team resulted in the Nursing Outcomes Classification (NOC), a comprehensive, standardized classification of patient outcomes that can be used to evaluate the results of nursing interventions.

Patient outcomes serve as the criteria against which to judge the success of a nursing intervention. Outcomes describe a patient's state, behaviors, responses, and feelings in response to the care provided. It is recognized that a number of variables, in addition to the intervention, influence patient outcomes. These variables range from the process used in providing the care, including the actions of other health care providers, to organizational and environmental variables that influence how interventions are selected and provided to patient characteristics, including the patient's physical and emotional health, as well as the life circumstances being experienced by the patient. The task for nursing is to define which patient outcomes are sensitive to nursing care; that is, those outcomes that are most influenced by nursing interventions for each patient, each family, or group of patients.

NOC contains individual, family, and community outcomes that are influenced by both independent and collaborative nursing interventions. An outcome is stated as "a variable patient or family caregiver state, behavior, or perception that is responsive to nursing interventions and conceptualized at middle levels of abstraction" (Johnson, Maas, & Moorhead, 2000, p. 24). Since the outcomes describe the status of the patient, other disciplines may find them useful for the evaluation of their interventions.

Each NOC outcome has a label name, a definition, a list of indicators to evaluate patient status in relation to the outcome, a five-point Likert scale to measure patient status, and a short list of references used in the development of the outcome, as illustrated in Table 1-3. Examples of scales used with the outcomes are as follows:

- 1 = extremely compromised to 5 = not compromised
- 1 = never demonstrated to 5 = consistently demonstrated

The scales allow measurement of the outcome status at any point on a continuum from most negative to most positive, as well as identification of changes in patient status at different points in time. The scales can be used to measure patient status with each of the indicators and with the outcome. In contrast to the information provided by a goal statement, that is, whether a goal is met or not met, NOC outcomes can be used to monitor progress, or lack of progress, throughout an episode of care and across different care settings. The outcomes have been developed to be used in all settings, all specialties, and across the care continuum. The original classification, first published in 1997, contained 190 outcomes (Johnson & Maas, 1997); the second edition, published in 2000, contains 260 outcomes (Johnson, Maas, & Moorhead, 2000).

The 260 outcomes in the second edition are grouped into 29 classes and 7 domains for ease of use. The seven domains are (1) Functional Health, (2) Physiologic Health, (3) Psychosocial Health, (4) Health Knowledge & Behavior, (5) Perceived Health, (6) Family Health, and (7) Community Health. Each outcome is in only one class and has a unique code number that facilitates the use of the outcomes in computerized clinical information systems. Each outcome indicator and measurement scale also has a unique code number that is related to the code number for the outcome. The classification is continually updated to include new outcomes and to revise older outcomes based on new research or user feedback.

The development of the outcomes and the taxonomy used research methods similar to those described for the development of NIC. Questionnaires sent to clinically expert nurses asked nurses to respond to the importance of the indicators for determining the outcome and the influence of nursing on the outcome. Approximately 1200 nurses representing 21 specialties have responded to these questionnaires. The outcomes are currently being evaluated in nine clinical sites representing hospitals, long-term institutional care, home care, parish nursing, and nursing centers. The focus of the evaluation is on the reliability and validity of the measurement scales when used by nurses in a variety of practice sites.

The outcomes have been linked to NANDA diagnoses, to Omaha System problems, to the Long-Term Care Minimum Data Set, to the Resident Assessment Instrument used in nursing homes, and to NIC interventions. Interest in NOC has been demonstrated in other countries as evidenced by increasing requests to translate the book. The NOC classification has been translated in four languages, and four other translations are in progress. NOC is being adopted in a number of clinical sites for the evaluation of nursing practice and is being used in educational settings to structure curricula and teach students clinical evaluation. Current information about NOC is available on the Center for Nursing Classification web page: http://www.nursing.uiowa.edu/cnc.

TABLE 1-3 ONE EXAMPLE OF A **NOC** OUTCOME

Anxiety Control

Definition: Personal actions to eliminate or reduce feelings of apprehension and tension from an unidentifiable source

Anxiety Control	Never Demonstrated 1	Rarely Demonstrated 2	Sometimes Demonstrated 3	Often Demonstrated 4	Consistently Demonstrated 5
Monitors intensity of anxiety	1	2	3	4	5
Eliminates precursors of anxiety	1	2	3	4	5
Decreases environmental stimuli when anxious	1	2	3	4	5
Seeks information to reduce anxiety	1	2	3	4	5
Plans coping strategies for stressful situations	1	2	3	4	5
Uses effective coping strategies	1	2	3	4	5
Uses relaxation techniques to reduce anxiety	1	2	3	4	5
Reports decreased duration of episodes	1	2	3	4	5
Reports increased length of time between episodes	1	2	3	4	5
Maintains role performance	1	2	3	4	5
Maintains social relationships	1	2	3	4	5
Maintains concentration	1	2	3	4	5
Reports absence of sensory perceptual distortions	1	2	3	4	5
Reports adequate sleep	1	2	3	4	5
Reports absence of physical manifestations of anxiety	1	2	3	4	5
Behavioral manifestations of anxiety absent	1	2	3	4	5
Controls anxiety response	1	2	3	4	5
Other _____ (Specify)	1	2	3	4	5

From M. Johnson, M. Maas, & S. Moorhead (Eds.). (2000). *Nursing outcomes classification (NOC)* (2nd ed.). St. Louis: Mosby.

NANDA, NIC, and NOC can be used together or separately. Together they represent the domain of nursing in all settings and specialties. They have been recognized by the ANA, included in the National Library of Medicine's Metathesaurus for a Unified Medical Language System (UMLS), and included in the Cumulative Index to Nursing Literature (CINAHL). Multiple clinical agencies and educational settings are using one or more of these nursing languages for the documentation of patient care and for the education of nursing students. Linking the three languages provides a template for how the languages can be used together and facilitates their use.

REFERENCES

American Nurses Association. (1980). *Nursing: A social policy statement*. Kansas City, MO: Author.

American Nurses Association. (1995). *Nursing's social policy statement*. Washington, DC: Author.

Craft-Rosenberg, M., & Delaney, C. (1997). Nursing diagnosis extension and classification (NDEC). In M. Rantz & P. Lemone (Eds.), *Classification of nursing diagnoses: Proceedings of the Twelfth Conference* (pp. 26-31). Glendale, CA: CINAHL.

Fehring, R. J. (1986). Validating diagnostic labels: Standardized methodology. In M. E. Hurley (Ed.), *Classification of nursing diagnoses: Proceedings of the Sixth Conference* (pp. 183-190). St. Louis: Mosby.

Fitzpatrick, J. J. (1998). The translation of NANDA taxonomy I into ICD code. *Nursing Diagnosis*, 9(2), 34-36.

Horn, B. J., & Swain, M. A. (1978). *Criterion measures of nursing care* (DHEW Pub. No. PHS 78-3187). Hyattsville, MD: National Center for Health Services Research.

Hoskins, L. (1997). How to do a validations study. In M. Rantz & P. Lemone (Eds.), *Classification of nursing diagnoses: Proceedings of the Twelfth Conference* (pp. 78-86). Glendale, CA: CINAHL.

Johnson, M., & Maas, M. (Eds.). (1997). *Nursing outcomes classification (NOC)*. St. Louis: Mosby.

Johnson, M., Maas, M., & Moorhead, S. (Eds.). (2000). *Nursing outcomes classification (NOC)* (2nd ed.). St. Louis: Mosby.

Jones, D. L. (1997). Building the information infrastructure required for managed care. *Image: Journal of Nursing Scholarship*, 29(4), 377-382.

Keenan, G., & Aquilino, M. L. (1998). Standardized nomenclatures: Keys to continuity of care, nursing accountability, and nursing effectiveness. *Outcomes Management for Nursing Practice*, 2(2), 81-85.

Maas, M. L.(1985). Nursing diagnosis: A leadership strategy for nursing administrators. *Journal of Nursing Administration*, 1(6), 39-42.

McCloskey, J. C., & Bulechek, G. M. (Eds.). (1992). *Nursing interventions classification (NIC)*. St. Louis: Mosby.

McCloskey, J. C., & Bulechek, G. M. (1994). Standardizing the language for nursing treatments: An overview of the issues. *Nursing Outlook*, 42(2), 56-63.

McCloskey, J. C., & Bulechek, G. M. (Eds.). (1996). *Nursing interventions classification (NIC)* (2nd ed). St. Louis: Mosby.

McCloskey, J. C., & Bulechek, G. M. (Eds.). (2000). *Nursing interventions classification (NIC)* (3rd ed). St. Louis: Mosby.

McCormick, K. A. (1991). Future data needs for quality of care monitoring, DRG considerations, reimbursement, and outcome measurement. *Image: Journal of Nursing Scholarship*, 23(1), 29-32.

Marek, K. D. (1989). Outcomes measurement in nursing. *Journal of Nursing Quality Assurance*, 4(1), 1-9.

Martin, K. S., & Scheet, N. J. (1992). *The Omaha system: Applications for community health nursing*. Philadelphia: W.B. Saunders.

North American Nursing Diagnosis Association. (1995). *Nursing diagnoses: Definitions & classifications 1995-1996.* Philadelphia: Author.

North American Nursing Diagnosis Association. (1999). *Nursing diagnoses: Definitions & classification 1999-2000.* Philadelphia: Author.

Parker, L., & Lunney, M. (1998). Moving beyond content validation of nursing diagnoses. *Nursing Diagnosis, 9*(4), 144-150.

Waltz, C. F. & Strickland, O. L. (Eds.). (1988). *Measurement of nursing outcomes.* Vol. 1. *Measuring client outcomes.* New York: Springer Publishing Company.

Whitley, G. G. (1999). Processes and methodologies for research validation of nursing diagnoses. *Nursing Diagnosis, 10*(1), 5-14.

Zielstorff, R. D. (1994). National data bases: Nursing's challenge, classification of nursing diagnoses. In R. M. Carroll-Johnson & M. Paquette (Eds.), *Classification of nursing diagnoses: Proceedings of the Tenth Conference* (pp. 34-42). Philadelphia: J.B. Lippincott.

CHAPTER 2

The Linkages

Part II of this book links NANDA diagnoses, NIC interventions, and NOC outcomes. The work represents the judgment of selected members of the NIC and NOC research teams, including academicians, clinicians, and students. *The linkages are not meant to be prescriptive and do not replace the clinical judgment of the practitioner.* In addition to the linkages provided in this book, users may select other outcomes and interventions for a particular diagnosis. The linkages presented here illustrate how three distinct nursing languages can be connected and used together when planning care for an individual patient or a group of patients.

DESCRIPTION OF THE LINKAGES

The linkages provided in this book are between the North American Nursing Diagnosis Association's (NANDA) diagnoses, the Nursing Interventions Classification (NIC) interventions and the Nursing Outcomes Classification (NOC) outcomes. A linkage can be defined as that which directs the relationship or association of concepts. The links between the NANDA diagnoses and the NOC outcomes suggest the relationships between the patient's problem or current status and those aspects of the problem or status that are expected to be resolved or improved by an intervention. The links between the NANDA diagnoses and the NIC interventions suggest the relationship between the patient's problem and the nursing actions that will resolve or decrease the problem. The links between the NOC outcomes and the NIC interventions suggest a similar relationship, that between the resolution of a problem and the nursing actions directed at problem resolution or the outcome state that an intervention is expected to influence.

The concept names and definitions used in the linkages are those in the 1999-2000 edition of *Nursing Diagnoses: Definitions & Classification* (North American Nursing Diagnosis Association, 1999), the third edition of *Nursing Interventions Classification (NIC)* (McCloskey & Bulechek, 2000), and the second edition of *Nursing Outcomes Classification (NOC)* (Johnson, Maas, & Moorhead, 2000). The NANDA diagnosis is the entry point for the linkages. The diagnoses are listed in alphabetical order except for the risk diagnoses that appear altogether in one section at the end of the linkages. However, the NANDA diagnostic name wording has been reordered when the beginning term does not specify the concept of concern in the diagnostic label; for example, *Ineffective Thermoregulation* is presented in these linkages as *Thermoregulation: Ineffective*. This was done to facilitate the ease with which a diagnosis can be found. Each diagnosis contains the diagnostic name and the definition. Suggested NOC outcomes with associated NIC interventions are also provided for each diagnosis. The interventions are identified as major, suggested, and optional interventions for achieving each of the suggested outcomes for a diagnosis. Definitions of the NIC interventions and NOC outcomes used in the linkages are in Appendixes A and B.

The alphabetical ordering of the diagnoses does not reflect the taxonomic structure used by NANDA. Likewise, the taxonomic and coding structures of NIC and NOC are not reflected in these linkages. The current taxonomic structure for each of these languages can be found in the books describing each language.

Development of the Linkages

Development of links between NANDA diagnoses and NIC interventions, NANDA diagnoses and NOC outcomes, and NIC interventions and NOC outcomes preceded the work of linking the three languages. Suggested interventions for each NANDA diagnosis are provided in the third edition of the *Nursing Interventions Classification (NIC)* (McCloskey & Bulechek, 2000), and suggested interventions for each NOC outcome are available in a monograph (Iowa Interventions Project, 1998) from the Center for Nursing Classification. Suggested outcomes for each NANDA diagnosis are in the second edition of the *Nursing Outcomes Classification (NOC)* (Johnson, Maas, & Moorhead, 2000). All of the linkage work mentioned above is comprehensive and provides multiple links for each of the diagnoses or outcomes. The methods used in the development of each linkage are described in the publications in which they appear. As with the preceding linkage work, the current work is based on expert judgment and is not intended to be prescriptive. The previous linkage work was used as the basis for the development of the NANDA-NOC-NIC links in this book.

Development of the NANDA-NOC-NIC links presented in this book proceeded in the following three phases: (1) creating an initial list of linkages, (2) first level linkage refinement, and (3) second level linkage refinement. Creating the initial list required that the format for presenting the links be determined. Diagnoses were selected as the entry point for the linkages because traditionally they are considered the second step in the nursing process, following assessment and preceding the selection of interventions and outcomes. Although nursing interventions can be initiated on the basis of patient symptoms prior to the identification of a nursing or medical diagnosis, interventions and outcomes are generally considered in conjunction with a diagnosis.

Suggested outcomes from the NANDA-NOC linkages (Johnson, Maas, & Moorhead, 2000) were linked to each diagnosis. The diagnosis can be thought of as a standardized term that represents the initial condition or present state of the patient and the outcome as the desired or end state that results from nursing interventions (Pesut & Herman, 1999). Thus, the desired outcome is selected prior to the selection of nursing interventions. Bulechek and McCloskey identify the desired patient outcome and the characteristics of the diagnosis as two of the factors to be considered when selecting a nursing intervention (Bulechek & McCloskey, 1999). After the suggested outcomes were linked to the diagnosis, the related interventions from the NOC-NIC linkages (Iowa Intervention Project, 1998) were linked to the outcomes. The interventions for an outcome were used as they appear in the NOC-NIC linkage work, including the identification of an intervention as major, suggested, and optional for each outcome.

In general, the outcomes and interventions are not linked to the defining characteristics (signs and symptoms) or the related factors (etiologies) of each diagnosis because this would generate multiple repetitive linkages for each diagnosis. However, when the NANDA diagnosis is related to a specific etiological factor, such as with functional or stress urinary incontinence, the suggested outcomes and interventions for that diagnosis are specific for the etiology. When the NANDA diagnosis requires further specification, such as the type of altered tissue perfusion or sensory deficit, a diagnosis with associated outcomes and interventions was provided for each diagnostic type presented in NANDA. In all instances, the defining characteristics and related factors were considered when the initial links between the diagnoses and interventions or outcomes were developed.

In summary, the initial links were derived by linking the suggested outcomes from the second edition of *NOC* with the NANDA diagnosis, and then linking the major, suggested, and optional interventions from the NOC-NIC linkage work with each of the outcomes. The work then moved into the second phase, the initial refinement of the linkage work. This was done by one of the authors using the following steps:

1. The relevance of the interventions associated with each outcome for the specific diagnosis was evaluated, and interventions linked to and appropriate for the outcome but not appropriate for the diagnosis were eliminated. The decision to eliminate an intervention was based on the clinical judgment of the reviewer and the comparison of the interventions with those in the NANDA-NIC linkage work. For example, *Tissue Integrity: Skin & Mucous Membranes* is a suggested outcome for the diagnosis *Oral Mucous Membrane, Altered*. However, some of the interventions such as *Bathing, Foot Care,* and *Pressure Ulcer Prevention,* although appropriate interventions for the outcome *Tissue Integrity: Skin & Mucous Membranes,* are not appropriate for the diagnosis, *Oral Mucous Membrane, Altered*.

2. The interventions previously linked to the diagnosis (NANDA-NIC linkages) were compared with the interventions associated with each of the outcomes selected for the diagnosis. If an intervention in the NANDA-NIC linkage was not linked to the diagnosis via one of the outcomes, the relevance of the intervention for each of the outcomes was considered and the missing intervention was linked to one of the outcomes if relevant to the outcome. This means that an intervention linked to an outcome for a specific diagnosis may not be linked to the NOC outcome in the NIC-NOC linkages (Iowa Interventions Project, 1998) and an intervention linked to the diagnosis in the NANDA-NIC linkages (McCloskey & Bulechek, 2000) may not be present in these linkages.

3. As the interventions linked to the outcomes for a diagnosis were compared with the interventions previously linked to the diagnosis, some discrepancies among the linkages became evident. In some instances the interventions previously linked to the suggested outcomes were quite different from the interventions previously linked to the diagnosis. When this occurred, the outcomes not associated with interventions recommended for the diagnosis were reviewed to determine if they should be retained or if other outcomes would be more appropriate. As a result of the decisions made at this step, some of the outcomes selected for the NANDA diagnoses in this book are not consistent with the suggested outcomes in the NANDA-NOC linkages in the second edition of the *Nursing Outcomes Classification (NOC)* book (Johnson, Mass, & Moorhead, 2000). However, these steps allowed for a comprehensive review of the previous linkage work and resulted in overall consistency between the interventions in the NANDA-NIC linkages and the ones recommended here for each of the diagnoses.

4. As the previous steps were being carried out, the placement of each intervention as major, suggested, and optional was evaluated for appropriateness for the particular diagnosis. In some cases the placement of the interventions remained the same as in the previous NOC-NIC linkages (Iowa Interventions Project, 1998), and at other times the interventions were moved to a different level of importance for the diagnosis. This has resulted in some differences between the placement of the interventions in this book and the NOC-NIC linkages. One of the factors used to determine the appropriate placement of an intervention was the placement of the intervention when linked to the diagnosis. Was the intervention identified as major, suggested or optional in the NANDA-NIC linkages (McCloskey & Bulechek, 2000)? However, since the NANDA-NIC linkages were used to review the placement of the interventions as major, suggested, and optional rather than to make the initial links, there are differences in the placement of the interventions in the NANDA-NIC linkage work and the linkage work represented here.

The final phase in the development of the linkages was the second level refinement accomplished through reviews of the work. Since the initial links were completed by one person, it was important that the linkage work be reviewed by others. Reviewers were the other authors of the book and, in some instances, selected clinicians and graduate students. Changes suggested by the reviewers were made in the linkages if there was agreement among the reviewers. If reviewer agreement was not reached, the suggested changes were brought to the authors for discussion and for a final decision. A final review of the outcomes and interventions linked to each diagnosis was the final step in the review process.

The development of the linkages for this book required scrutiny of the linkage work that preceded the development of the NANDA-NOC-NIC links. As a result, the linkages in this book, although similar to the previous linkage work, are not identical to the linkages found in the third edition of the *Nursing Interventions Classification (NIC)* or the second edition of the *Nursing Outcomes Classification (NOC)*. The discrepancies may occur because a particular link is not appropriate for a specific diagnosis or outcome, and yet the previous work does not need to be changed, or the discrepancy may reflect, indeed, the need for changes in the previous linkage work. Feedback from clinicians and others using the work will assist the authors to further refine the linkage work.

REFERENCES

Bulechek, G. M., & McCloskey, J. C. (Eds.). (1999). *Nursing interventions: Effective nursing treatments* (3rd ed.). Philadelphia: W.B. Saunders.

Iowa Interventions Project. (1998). *NIC interventions linked to NOC outcomes.* Iowa City, IA: Center for Nursing Classification.

Johnson, M., Maas, M., & Moorhead, S. (Eds.). (2000). *Nursing outcomes classification (NOC)* (2nd ed.). St. Louis: Mosby.

McCloskey, J. C., & Bulechek, G. M. (Eds.). (2000). *Nursing interventions classification (NIC)* (3rd ed.). St. Louis: Mosby.

North American Nursing Diagnosis Association. (1999). *Nursing diagnoses: Definitions & classification 1999-2000.* Philadelphia: Author.

Pesut, D. J., & Herman, J. (1999). *Clinical reasoning: The art & science of critical & creative thinking.* Boston: Delmar Publishers.

CHAPTER 3

Linkage Applications

The linkages provided in this book have a number of uses. They can be used for the development of care plans and critical paths for patient populations or for individual patients. They can facilitate software development for electronic nursing information systems. They can assist educators in teaching clinical decision making and developing curricula and can be used by researchers to test nursing interventions, to evaluate the connections suggested in the linkages, and to develop mid-range nursing theories.

CARE PLANNING

Nurses use a decision-making process to determine a nursing diagnosis, project a desired outcome, and select interventions to achieve the desired outcome. That process may be assisted by the linkages provided in this book. It is important to keep in mind that the linkages are only guides; the nurse must continually evaluate the situation and adjust the diagnoses, outcomes, and interventions to fit each patient's or population's unique needs. The use of suggested links does not alter the skills that nurses need and use in making decisions about patient care. "The skills the nurse must have to use the nursing process are: intellectual, interpersonal, and technical. Intellectual skills entail problem solving, critical thinking, and making nursing judgments" (Yura & Walsh, 1973, p. 69). When using the linkages, these intellectual skills are directed toward the evaluation and selection or rejection of the outcomes and interventions provided for each nursing diagnosis.

The first judgment the nurse must make when using the linkages is to determine the nursing diagnosis. There is general agreement that prior to making a nursing diagnosis, an assessment of the patient status must be made. Rubenfeld and Scheffer (1999) state that assessment includes both data collection and data analysis or, as they describe it, "finding clues" and "making sense of the clues" (p. 130). They detail a number of steps used in assessment that enable the nurse to draw conclusions about the patient's strengths and health concerns, that is, to make a diagnosis. They further suggest categorizing health concerns as (1) problems for referral (issues addressed by other health providers), (2) interdisciplinary problems addressed collaboratively with other providers, and (3) nursing diagnoses for which the nurse has primary responsibility for treating the patient.

Pesut and Herman (1999) use terms other than assessment to describe the stage of data gathering. They indicate that the nurse listens to the client's story and then uses "cue logic" to discern the meaning of the story and "framing" to connect cues and discern between the central issue or problem and peripheral problems. This allows the nurse to develop a description of the initial condition of the patient, referred to as the present state, and select a desired end state, or the outcome. The present state can then be compared with the end state after a nursing intervention to determine the effectiveness of that intervention. Both the present state and end state can be defined by standardized terms, for example, a NANDA diagnosis and a NOC outcome. The present state may be *Altered Thought Processes* and possible outcomes might be *Cognitive Ability, Distorted Thought Control, or Memory,* depending upon the etiology and type of thought alteration.

Determining a nursing diagnosis is an essential first step for accessing the links in this book. This is true when planning the care for one patient (an individual care plan) or for a group of patients (a critical path). However, identification of the nursing diagnosis for a group of patients requires an additional step: the collection and analysis of data to determine the diagnoses that occur most frequently and are important to address for the entire population. Once a nursing diagnosis is determined, the nurse can locate the diagnosis in the linkages and determine if any of the suggested outcomes are appropriate for the individual patient or patient group. When selecting the outcome, the nurse should consider the following factors: (1) the defining characteristics of the diagnosis, (2) the related factors of the diagnosis, (3) the patient characteristics that can affect outcome achievement, (4) the outcomes generally associated with the diagnosis, and (5) the preferences of the patient. It is important to note that the outcomes presented in the linkage work reflect an overall outcome related to the patient state to be achieved. For example, the suggested outcomes for *Noncompliance* are *Adherence Behavior, Compliance Behavior,* and *Treatment Behavior: Illness or Injury.* However, intermediate outcomes that address the related factors (etiologies) in a NANDA diagnosis must often be met before the general outcome is achieved. For example, if *Noncompliance* is related to inadequate knowledge of the disease process, the nurse might want to select the outcome *Knowledge: Disease Process* as well as the outcome *Compliance Behavior.*

The nurse can then use the interventions suggested in the linkage work to assist in the selection of an intervention(s) for the individual or group. The major intervention is the most obvious intervention and should be considered first. If the major intervention is not selected, consideration should be given to the suggested interventions and then to the optional interventions. Bulechek and McCloskey (1992) identify six factors to consider when selecting a nursing intervention. They are (1) the desired patient outcome, (2) the characteristics of the nursing diagnosis, (3) the research base associated with the intervention, (4) the feasibility of implementing the intervention, (5) the acceptability of the intervention to the patient, and (6) the capability of the nurse. These factors should be considered when using the linkage work; the linkages can assist the nurse by suggesting interventions associated with both the outcome and the diagnosis, but cannot replace the nurse's judgment when selecting an intervention.

The use of the NANDA-NOC-NIC linkages in the development of individualized care plans is illustrated in the following case studies developed by registered nurse students in the RN-BSN nursing program. Although each case study could have a number of NANDA diagnoses, only the major diagnosis has been selected. The diagnosis is presented with the major NOC outcome(s) and NIC intervention(s). The outcome includes the major outcome indicators pertinent for the patient, but does not include the scale that would be used to measure patient status. Likewise, the NIC intervention includes selected activities appropriate for the patient.

Text continued on p. 28

CASE STUDY I

Mrs. C, a 38-year-old female, is married and has two adult stepchildren. She maintains a healthy life style and has no family history of cancer. She performs breast self-exams routinely and has never identified a lump or any unusual finding during her monthly exam. Mrs. C works full-time as a magazine publisher. One day at work as she was going down a flight of stairs, her high heel caught on the rung of the step, and she fell to the next landing. She received multiple bruises, including one in the chest area where she hit a metal railing. Ignoring her injuries because she was embarrassed about the fall, she continued to work throughout the day. That evening she told her family about her fall at work. Everyone was concerned, but she downplayed the incident since she was still more embarrassed about falling than concerned about the injuries she sustained.

Subsequently Mrs. C experienced localized pain in her left breast. The pain started out as a dull ache and did not improve over time. For several days Mrs. C was aware of the breast pain but disregarded it as simply being a bruise resulting from the accident. The pain gradually became worse, and ultimately, Mrs. C could feel a lump in her breast at the site of the pain. She finally went to a doctor 2 months after her fall. Upon examination the doctor recommended a biopsy of the lump in her breast. The biopsy was done a week later and confirmed the presence of a malignant tumor. Mrs. C had a radical mastectomy of the left breast several days later.

Mr. C was at the hospital during the surgery but left for work after Mrs. C entered postanesthesia recovery. After work Mr. C, an alcoholic, decided to go to the bar for a few drinks. He phoned Mrs. C from the bar and told her he would call her again once he reached home. Mrs. C was concerned about her husband driving home from the bar and worried a great deal about this during the evening. Several hours later he phoned her from home. While talking to her he "passed out" on the other end, and she could not disconnect from him. This upset Mrs. C because she knew he was not dealing well with the mastectomy. She needed his support to deal with her recovery, and he needed her to help him cope with her surgery. Mrs. C relied on the nursing staff for support with accepting her body image changes and also for emotional support. The staff located Reach for Recovery, a breast cancer support group, to help Mrs. C through this difficult time in her life. Table 3-1 provides a summary of the information in this case showing the linkages among NANDA, NOC, and NIC.

(Courtesy of Kimberly Albright, BSN.)

TABLE 3-1 PLAN OF CARE FOR MRS. C		
Nursing Diagnosis	**Nursing Outcome**	**Nursing Intervention**
BODY IMAGE DISTURBANCE	BODY IMAGE	BODY IMAGE ENHANCEMENT
DEFINING CHARACTERISTICS Nonverbal response to actual or perceived change in structure and/or function; verbalization of feelings that reflect an altered view of one's body in appearance, structure, or function **Objective:** Missing body part; not touching body part; not looking at body part **Subjective:** Negative feelings about body; fear of rejection or of reaction by others **Related Factors** Surgery; illness treatment	**INDICATORS** Congruence between body reality, body ideal, and body presentation Description of affected body part Willingness to touch affected body part Satisfaction with body appearance Adjustment to changes in physical appearance Adjustment to changes in health status Willingness to use strategies to enhance appearance and function	**NURSING ACTIVITIES** Assist patient to discuss changes caused by illness or surgery Assist patient to separate physical appearance from feelings of personal worth Assist the patient to discuss stressors affecting body image due to surgery Monitor frequency of statements of self-criticism Monitor whether patient can look at the changed body part Monitor for statements that identify body image perceptions concerned with body shape and body weight Determine patient's and family's perception of the alteration in body image versus reality Determine if a change in body image has contributed to increased social isolation Assist patient to identify actions that will enhance appearance Facilitate contact with individuals with similar changes in body image Identify support groups available to patient

CASE STUDY 2

Mrs. S is a 33-year-old married white female. She has three school-age children under the age of 8: one daughter, age 6, and two sons, ages 8 and 5. All of the children ride the school bus to attend a local elementary school. The family dwelling is a two-story home with two bedrooms upstairs and one downstairs, a living room, kitchen, dining room, one bathroom, and laundry facilities located on the back porch. There are two entry doors to the home, both with four steps. Her husband is employed full-time as a mechanic with a local company. Mrs. S has been employed full-time as a secretary/receptionist with a local construction company for the last 3 years. Both Mrs. S and her husband work normal daytime business hours. Mrs. S has a history of chronic back and neck pain.

Mrs. S initially arrived at the health care agency complaining of severe head, neck, shoulder, upper back, and upper arm pain. She stated that she was riding as a passenger in a truck involved in an accident several days ago; the truck hit a large deer. At the time of the accident she was wearing a lap seatbelt. The truck was traveling 45 to 55 miles per hour at the time of impact. Mrs. S did not have an evaluation at the time of the accident, stating that she had not felt it was necessary. She did experience some discomfort initially and expected to have stiffness and soreness for several days after the accident; however, the pain continued to increase in severity, affecting all aspects of her daily activities and sleep. Mrs. S rated her pain at 9 to 10 on a scale of 0 to 10, with 10 representing the most severe pain.

Mrs. S has received follow-up treatment since the accident for cervical/dorsal strain and degenerative joint disease of the cervical spine. The focus of treatment is on the management of the chronic nonmalignant pain. Treatment included limiting and restructuring home/daily activities, use of a TENS unit, relaxation therapy, stress reduction education, and medication as follows: Daypro, 1200 mg qd; Prozac, 20 mg qd; and Baclofen, 10 mg hs. Mrs. S states that she is now experiencing somewhat less pain (rated 5 to 6 on a scale of 0 to 10), but her normal activities of daily living and sleep pattern remain affected and have not returned to her normal preaccident status. She states that she experiences continual around-the-clock pain rated at 5 to 6 on a scale of 0 to 10. Table 3-2 provides a summary of the information in this case, showing the linkages among NANDA, NOC, and, NIC.

(Courtesy of Sileen Heston, BSN.)

TABLE 3-2 PLAN OF CARE FOR MRS. S

Nursing Diagnosis	Nursing Outcomes	Nursing Intervention
PAIN, CHRONIC	PAIN CONTROL	PAIN MANAGEMENT
DEFINING CHARACTERISTICS	**INDICATORS**	**NURSING ACTIVITIES**
Verbal or coded report or observed evidence of protective behavior; verbal or coded report or observed evidence of guarding behavior; verbal or coded report or observed evidence of facial mask; verbal or coded report or observed evidence of self-focusing; verbal or coded report or observed evidence of restlessness; verbal or coded report or observed evidence of depression; changes in sleep pattern; altered ability to continue previous activities	Recognizes causal factors Recognizes pain onset Uses analgesics appropriately Reports symptoms to health care professional Recognizes symptoms of pain Reports pain controlled	Determine the impact of the pain experience on quality of life (e.g., sleep, appetite, activity, cognition, mood, relationships, performance of job, and role responsibilities) Evaluate past experiences with pain to include individual or family history of chronic pain or resulting disability, as appropriate
	PAIN: DISRUPTIVE EFFECTS	Evaluate, with the patient and the health care team, the effectiveness of past pain control measures that have been used
	INDICATORS	
	Impaired role performance Compromised work Impaired mood Disrupted sleep Impaired physical mobility Impaired self-care Lack of appetite	Select and implement a variety of measures (e.g., pharmacological, nonpharmacological, interpersonal) to facilitate pain relief as appropriate
Related Factors Chronic physical disability		
	PAIN LEVEL	Consider type and source of pain when selecting pain relief strategy
	INDICATORS	Encourage patient to monitor own pain and to intervene appropriately
	Reported pain Frequency of pain Length of pain episodes Oral expressions of pain Facial expressions of pain Protective body positions Restlessness Appetite loss	Teach the use of nonpharmacological techniques (e.g., biofeedback, TENS, hypnosis, relaxation, guided imagery, music therapy, distraction, play therapy, activity therapy, acupressure, hot/cold application, and massage) before and after and, if possible, during painful activities; before pain occurs or increases; and along with other pain relief measures

TENS, Transcutaneous electrical nerve stimulation.

TABLE 3-2	PLAN OF CARE FOR MRS. S—cont'd	
Nursing Diagnosis	**Nursing Outcomes**	**Nursing Intervention**
PAIN, CHRONIC	PAIN CONTROL	PAIN MANAGEMENT
		NURSING ACTIVITIES—CONT'D Use pain control measures before pain becomes severe Institute and modify pain control measures on the basis of the patient's response Promote adequate rest/sleep to facilitate pain relief Encourage patient to discuss his/her pain experience Incorporate the family in the pain relief modality, if possible Monitor patient satisfaction with pain management at specified intervals.

Case Study 3

Mr. B, a 61-year-old male patient, was admitted to the emergency room at the hospital with severe chest pain and pain in both arms at his elbows. He complained of having difficulty catching his breath and feeling nauseated. He was pale and diaphoretic. Auscultation of his chest revealed clear lungs and a regular heart rate of 70. The patient was started on oxygen (O_2) at 5 liters per nasal cannula and hooked up to the cardiac monitor. The cardiac monitor showed a sinus rhythm with elevated ST segments. His blood pressure was 108/62; respiratory rate, 32; and O_2 saturation, 86% before O_2 was started. Two IVs were started, both normal saline, running at a keep-open rate. A third IV was inserted and made into a saline lock. Mr. B received one nitroglycerin tablet sublingually, and his blood pressure dropped to 80/42. A total of 5 mg of morphine sulfate was given IV but did not eliminate his chest pain. A baby aspirin and IV Cardiazem were also given. An electrocardiogram (ECG) and chest x-ray were done. Labs drawn included cardiac enzymes including troponin level, sedimentation rate, electrolytes, blood urea nitrogen (BUN), creatinine, blood sugar, and arterial blood gases (ABGs). Mr. B appeared anxious, apprehensive, and expressed a fear of dying.

Mr. B's history includes previous episodes of chest pain during exertion, which lasted no longer than a few minutes when he stopped to rest. This time his pain started while he was mowing his lawn and did not subside with rest. He came to the emergency room within 45 minutes of when the pain began. He does not exercise routinely and has smoked two packs of cigarettes a day for the last 35 years. He weighs 260 pounds and is 5 feet, 11 inches tall. His family history is positive for cardiac problems. His father died from a myocardial infarction (MI) at age 62, and his brother has coronary artery disease. He had two uncles who died from MIs when they were in their early 60s.

The blood tests and electrocardiogram revealed that Mr. B was experiencing myocardial infarction, creatine kinase (CK), 682; creatine kinase isoenzyme containing M and B subunits (MB-CK), 20; relative index, 8; and his troponin level was positive. ABGs showed a PO_2 level of 68. All other laboratory test results were within normal limits. The ECG showed Q waves and ST segment elevation. A cardiologist was consulted, and the ECG was faxed to him. The patient received streptokinase and was started on Tridil drip. His blood pressure did come up to 110/56. Mr. B remained stable and his chest pain subsided slowly. He developed premature ventricular contractions (PVCs) unifocal and multifocal and had short runs of ventricular tachycardia (V tach). The irregular heart beats were monitored, and Mr. B remained symptomatic. His O_2 saturation remained in the low 90s after oxygen and medications were given. He appeared less anxious, less diaphoretic, and his color was better after his chest pain was relieved. Mr. B remained pain-free and was airlifted to another hospital where he was taken to the cardiac cath lab and had angioplasty done. He sustained minimal cardiac muscle damage. Table 3-3 provides a summary of the information in this case showing the linkages among NANDA, NOC, and NIC.

(Courtesy of Shelley McShane, BSN.)

TABLE 3-3	PLAN OF CARE FOR MR. B	
Nursing Diagnosis	**Nursing Outcome**	**Nursing Intervention**
CARDIAC OUTPUT, DECREASED	CARDIAC PUMP EFFECTIVENESS	CARDIAC CARE: ACUTE
DEFINING CHARACTERISTICS	**INDICATORS**	**NURSING ACTIVITIES**
Fatigue; variations in blood pressure readings; restlessness; dyspnea; cold clammy skin; arrhythmias; skin color changes; chest pain; increased respiratory rate; ECG changes; abnormal cardiac enzymes	BP IER	Evaluate chest pain
	Heart rate IER	Monitor cardiac rhythm and rate
	Cardiac index IER	Auscultate heart sounds
	Activity tolerance IER	Auscultate lungs for crackles or other adventitious sounds
	Heart size normal	Monitor intake/output, urine output, and daily weight, if appropriate
	Skin color normal	
	Neck vein distention not present	Select best ECG lead for continuous monitoring
	Dysrhythmia not present	Obtain 12-lead ECG
	Abnormal heart sounds not present	Draw serum, CK, LDH, and AST levels
	Angina not present	Monitor renal function
	Peripheral edema not present	Monitor lab values for electrolytes, which may increase risk of dysrhythmias
	Nausea not present	
	Extreme fatigue not present	Obtain chest x-ray
		Monitor trends in blood pressure and hemodynamic parameters
		Monitor the effectiveness of oxygen therapy
		Monitor determinants of oxygen delivery
		Maintain an environment conducive to rest and healing
		Instruct the patient to avoid activities that result in the Valsalva maneuver
		Administer medications to relieve/prevent pain and ischemia
		Monitor effectiveness of medication

ECG, Electrocardiogram; *BP*, blood pressure; *IER*, in expected range; *CK*, creatine kinase; *LDH*, lactate dehydrogenase; *AST*, aspartate aminotransferase.

Case Study 4

Mr. M, a 79-year-old white male, lives in a retirement living center. He has been widowed for 9 years. His only child, a son, lives in the same city and visits him every week. His son sets up his medications in a 7-day pill container during his visits. He has one nephew who maintains contact by phone once or twice a month. Mr. M has a history of atrial fibrillation controlled by medication and has moderate-to-severe venous insufficiency.

Over the past 6 months, Mr. M has developed multiple leg ulcers on both legs, but predominantly on the left leg. Vesicles, crusts, and eroded areas are noted over the lower half of the left leg, and the tissue around and between the toes on his left foot is sloughing off. At times the serous drainage is heavy enough to wet his trousers legs. There is a foul odor when Mr. M's stockings are removed.

Mr. M receives skilled nursing visits daily for assessment and wound care to his legs. On most visits the elastic stockings have to be soaked off of Mr. M's legs because of the large amounts of crusted serous drainage that sticks to the stockings. Even when his legs are soaked, there are times when the crusted areas of the wound adhere to the stockings, and tissue is pulled off as the stockings are removed. When asked if there is any pain or discomfort associated with touch to his left leg, Mr. M denies any, but winces and tenses his muscles when his legs are touched.

His physician has ordered elevation of Mr. M's legs above his hips and warm soaks of his legs using wet towels for 20 minutes and then air drying for 20 to 30 minutes. Elastic stockings are to be reapplied after legs are dry. Excessive crusts are to be washed off using an antibacterial soap and tap water. No medication is to be applied to the legs topically. Oral antibiotic therapy has been initiated. Reinforcement and teaching regarding the importance of elevating his legs when he is sitting down, not crossing his legs, and wearing his elastic stockings at all times when he is out of bed is done with each nursing visit.

Although there has been improvement in the condition of Mr. M's legs, it has not been significant enough for Mr. M to resume his previous level of self-care. In addition, he has started to use a wheelchair for transportation to and from the dining area for meals. Because of the use of the wheelchair, Mr. M is having difficulty making it to meals and caring for his own needs. If Mr. M cannot meet the minimum self-care standards for the retirement center, he may have to move from the center. When asked if he understands the impact of the current situation related to his ability to care for himself, he states that his legs "really don't feel so bad," and he does not think the concern expressed by those caring for him is warranted. He does not feel his ability to perform his activities of daily living has declined, nor does he feel the condition of his legs is impacting his performance of these activities. Table 3-4 provides a summary of the information in this case showing the linkages among NANDA, NOC, and NIC.

(Courtesy of Pamela Gedney, BSN.)

TABLE 3-4	PLAN OF CARE FOR MR. M	
Nursing Diagnosis	**Nursing Outcomes**	**Nursing Interventions**
SKIN INTEGRITY, IMPAIRED	**WOUND HEALING: SECONDARY INTENTION**	**WOUND CARE**
DEFINING CHARACTERISTICS	**INDICATORS**	**NURSING ACTIVITIES**
Destruction of the skin layers; disruption of skin surface	Granulation Resolution of purulent drainage Resolution of serous drainage	Note characteristics of the wound Note characteristics of any drainage
Related Factors	Resolution of surrounding skin erythema	Clean with antibacterial soap, as appropriate
Altered circulation; altered sensation	Resolution of blistered skin Resolution of necrosis Resolution of sloughing Resolution of wound odor Resolution of wound size	Administer skin ulcer care, as needed Bandage appropriately Inspect the wound with each dressing change Compare and record any changes in the wound
	CIRCULATION STATUS	**CIRCULATORY CARE: VENOUS INSUFFICIENCY**
	INDICATORS	**NURSING ACTIVITIES**
	Peripheral perfusion Peripheral edema not present Cognitive status IER	Evaluate peripheral edema and pulses Palpate limb with caution Monitor degree of discomfort or pain Apply antiembolism stockings Elevate affected limb 20 degrees or greater above the level of the heart Instruct patient on importance of prevention of venous stasis Protect extremity from injury

IER, In expected range.

ELECTRONIC INFORMATION SYSTEMS

Computerized clinical information systems are becoming more prevalent in health care organizations as the need to capture and evaluate clinical data has increased. Health care purchasers and managed care entities rely on statistical information derived from these systems to determine how health care dollars will be spent. As one author so aptly noted, "if nurses do not develop and adopt the tools needed to participate in this information-driven environment, opportunities to provide nursing services may significantly diminish in the future" (Jones, 1997, p. 377). Although the development of nursing information systems was identified as a high priority as early as 1988 (National Center for Nursing Research, 1988), the development of systems that use standardized data elements is in its infancy. As health care information systems expand, each discipline must identify the data elements required to evaluate the processes and outcomes of care.

Data base development requires a common language and a standard way to organize data. A uniform data set establishes standard measurements, definitions, and classifications (Murnaghan, 1978) for use in electronic information systems. The NANDA-NOC-NIC linkages are a beginning step in the organization of nursing information and provide meaningful categories of data for analysis. In an effort to move nursing forward in preparation for an electronic patient record, the American Nurses Association (ANA) has developed a set of standards for nursing data sets in information systems. Standards include those related to nomenclatures, clinical content linkages, the data repository, and general system requirements (American Nurses Association, 1997). The NANDA, NOC, and NIC vocabularies are recognized as approved nomenclatures, and the linkage work will provide beginning clinical content linkages.

Nurses' documentation of the diagnoses they treat, the interventions used to treat the diagnoses, and the resulting outcome responses to interventions in computerized information systems is necessary for the development of large local, regional, national, and international nursing data bases (Iowa Intervention Project, 1997). Large clinical data bases are needed to assess nursing effectiveness, generate hypotheses for testing with controlled research designs, and refine the linkages among diagnoses, interventions, and outcomes based on clinical and research evidence. These data base uses are essential for nursing knowledge development, for research-based practice, and to influence health policy. Busy clinicians, however, cannot afford the time to repeatedly sort through each standardized language in alphabetical form in a computerized system. Nurses also are reluctant to fully document their data if they must access a large number of computer screens for recording. The NANDA-NOC-NIC linkages presented in this book assist with the organization and structuring of nursing clinical information systems that are the most efficient for nurses' documentation of their practice. The taxonomies provide an organizing scheme for the arrangement of computer screens that ease clinicians' access for documentation. Likewise, the linkages offer greater efficiency by supplying groupings of diagnoses, interventions, and outcomes with a high probability of effective relationships for patient care.

Although not specifically prescriptive, the linkages also offer some decision support. A review of the outcomes and interventions that are most likely associated with a diagnosis by experienced nurses will help them consider possible treatments and responses that might be overlooked in the context of hectic and demanding clinical decision making. This decision support is sure to be even more helpful to novice nurses who also need clinical reasoning options available for review, but who often have difficulty identifying the critical and priority outcomes and interventions for a diagnosis.

TEACHING CLINICAL DECISION MAKING

The linkages can be used in conjunction with the three languages (NANDA, NOC, and NIC) to assist students in developing the skills necessary for clinical decision making. Case studies and computer simulations can be developed using the linkages in this book. Discussion of the cases can focus on the adequacy of the diagnosis selected to address the problem, the appropriateness of the outcomes and interventions selected, the rationale for their selection, and the identification of other outcomes or interventions that might be more appropriate in a given situation. A data base with the linkages can be made available for students to use when planning care for a patient or a group of patients. Students can use the linkages to evaluate the relationship between the patient's signs and symptoms, the defining characteristics and related factors of the diagnosis, the outcome and its indicators, and the intervention and its activities. They can select the outcome indicators and intervention activities for a patient based on the patient's status and the elements of the nursing diagnosis. The linkages will facilitate the teaching of clinical decision making through the application of teaching strategies such as the Outcome-Present State Test (OPT) model (Pesut & Herman, 1999).

The linkages also can be used in planning content for the curriculum. They can assist the faculty in selecting a body of content and distributing the content among the various courses. The linkages between diagnoses, outcomes, and interventions can be a starting point to identify a body of content related to the nursing diagnoses that will be taught in the curriculum. For example, the faculty may choose to teach content related to the diagnosis *Anxiety* and the outcome *Anxiety Control*. Although these concepts may be covered in a number of courses, the interventions might be most appropriately distributed among courses. For example, *Active Listening*, *Calming Technique*, and *Exercise Promotion* might be taught early in the curriculum whereas *Hypnosis, Simple Guided Imagery*, and *Therapeutic Touch* might be taught later in the curriculum or even in a graduate program.

There are a number of advantages to using NANDA-NOC-NIC vocabularies and linkages in a nursing curriculum. The vocabularies are comprehensive and can be used for patients across the continuum of care and in all settings in which care is provided. The terminology is useful for nurses in all nursing specialties and in various nursing roles. This makes the vocabularies and associated linkage work useful in both undergraduate and graduate curricula.

RESEARCH AND KNOWLEDGE DEVELOPMENT

The development of nursing knowledge requires evaluation of the effectiveness of various nursing interventions and the appropriateness of the decision-making process in selecting interventions to resolve a nursing diagnosis or to achieve a particular outcome. The linkage work contained in this book provides numerous relationships that require testing and evaluation in a clinical setting. Questions about which of the suggested interventions achieve the best outcome for a particular diagnosis, which of the outcomes are most achievable for a particular patient population, and what diagnoses and interventions are associated with specific medical diagnoses are just a sample of the questions that can be addressed.

Empirical work, as just described, will build mid-range theories unique to nursing (Blegen & Tripp-Reimer, 1997a; 1997b). The labels as defined in the taxonomies provide the concepts; the linkages between the diagnoses, interventions, and outcomes provide the connections between the concepts. As this work unfolds, we will have a clear articulation between theory, practice, and research and will build the body of knowledge unique to the discipline.

As well as studying the relationships between interventions and outcomes, the relationships among the environment, the structure of the health care organization, the processes of care, and the patient outcomes need to be studied. Without this type of data, organizations have little information on which to adjust staff mix or determine the cost-effectiveness of structural or process changes in the nursing care delivery system. Issues related to the study of organizational factors that influence patient outcomes have gained increased emphasis in recent literature. The November 1997 supplement (Vol. 35, No. 11) of *Medical Care*, the journal of the American Public Health Association, is devoted to a discussion of these factors.

Identification of patient factors that influence outcome attainment, referred to as risk factors, is another area that needs to be studied to carry out effectiveness research related to nursing interventions. These factors need to be identified to reduce or remove the effects of confounding factors in studies where the cases are not randomly assigned to different treatments, as is typical in most effectiveness research (Iezzoni, 1997). Identification of the personal factors that influence outcome achievement for a particular diagnosis or the effectiveness of an intervention for patients with varying personal characteristics and life circumstances will add to the body of nursing knowledge and allow nurses to provide the highest quality care possible.

Professional practice languages and classification systems are the fundamental categories of thought that define a profession and its scope of practice. While the nursing profession has made considerable progress in developing languages and classification systems, there is a need to use the languages to promote knowledge development. It is hoped that these linkages will suggest questions for study, including comparisons of the various languages currently used in nursing.

Development of the linkages in this book began with previous linkage work to link NANDA-NIC terms, NANDA-NOC terms, and NOC-NIC terms. This work relied on the previous work in the development of the linkages provided in Part II of this book. Requests to link NANDA diagnoses, NIC interventions, and NOC outcomes have come from practicing nurses, nurse educators, and software developers for clinical information systems. The linkages serve a number of uses for practice, education, and research. They are, however, just a beginning; their development is based on expert opinion, and further testing in clinical settings is needed.

REFERENCES

American Nurses Association. (1997). *Nursing informatics & data set evaluation center (NIDSEC) standards and scoring guidelines.* Washington, DC: Author.

Blegen, M. A., & Tripp-Reimer, T. (1997a). Implications of nursing taxonomies for middle-range theory development. *Advances in Nursing Science,* 19(3), 37-49.

Blegen, M. A., & Tripp-Reimer T. (1997b). Nursing theory, nursing research, and nursing practice: Connected or separate? In J. C. McCloskey & H. K. Grace (Eds.), *Current issues in nursing* (5th ed., pp. 68-74). St. Louis: Mosby.

Bulechek, G. M., & McCloskey, J. C. (Eds.). (1992). *Nursing interventions: Essential nursing treatments* (2nd ed.). Philadelphia: W.B. Saunders.

Iezzoni, L.I. (1997). Dimensions of risk. In L. I. Iezzoni (Ed.), *Risk adjustment for measuring healthcare outcomes* (2nd ed., pp. 43-115). Chicago: Health Administration Press.

Iowa Intervention Project. (1997). Proposal to bring nursing into the information age. *Image: Journal of Nursing Scholarship, 29*(3), 275-281.

Jones, D. L. (1997). Building the information infrastructure required for managed care. *Image: Journal of Nursing Scholarship, 29*(4), 377-382.

Murnaghan, H. (1978). Uniform basic data sets for health statistical systems. *International Journal of Epidemiology, 7*, 263-269.

National Center for Nursing Research. (1988, January 27-29). *Report on the national nursing research agenda for the participants in the conference on research priorities in nursing science.* Washington, DC: Author.

Pesut, D. J., & Herman, J. (1999). *Clinical reasoning: The art & science of critical & creative thinking.* Boston: Delmar Publishers.

Rubenfeld, M. G., & Scheffer, B. K. (1999). *Critical thinking in nursing: An interactive approach* (2nd ed.). Philadelphia: Lippincott.

Yura, H., & Walsh, M.B. (1973). *The nursing process: Assessing, planning, implementing, evaluating* (2nd ed.). New York: Appleton-Century-Crofts.

PART II

NANDA, NOC, and NIC Linkages

Introduction

This section of the book contains the linkages described in the preceding chapters. Entry to the linkages is through a NANDA diagnosis. The user will locate the diagnosis of interest, and the associated outcomes and interventions will appear with that diagnosis. The diagnoses are in alphabetical order; however, the first word represents the major concept in the diagnosis. For example, when looking for the diagnosis *Impaired Gas Exchange*, look for *Gas Exchange, Impaired*. When the NANDA diagnosis begins with impaired, ineffective, or altered, those terms will appear at the end of the label name rather than at the beginning. The diagnoses that capture the risk for developing a problem are not included in the alphabetical list of diagnoses that represent an altered patient/client state but, instead, appear as a group following those diagnoses that capture existing patient problems or the potential for improvement.

The "risk for" diagnoses are also listed in alphabetical order, with the major concept at the beginning and the term *risk for* following. For example, *Risk for Fluid Volume Imbalance* is presented as *Fluid Volume Imbalance, Risk for*. The NANDA diagnoses that capture risk do not include the same elements as the diagnoses that capture existing problem states or the potential to enhance patient states. Diagnoses that represent existing problems include a definition, defining characteristics, and related factors; *risk for* diagnoses include a definition and risk factors. The outcomes linked with the risk diagnoses are the outcomes that would be evaluated to determine if the state that the patient/client is at risk for has occurred. For example, the suggested outcomes for *Activity Intolerance, Risk for* include *Activity Tolerance, Endurance,* and *Energy Conservation*. The interventions that are linked to the outcome are those associated with promoting the patient state represented by the outcome. The major interventions for *Activity Tolerance* include *Energy Management* and *Exercise Promotion: Strength Training*. However, the authors recognize that to address the risk, interventions that treat the underlying risk factors must be selected. Since the risk factors associated with each diagnosis vary from a few to a lengthy list, the authors chose not to address each of the risk factors when providing linkages in this book. To assist the user, NANDA diagnoses that represent specific risk factors are identified at the end of each linkage. Outcomes and interventions linked to those diagnoses can be found by looking up the diagnosis of interest. NANDA diagnoses suggested for *Activity Intolerance, Risk for* include *Breathing Pattern, Ineffective; Cardiac Output, Deceased; Failure to Thrive, Adult; Fatigue; Gas Exchange, Impaired;* and *Health Maintenance, Altered*. Although these NANDA diagnoses were identified from the list of NANDA risk factors, the authors selected those that in their opinion reflected the identified risk factors. It is important to note that in some instances the suggested diagnoses may not encompass all of the risk factors if there is not a NANDA diagnosis for a particular risk factor. For example, *Altered Parenting, Risk for* includes a number of patient characteristics that the nurse must consider, but for which NANDA does not propose a specific diagnosis. Some of the characteristics identified as risk factors include legal difficulties, single parent, low educational level, and multiple births.

NANDA, NOC, and NIC Linkages

Activity Intolerance
Adjustment, Impaired
Airway Clearance, Ineffective
Anxiety
Body Image Disturbance
Breastfeeding, Effective
Breastfeeding, Ineffective
Breastfeeding, Interrupted
Breathing Pattern, Ineffective
Cardiac Output, Decreased
Caregiver Role Strain
Communication, Impaired Verbal
Community Coping, Ineffective
Community Coping, Potential for Enhanced
Community Management of Therapeutic Regimen, Ineffective
Confusion, Acute
Confusion, Chronic
Constipation
Constipation, Perceived
Death Anxiety
Decisional Conflict (Specify)
Defensive Coping
Denial, Ineffective
Dentition, Altered
Diarrhea
Diversional Activity Deficit
Dysreflexia
Energy Field Disturbance
Environmental Interpretation Syndrome, Impaired
Failure to Thrive, Adult
Families Management of Therapeutic Regimen, Ineffective
Family Coping: Compromised, Ineffective
Family Coping: Disabling, Ineffective
Family Coping: Potential for Growth
Family Processes, Altered
Family Processes, Altered: Alcoholism
Fatigue
Fear
Fluid Volume Deficit
Fluid Volume Excess
Gas Exchange, Impaired
Grieving, Anticipatory
Grieving, Dysfunctional
Growth and Development, Altered
Health Maintenance, Altered
Health-Seeking Behaviors (Specify)
Home Maintenance Management, Impaired
Hopelessness
Hyperthermia

Hypothermia
Incontinence: Bowel
Individual Coping, Ineffective
Individual Management of Therapeutic Regimen, Effective
Individual Management of Therapeutic Regimen, Ineffective
Infant Behavior, Disorganized
Infant Behavior, Organized, Potential for Enhanced
Infant Feeding Pattern, Ineffective
Intracranial Adaptive Capacity, Decreased
Knowledge Deficit (Specify)
Latex Allergy Response
Memory, Impaired
Mobility, Impaired Bed
Nausea
Noncompliance (Specify)
Nutrition, Altered: Less than Body Requirements
Nutrition, Altered: More than Body Requirements
Oral Mucous Membrane, Altered
Pain
Pain, Chronic
Parental Role Conflict
Parenting, Altered
Personal Identity Disturbance
Physical Mobility, Impaired
Post-Trauma Syndrome
Powerlessness
Protection, Altered
Rape-Trauma Syndrome
Rape-Trauma Syndrome: Compound Reaction
Rape-Trauma Syndrome: Silent Reaction
Relocation Stress Syndrome
Role Performance, Altered
Self-Care Deficit: Bathing/Hygiene
Self-Care Deficit: Dressing/Grooming
Self-Care Deficit: Feeding
Self-Care Deficit: Toileting
Self-Esteem, Chronic Low
Self-Esteem Disturbance
Self-Esteem, Situational Low
Sensory/Perceptual Alterations: Auditory
Sensory/Perceptual Alterations: Gustatory
Sensory/Perceptual Alterations: Kinesthetic
Sensory/Perceptual Alterations: Olfactory
Sensory/Perceptual Alterations: Tactile
Sensory/Perceptual Alterations: Visual
Sexual Dysfunction
Sexuality Patterns, Altered
Skin Integrity, Impaired
Sleep Deprivation
Sleep Pattern Disturbance
Social Interaction, Impaired

Social Isolation
Sorrow, Chronic
Spiritual Distress (Distress of the Human Spirit)
Spiritual Well-Being, Potential for Enhanced
Surgical Recovery, Delayed
Swallowing, Impaired
Thermoregulation, Ineffective
Thought Processes, Altered
Tissue Integrity, Impaired
Tissue Perfusion, Altered: Cardiopulmonary
Tissue Perfusion, Altered: Cerebral
Tissue Perfusion, Altered: Gastrointestinal
Tissue Perfusion, Altered: Peripheral
Tissue Perfusion, Altered: Renal
Transfer Ability, Impaired
Unilateral Neglect
Urinary Elimination, Altered
Urinary Incontinence, Functional
Urinary Incontinence, Stress
Urinary Incontinence, Total
Urinary Incontinence, Urge
Urinary Retention
Ventilation, Inability to Sustain Spontaneous
Ventilatory Weaning Response, Dysfunctional
Walking, Impaired
Wheelchair Mobility, Impaired

NANDA, NOC, and NIC Linkages (Risk for Developing)

Activity Intolerance, Risk for
Aspiration, Risk for
Autonomic Dysreflexia, Risk for
Body Temperature, Risk for Altered
Caregiver Role Strain, Risk for
Constipation, Risk for
Development, Risk for Altered
Disuse Syndrome, Risk for
Fluid Volume Deficit, Risk for
Fluid Volume Imbalance, Risk for
Growth, Risk for Altered
Infant Behavior, Disorganized, Risk for
Infection, Risk for
Injury, Risk for
Latex Allergy Response, Risk for
Loneliness, Risk for
Nutrition, Altered: Risk for More than Body Requirements
Parent/Infant/Child Attachment, Risk for Altered
Parenting, Risk for Altered
Perioperative Positioning Injury, Risk for
Peripheral Neurovascular Dysfunction, Risk for
Poisoning, Risk for

Post-Trauma Syndrome, Risk for
Self-Mutilation, Risk for
Skin Integrity, Risk for Impaired
Spiritual Distress, Risk for
Suffocation, Risk for
Trauma, Risk for
Urinary Urge Incontinence, Risk for
Violence, Risk for: Directed at Others
Violence, Risk for: Self-Directed

Nursing Diagnosis: ACTIVITY INTOLERANCE

DEFINITION: A state in which an individual has insufficient physiological or psychological energy to endure or complete required or desired daily activities.

Outcome: ACTIVITY TOLERANCE

MAJOR INTERVENTIONS	SUGGESTED INTERVENTIONS	OPTIONAL INTERVENTIONS

Activity Therapy
Energy Management
Exercise Promotion:
  Strength Training
	Animal-Assisted
	  Therapy
	Body Mechanics
	  Promotion
	Cardiac Care:
	  Rehabilitative
	Environmental
	  Management
	Exercise Promotion
	Exercise Promotion:
	  Stretching
	Exercise Therapy:
	  Ambulation
	Exercise Therapy:
	  Balance
	Exercise Therapy: Joint
	  Mobility
	Exercise Therapy:
	  Muscle Control
	Music Therapy
	Pain Management
	Teaching: Prescribed
	  Activity/Exercise
		Art Therapy
		Autogenic Training
		Biofeedback
		Environmental
		  Management: Comfort
		Hypnosis
		Medication Management
		Meditation Facilitation
		Mutual Goal Setting
		Nutrition Management
		Oxygen Therapy
		Progressive Muscle
		  Relaxation
		Sleep Enhancement
		Smoking Cessation
		  Assistance
		Spiritual Support
		Therapeutic Touch
		Visitation Facilitation
		Weight Management

Continued

Outcome: ENDURANCE

MAJOR INTERVENTIONS	SUGGESTED INTERVENTIONS	OPTIONAL INTERVENTIONS

Activity Therapy
Energy Management
Exercise Promotion:
  Strength Training
	Exercise Promotion
	Nutrition Management
	Sleep Enhancement
	Teaching: Prescribed
	  Activity/Exercise
		Cardiac Care:
		  Rehabilitative
		Eating Disorders
		  Management
		Environmental
		  Management
		Environmental
		  Management: Comfort
		Exercise Therapy:
		  Ambulation
		Exercise Therapy:
		  Balance
		Exercise Therapy: Joint
		  Mobility
		Exercise Therapy:
		  Muscle Control
		Mutual Goal Setting
		Oxygen Therapy
		Pain Management
		Visitation Facilitation
		Weight Management

Outcome: ENERGY CONSERVATION

MAJOR INTERVENTIONS	SUGGESTED INTERVENTIONS	OPTIONAL INTERVENTIONS

Energy Management
Nutrition Management
	Activity Therapy
	Body Mechanics
	  Promotion
	Environmental
	  Management
	Environmental
	  Management: Comfort
	Exercise Promotion
	Sleep Enhancement
	Teaching: Prescribed
	  Activity/Exercise
		Exercise Therapy:
		  Ambulation
		Exercise Therapy:
		  Balance
		Exercise Therapy: Joint
		  Mobility
		Exercise Therapy:
		  Muscle Control
		Meditation Facilitation
		Music Therapy
		Weight Management

Outcome: SELF-CARE: ACTIVITIES OF DAILY LIVING (ADL)

MAJOR INTERVENTIONS	SUGGESTED INTERVENTIONS	OPTIONAL INTERVENTIONS
Self-Care Assistance	Case Management Exercise Promotion: Stretching Exercise Therapy: Ambulation Exercise Therapy: Balance Exercise Therapy: Joint Mobility Self-Care Assistance: Bathing/Hygiene Self-Care Assistance: Dressing/Grooming Self-Care Assistance: Feeding Self-Care Assistance: Toileting Teaching: Prescribed Activity/Exercise	Body Mechanics Promotion Energy Management Exercise Promotion Exercise Therapy: Muscle Control

Outcome: SELF-CARE: INSTRUMENTAL ACTIVITIES OF DAILY LIVING (IADL)

MAJOR INTERVENTIONS	SUGGESTED INTERVENTIONS	OPTIONAL INTERVENTIONS
Home Maintenance Assistance	Consultation Energy Management Environmental Management Environmental Management: Home Preparation Financial Resource Assistance Referral	Body Mechanics Promotion

Nursing Diagnosis: ADJUSTMENT, IMPAIRED

DEFINITION: Inability to modify life style/behavior in a manner consistent with a change in health status.

Outcome: ACCEPTANCE: HEALTH STATUS

MAJOR INTERVENTIONS	SUGGESTED INTERVENTIONS	OPTIONAL INTERVENTIONS

Coping Enhancement
Emotional Support
	Behavior Modification
	Body Image
	  Enhancement
	Counseling
	Crisis Intervention
	Decision-Making
	  Support
	Hope Instillation
	Presence
	Spiritual Support
	Support Group
	Support System
	  Enhancement
	Values Clarification
		Anxiety Reduction
		Self-Awareness
		  Enhancement
		Teaching: Disease
		  Process
		Truth Telling

Outcome: COMPLIANCE BEHAVIOR

MAJOR INTERVENTIONS	SUGGESTED INTERVENTIONS	OPTIONAL INTERVENTIONS

Behavior Modification
Mutual Goal Setting
Patient Contracting
	Coping Enhancement
	Counseling
	Decision-Making
	  Support
	Health System Guidance
	Learning Readiness
	  Enhancement
	Self-Modification
	  Assistance
	Self-Responsibility
	  Facilitation
	Support System
	  Enhancement
	Values Clarification
		Culture Brokerage
		Family Involvement
		  Promotion
		Family Mobilization
		Family Support
		Patient Rights Protection
		Teaching: Individual
		Teaching: Prescribed
		  Activity/Exercise
		Teaching: Prescribed
		  Diet
		Teaching: Prescribed
		  Medication
		Teaching: Procedure/
		  Treatment
		Teaching: Psychomotor
		  Skill

Outcome: COPING

MAJOR INTERVENTIONS	SUGGESTED INTERVENTIONS	OPTIONAL INTERVENTIONS

Coping Enhancement
Counseling
Crisis Intervention
	Anticipatory Guidance
	Anxiety Reduction
	Decision-Making
	  Support
	Emotional Support
	Family Support
	Health System Guidance
	Hope Instillation
	Mutual Goal Setting
	Pain Management
	Recreation Therapy
	Role Enhancement
	Spiritual Support
	Support Group
	Values Clarification
		Behavior Modification
		Body Image
		  Enhancement
		Caregiver Support
		Cognitive Restructuring
		Family Therapy
		Mood Management
		Reminiscence Therapy
		Sibling Support
		Simple Relaxation
		  Therapy
		Support System
		  Enhancement
		Surveillance
		Therapy Group
		Truth Telling

Outcome: GRIEF RESOLUTION

MAJOR INTERVENTIONS	SUGGESTED INTERVENTIONS	OPTIONAL INTERVENTIONS

Grief Work Facilitation	Active Listening
	Anticipatory Guidance
	Coping Enhancement
	Counseling
	Dying Care
	Emotional Support
	Hope Instillation
	Support Group
	Support System
	  Enhancement
		Animal-Assisted
		  Therapy
		Bibliotherapy
		Decision-Making
		  Support
		Guilt Work Facilitation
		Music Therapy
		Presence
		Sibling Support
		Spiritual Support
		Touch

Continued

Outcome: HEALTH SEEKING BEHAVIOR

MAJOR INTERVENTIONS	SUGGESTED INTERVENTIONS	OPTIONAL INTERVENTIONS
Decision-Making Support Health Education Values Clarification	Anticipatory Guidance Counseling Emotional Support Health System Guidance Learning Facilitation Learning Readiness Enhancement Mutual Goal Setting Patient Contracting Referral Self-Awareness Enhancement Self-Modification Assistance Self-Responsibility Facilitation Support Group	Bibliotherapy Culture Brokerage Smoking Cessation Assistance Substance Use Prevention Teaching: Safe Sex Weight Management

Outcome: PARTICIPATION: HEALTH CARE DECISIONS

MAJOR INTERVENTIONS	SUGGESTED INTERVENTIONS	OPTIONAL INTERVENTIONS
Decision-Making Support Health System Guidance	Active Listening Anticipatory Guidance Assertiveness Training Counseling Culture Brokerage Self-Responsibility Facilitation Values Clarification	Anxiety Reduction Behavior Modification Coping Enhancement Family Involvement Promotion Health Care Information Exchange

Outcome: PSYCHOSOCIAL ADJUSTMENT: LIFE CHANGE

MAJOR INTERVENTIONS	SUGGESTED INTERVENTIONS	OPTIONAL INTERVENTIONS
Anticipatory Guidance Coping Enhancement	Behavior Modification Cognitive Restructuring Counseling Crisis Intervention Dying Care Emotional Support Health Education Role Enhancement	Decision-Making Support Humor Spiritual Support

Outcome: TREATMENT BEHAVIOR: ILLNESS OR INJURY

MAJOR INTERVENTIONS	SUGGESTED INTERVENTIONS	OPTIONAL INTERVENTIONS

Self-Responsibility
  Facilitation
Teaching: Disease
  Process
	Behavior Modification
	Counseling
	Environmental
	  Management
	Health Education
	Health System Guidance
	Mutual Goal Setting
	Patient Contracting
	Surveillance
		Behavior Management
		Cognitive Restructuring
		Self-Care Assistance

Nursing Diagnosis: AIRWAY CLEARANCE, INEFFECTIVE

Definition: Inability to clear secretions or obstructions from the respiratory tract to maintain a clear airway.

Outcome: ASPIRATION CONTROL

MAJOR INTERVENTIONS	SUGGESTED INTERVENTIONS	OPTIONAL INTERVENTIONS
Airway Management Airway Suctioning Aspiration Precautions Positioning	Cough Enhancement Resuscitation: Neonate Surveillance Swallowing Therapy Vomiting Management	Chest Physiotherapy Emergency Care Endotracheal Extubation

Outcome: RESPIRATORY STATUS: AIRWAY PATENCY

MAJOR INTERVENTIONS	SUGGESTED INTERVENTIONS	OPTIONAL INTERVENTIONS

Airway Management
Airway Suctioning
Cough Enhancement
	Airway Insertion and
	  Stabilization
	Artificial Airway
	  Management
	Aspiration Precautions
	Chest Physiotherapy
	Positioning
	Surveillance
	Vital Signs Monitoring
		Allergy Management
		Anaphylaxis
		  Management
		Emergency Care

Outcome: RESPIRATORY STATUS: GAS EXCHANGE

MAJOR INTERVENTIONS	SUGGESTED INTERVENTIONS	OPTIONAL INTERVENTIONS

Acid-Base Monitoring
Oxygen Therapy
Respiratory Monitoring
Ventilation Assistance
	Acid-Base Management:
	  Respiratory Acidosis
	Acid-Base Management:
	  Respiratory Alkalosis
	Airway Management
	Anxiety Reduction
	Chest Physiotherapy
	Positioning
	Vital Signs Monitoring
		Airway Insertion and
		  Stabilization
		Airway Suctioning
		Artificial Airway
		  Management
		Aspiration Precautions
		Cough Enhancement
		Embolus Care:
		  Pulmonary
		Laboratory Data
		  Interpretation
		Mechanical Ventilation
		Phlebotomy: Arterial
		  Blood Sample

Outcome: **RESPIRATORY STATUS: VENTILATION**		
MAJOR INTERVENTIONS	**SUGGESTED INTERVENTIONS**	**OPTIONAL INTERVENTIONS**

Airway Management
Respiratory Monitoring
Ventilation Assistance
	Airway Insertion and
	  Stabilization
	Airway Suctioning
	Allergy Management
	Artificial Airway
	  Management
	Aspiration Precautions
	Energy Management
	Infection Control
	Mechanical Ventilation
	Medication
	  Administration:
	  Inhalation
	Positioning
		Acid-Base Monitoring
		Anxiety Reduction
		Chest Physiotherapy
		Cough Enhancement
		Fluid Monitoring
		Mechanical Ventilatory
		  Weaning
		Oxygen Therapy

Nursing Diagnosis: **ANXIETY**

DEFINITION: A vague uneasy feeling of discomfort or dread accompanied by an autonomic response; the source is often nonspecific or unknown to the individual; a feeling of apprehension caused by anticipation of danger. It is an altering signal that warns of impending danger and enables the individual to take measures to deal with threat.

Outcome: **AGGRESSION CONTROL**

MAJOR INTERVENTIONS	SUGGESTED INTERVENTIONS	OPTIONAL INTERVENTIONS
Anger Control Assistance Impulse Control Training	Anxiety Reduction Area Restriction Calming Technique Coping Enhancement Counseling Crisis Intervention Family Process Maintenance Fire-Setting Precautions Limit Setting Patient Contracting Surveillance: Safety	Art Therapy Behavior Management: Self-Harm Environmental Management Environmental Management: Safety Music Therapy Self-Modification Assistance Self-Responsibility Facilitation Socialization Enhancement Therapeutic Play Therapy Group

Outcome: **ANXIETY CONTROL**		
MAJOR INTERVENTIONS	**SUGGESTED INTERVENTIONS**	**OPTIONAL INTERVENTIONS**
Anxiety Reduction	Active Listening Anticipatory Guidance Behavior Management Calming Technique Childbirth Preparation Coping Enhancement Counseling Dementia Management Examination Assistance Exercise Promotion Medication Administration Medication Prescribing Preparatory Sensory Information Presence Security Enhancement Telephone Consultation	Animal-Assisted Therapy Art Therapy Autogenic Training Biofeedback Distraction Environmental Management Guilt Work Facilitation Humor Hypnosis Meditation Facilitation Music Therapy Progressive Muscle Relaxation Simple Guided Imagery Simple Relaxation Therapy Support Group Teaching: Preoperative Therapeutic Play Therapy Group

Continued

Outcome: COPING

MAJOR INTERVENTIONS	SUGGESTED INTERVENTIONS	OPTIONAL INTERVENTIONS
Anticipatory Guidance Coping Enhancement	Anxiety Reduction Calming Technique Counseling Crisis Intervention Emotional Support Family Process Maintenance Grief Work Facilitation Grief Work Facilitation: Perinatal Death Guilt Work Facilitation Hope Instillation Humor Meditation Facilitation Presence Progressive Muscle Relaxation Simple Relaxation Therapy Spiritual Support Support Group	Animal-Assisted Therapy Art Therapy Childbirth Preparation Distraction Genetic Counseling Preparatory Sensory Information Recreation Therapy Reminiscence Therapy Sibling Support Therapeutic Play Therapy Group

Outcome: IMPULSE CONTROL

MAJOR INTERVENTIONS	SUGGESTED INTERVENTIONS	OPTIONAL INTERVENTIONS
Impulse Control Training	Anger Control Assistance Anxiety Reduction Area Restriction Behavior Management Behavior Management: Self-Harm Coping Enhancement Elopement Precautions Environmental Management: Safety Limit Setting Milieu Therapy	Emotional Support Mood Management Security Enhancement Support Group Support System Enhancement Surveillance: Safety Teaching: Individual Therapy Group

Outcome: SELF-MUTILATION RESTRAINT

MAJOR INTERVENTIONS	SUGGESTED INTERVENTIONS	OPTIONAL INTERVENTIONS
Behavior Management: Self-Harm	Anger Control Assistance Anxiety Reduction Area Restriction Coping Enhancement Counseling Crisis Intervention Emotional Support Environmental Management: Safety Impulse Control Training Limit Setting Security Enhancement Suicide Prevention Surveillance: Safety	Elopement Precautions Mood Management Self-Modification Assistance Therapy Group

Outcome: SOCIAL INTERACTION SKILLS

MAJOR INTERVENTIONS	SUGGESTED INTERVENTIONS	OPTIONAL INTERVENTIONS
Behavior Modification: Social Skills Complex Relationship Building	Active Listening Anger Control Assistance Anxiety Reduction Assertiveness Training Counseling Family Process Maintenance	Calming Technique Coping Enhancement Guilt Work Facilitation Humor Impulse Control Training Therapy Group

Nursing Diagnosis: BODY IMAGE DISTURBANCE

DEFINITION: Confusion in mental picture of one's physical self.

Outcome: BODY IMAGE

MAJOR INTERVENTIONS	SUGGESTED INTERVENTIONS	OPTIONAL INTERVENTIONS
Body Image Enhancement	Active Listening Amputation Care Anxiety Reduction Coping Enhancement Counseling Emotional Support Grief Work Facilitation Pain Management Self-Awareness Enhancement Self-Care Assistance Self-Esteem Enhancement Support Group Support System Enhancement Therapy Group Values Clarification Weight Management	Anticipatory Guidance Cognitive Restructuring Eating Disorders Management Nutritional Counseling Ostomy Care Pain Management Postpartal Care Prenatal Care Self-Modification Assistance Unilateral Neglect Management

Outcome: CHILD DEVELOPMENT: 2 YEARS

MAJOR INTERVENTIONS	SUGGESTED INTERVENTIONS	OPTIONAL INTERVENTIONS
Developmental Enhancement: Child Parent Education: Childrearing Family	Anticipatory Guidance Body Image Enhancement Family Involvement Promotion Nutrition Management Security Enhancement Socialization Enhancement	Abuse Protection Support: Child Behavior Management Bowel Training Nutritional Counseling Nutritional Monitoring Sibling Support Support System Enhancement Therapeutic Play Urinary Habit Training

Outcome: CHILD DEVELOPMENT: 3 YEARS

MAJOR INTERVENTIONS	SUGGESTED INTERVENTIONS	OPTIONAL INTERVENTIONS
Developmental Enhancement: Child Parent Education: Childrearing Family	Anticipatory Guidance Body Image Enhancement Bowel Management Bowel Training Family Involvement Promotion Nutrition Management Security Enhancement Socialization Enhancement Urinary Habit Training Urinary Incontinence Care: Enuresis	Abuse Protection Support: Child Behavior Management Nutritional Counseling Nutritional Monitoring Sibling Support Therapeutic Play

Outcome: CHILD DEVELOPMENT: 4 YEARS

MAJOR INTERVENTIONS	SUGGESTED INTERVENTIONS	OPTIONAL INTERVENTIONS
Developmental Enhancement: Child Parent Education: Childrearing Family	Anticipatory Guidance Body Image Enhancement Family Involvement Promotion Nutrition Management Security Enhancement Self-Care Assistance Socialization Enhancement	Abuse Protection Support: Child Behavior Management Behavior Modification Bowel Incontinence Care: Encopresis Counseling Nutritional Counseling Nutritional Monitoring Sibling Support Therapeutic Play Urinary Habit Training Urinary Incontinence Care: Enuresis

Continued

Outcome: Child Development: 5 Years

MAJOR INTERVENTIONS	SUGGESTED INTERVENTIONS	OPTIONAL INTERVENTIONS
Developmental Enhancement: Child Parent Education: Childrearing Family	Anticipatory Guidance Body Image Enhancement Family Involvement Promotion Nutrition Management Security Enhancement Self-Care Assistance Socialization Enhancement	Abuse Protection Support: Child Behavior Management Behavior Modification Counseling Nutritional Counseling Nutritional Monitoring Sibling Support Therapeutic Play Urinary Habit Training Urinary Incontinence Care: Enuresis

Outcome: Child Development: Middle Childhood (6-11 Years)

MAJOR INTERVENTIONS	SUGGESTED INTERVENTIONS	OPTIONAL INTERVENTIONS
Development Enhancement: Child Parent Education: Childrearing Family Risk Identification	Anticipatory Guidance Body Image Enhancement Exercise Promotion Family Involvement Promotion Mutual Goal Setting Nutrition Management Nutritional Counseling Nutritional Monitoring Patient Contracting Self-Awareness Enhancement Self-Esteem Enhancement Self-Modification Assistance Self-Responsibility Facilitation Socialization Enhancement Spiritual Support Substance Use Prevention Teaching: Sexuality Values Clarification	Abuse Protection Support: Child Behavior Management Behavior Modification Counseling Eating Disorders Management Sibling Support Therapeutic Play Urinary Incontinence Care: Enuresis Weight Management

Outcome: CHILD DEVELOPMENT: ADOLESCENCE (12-17 YEARS)

MAJOR INTERVENTIONS	SUGGESTED INTERVENTIONS	OPTIONAL INTERVENTIONS
Developmental Enhancement: Adolescent Parent Education: Adolescent Risk Identification Self-Esteem Enhancement	Anticipatory Guidance Body Image Enhancement Exercise Promotion Family Involvement Promotion Mutual Goal Setting Nutrition Management Nutritional Counseling Nutritional Monitoring Role Enhancement Self-Awareness Enhancement Self-Modification Assistance Socialization Enhancement Spiritual Support Substance Use Prevention Teaching: Individual Teaching: Safe Sex Teaching: Sexuality Values Clarification	Abuse Protection Support Behavior Management Behavior Modification Counseling Eating Disorders Management Sexual Counseling Sibling Support Support System Enhancement Weight Management

Outcome: GRIEF RESOLUTION

MAJOR INTERVENTIONS	SUGGESTED INTERVENTIONS	OPTIONAL INTERVENTIONS
Grief Work Facilitation	Active Listening Anticipatory Guidance Coping Enhancement Counseling Emotional Support Hope Installation Support Group Support System Enhancement	Bibliotherapy Decision-Making Support Guilt Work Facilitation Presence Sibling Support Spiritual Support

Continued

Outcome: Psychosocial Adjustment: Life Change

MAJOR INTERVENTIONS	SUGGESTED INTERVENTIONS	OPTIONAL INTERVENTIONS
Anticipatory Guidance Coping Enhancement	Childbirth Preparation Cognitive Restructuring Counseling Developmental Enhancement: Adolescent Developmental Enhancement: Child Dying Care Emotional Support Health Education	Decision-Making Support Family Process Maintenance Humor Lactation Counseling Spiritual Support

Outcome: Self-Esteem

MAJOR INTERVENTIONS	SUGGESTED INTERVENTIONS	OPTIONAL INTERVENTIONS
Self-Esteem Enhancement	Active Listening Body Image Enhancement Cognitive Restructuring Counseling Developmental Enhancement: Adolescent Developmental Enhancement: Child Emotional Support Self-Awareness Enhancement Socialization Enhancement Support Group	Assertiveness Training Behavior Modification Behavior Modification: Social Skills Bibliotherapy Complex Relationship Building Coping Enhancement Eating Disorders Management Family Mobilization Parent Education: Adolescent Parent Education: Childrearing Family Security Enhancement Self-Modification Assistance Spiritual Support Weight Management

Nursing Diagnosis: BREASTFEEDING, EFFECTIVE

DEFINITION: The state in which a mother-infant dyad/family exhibits adequate proficiency and satisfaction with breastfeeding process.

Outcome: BREASTFEEDING ESTABLISHMENT: INFANT

MAJOR INTERVENTIONS	SUGGESTED INTERVENTIONS	OPTIONAL INTERVENTIONS
Breastfeeding Assistance Lactation Counseling	Attachment Promotion Calming Technique Newborn Care Newborn Monitoring Parent Education: Infant Positioning Presence	Infant Care Kangaroo Care

Outcome: BREASTFEEDING ESTABLISHMENT: MATERNAL

MAJOR INTERVENTIONS	SUGGESTED INTERVENTIONS	OPTIONAL INTERVENTIONS

Lactation Counseling	Active Listening
	Anticipatory Guidance
	Emotional Support
	Fluid Management
	Infection Protection
	Nutrition Management
	Nutritional Counseling
	Positioning
	Skin Surveillance
		Body Mechanics
		  Promotion
		Heat/Cold Application
		Teaching: Individual
		Teaching: Psychomotor
		  Skill

Continued

Outcome: **BREASTFEEDING MAINTENANCE**

MAJOR INTERVENTIONS	SUGGESTED INTERVENTIONS	OPTIONAL INTERVENTIONS

Lactation Counseling	Active Listening
	Anticipatory Guidance
	Emotional Support
	Energy Management
	Family Involvement
	  Promotion
	Family Support
	Fluid Management
	Infant Care
	Infection Protection
	Nutrition Management
	Simple Relaxation
	  Therapy
	Skin Care: Topical
	  Treatments
	Skin Surveillance
	Sleep Enhancement
	Teaching: Infant
	  Nutrition
		Attachment Promotion
		Nutrition Therapy
		Support Group
		Weight Management

Outcome: **BREASTFEEDING WEANING**

MAJOR INTERVENTIONS	SUGGESTED INTERVENTIONS	OPTIONAL INTERVENTIONS

Lactation Counseling
Lactation Suppression
	Active Listening
	Anticipatory Guidance
	Emotional Support
	Family Involvement
	  Promotion
	Family Support
	Skin Surveillance
	Teaching: Infant
	  Nutrition
		Heat/Cold Application
		Infection Protection
		Pain Management

Nursing Diagnosis: BREASTFEEDING, INEFFECTIVE

DEFINITION: The state in which a mother, infant, or child experiences dissatisfaction or difficulty with the breastfeeding process.

Outcome: BREASTFEEDING ESTABLISHMENT: INFANT

MAJOR INTERVENTIONS	SUGGESTED INTERVENTIONS	OPTIONAL INTERVENTIONS
Breastfeeding Assistance Lactation Counseling	Attachment Promotion Calming Technique Newborn Care Newborn Monitoring Parent Education: Infant Positioning Presence Surveillance	Bottle Feeding Nutrition Therapy Fluid/Electrolyte Management Infant Care Kangaroo Care

Outcome: BREASTFEEDING ESTABLISHMENT: MATERNAL

MAJOR INTERVENTIONS	SUGGESTED INTERVENTIONS	OPTIONAL INTERVENTIONS

Breastfeeding Assistance
Lactation Counseling
	Active Listening
	Analgesic
	  Administration
	Anticipatory Guidance
	Anxiety Reduction
	Discharge Planning
	Emotional Support
	Environmental
	  Management:
	    Attachment Process
	Family Involvement
	  Promotion
	Family Support
	Fluid Management
	Infection Protection
	Nutritional Counseling
	Parent Education: Infant
	Positioning
	Simple Relaxation
	  Therapy
	Skin Care: Topical
	  Treatments
	Skin Surveillance
	Teaching: Infant
	  Nutrition
	Teaching:
	  Prescribed Diet
		Cesarean Section Care
		Coping Enhancement
		Heat/Cold Application
		Pain Management
		Sleep Enhancement
		Support Group
		Teaching: Individual
		Teaching: Psychomotor
		  Skill
		Telephone Consultation

Continued

Outcome: BREASTFEEDING MAINTENANCE

MAJOR INTERVENTIONS	SUGGESTED INTERVENTIONS	OPTIONAL INTERVENTIONS

Breastfeeding Assistance
Lactation Counseling
	Active Listening
	Coping Enhancement
	Emotional Support
	Energy Management
	Family Involvement
	  Promotion
	Family Support
	Fluid Management
	Infection Protection
	Nutritional Counseling
	Simple Relaxation
	  Therapy
	Skin Care: Topical
	  Treatments
	Skin Surveillance
	Sleep Enhancement
	Surveillance
	Teaching: Individual
		Attachment Promotion
		Support Group
		Sustenance Support
		Teaching: Infant Safety
		Teaching: Psychomotor
		  Skill

Outcome: BREASTFEEDING WEANING

MAJOR INTERVENTIONS	SUGGESTED INTERVENTIONS	OPTIONAL INTERVENTIONS

Lactation Counseling
Lactation Suppression
	Active Listening
	Anticipatory Guidance
	Emotional Support
	Family Involvement
	  Promotion
	Family Support
	Skin Surveillance
	Teaching: Infant
	  Nutrition
		Family Mobilization
		Heat/Cold Application
		Infection Protection
		Pain Management

Outcome: **KNOWLEDGE: BREASTFEEDING**		
MAJOR INTERVENTIONS	**SUGGESTED INTERVENTIONS**	**OPTIONAL INTERVENTIONS**

Breastfeeding Assistance
Lactation Counseling
	Learning Facilitation
	Learning Readiness
	  Enhancement
	Parent Education: Infant
	Teaching: Individual
	Teaching: Infant
	  Nutrition
		Anticipatory Guidance
		Bottle Feeding
		Environmental
		  Management:
		  Attachment Process
		Nonnutritive Sucking
		Postpartal Care
		Prenatal Care

Nursing Diagnosis: BREASTFEEDING, INTERRUPTED

Definition: A break in the continuity of the breastfeeding process as a result of inability or inadvisability to put baby to breast for feeding.

Outcome: BREASTFEEDING MAINTENANCE

MAJOR INTERVENTIONS	SUGGESTED INTERVENTIONS	OPTIONAL INTERVENTIONS
Bottle Feeding	Coping Enhancement	Active Listening
Emotional Support	Family Support	Anticipatory Guidance
Lactation Counseling	Fluid Management	Anxiety Reduction
	Health System Guidance	Attachment Promotion
	Infection Control	Behavior Modification
	Infection Protection	Referral
	Lactation Suppression	Simple Relaxation
	Medication Management	Therapy
	Nonnutritive Sucking	Support Group
	Skin Care: Topical	Wound Care
	Treatments	
	Skin Surveillance	
	Surveillance	
	Teaching: Individual	
	Teaching: Infant	
	Nutrition	

Outcome: KNOWLEDGE: BREASTFEEDING

MAJOR INTERVENTIONS	SUGGESTED INTERVENTIONS	OPTIONAL INTERVENTIONS
Lactation Counseling	Bottle Feeding	Anticipatory Guidance
Lactation Suppression	Learning Facilitation	Environmental
	Learning Readiness	Management:
	Enhancement	Attachment Process
	Parent Education: Infant	Health System Guidance
	Teaching: Individual	Nonnutritive Sucking
	Teaching: Infant	
	Nutrition	

Outcome: PARENT-INFANT ATTACHMENT

MAJOR INTERVENTIONS	SUGGESTED INTERVENTIONS	OPTIONAL INTERVENTIONS
Attachment Promotion	Bottle Feeding	Anticipatory Guidance
Environmental	Family Integrity	Anxiety Reduction
Management:	Promotion	Coping Enhancement
Attachment Process	Infant Care	Emotional Support
Kangaroo Care	Parent Education: Infant	Role Enhancement

Nursing Diagnosis: BREATHING PATTERN, INEFFECTIVE

DEFINITION: Inspiration and/or expiration that does not provide adequate ventilation.

Outcome: RESPIRATORY STATUS: AIRWAY PATENCY

MAJOR INTERVENTIONS	SUGGESTED INTERVENTIONS	OPTIONAL INTERVENTIONS
Airway Management Airway Suctioning	Airway Insertion and Stabilization Artificial Airway Management Aspiration Precautions Cough Enhancement Positioning Respiratory Monitoring Surveillance	Allergy Management Anaphylaxis Management Chest Physiotherapy Emergency Care Resuscitation

Outcome: RESPIRATORY STATUS: VENTILATION

MAJOR INTERVENTIONS	SUGGESTED INTERVENTIONS	OPTIONAL INTERVENTIONS
Airway Management Respiratory Monitoring Ventilation Assistance	Airway Insertion and Stabilization Airway Suctioning Anxiety Reduction Artificial Airway Management Aspiration Precautions Mechanical Ventilation Oxygen Therapy Positioning Progressive Muscle Relaxation Vital Signs Monitoring	Acid-Base Monitoring Allergy Management Chest Physiotherapy Cough Enhancement Energy Management Exercise Promotion Mechanical Ventilatory Weaning

Continued

Outcome: VITAL SIGNS STATUS

MAJOR INTERVENTIONS	SUGGESTED INTERVENTIONS	OPTIONAL INTERVENTIONS
Respiratory Monitoring Vital Signs Monitoring	Acid-Base Management Airway Management Anxiety Reduction Fluid Management Intravenous (IV) Insertion Intravenous (IV) Therapy Medication Management Medication Prescribing Surveillance Ventilation Assistance	Allergy Management Emergency Care Nutrition Management Oxygen Therapy Pain Management Postanesthesia Care Resuscitation Teaching: Prescribed Activity/Exercise Teaching: Prescribed Medication Teaching: Procedure/Treatment

Nursing Diagnosis: CARDIAC OUTPUT, DECREASED

DEFINITION: A state in which the blood pumped by the heart is inadequate to meet the metabolic demands of the body.

Outcome: CARDIAC PUMP EFFECTIVENESS

MAJOR INTERVENTIONS	SUGGESTED INTERVENTIONS	OPTIONAL INTERVENTIONS

Cardiac Care
Cardiac Care: Acute
Hemodynamic
  Regulation
Shock Management:
  Cardiac
	Acid-Base Management
	Acid-Base Monitoring
	Cardiac Care:
	  Rehabilitative
	Cardiac Precautions
	Code Management
	Electrolyte Management
	Electrolyte Monitoring
	Fluid Management
	Invasive Hemodynamic
	  Monitoring
	Medication
	  Administration
	Vital Signs Monitoring
		Bleeding Reduction
		Blood Products
		  Administration
		Dysrhythmia
		  Management
		Fluid Monitoring
		Intravenous (IV)
		  Therapy
		Patient Rights Protection
		Resuscitation
		Resuscitation: Fetus
		Resuscitation: Neonate
		Shock Management
		Shock Prevention

Outcome: CIRCULATION STATUS

MAJOR INTERVENTIONS	SUGGESTED INTERVENTIONS	OPTIONAL INTERVENTIONS

Circulatory Care:
  Arterial Insufficiency
Circulatory Care:
  Mechanical Assist
  Device
Circulatory Care: Venous
  Insufficiency
Shock Management:
  Cardiac
	Bleeding Precautions
	Bleeding Reduction
	Bleeding Reduction:
	  Antepartum Uterus
	Bleeding Reduction:
	  Gastrointestinal
	Bleeding Reduction:
	  Nasal
	Bleeding Reduction:
	  Postpartum Uterus
	Bleeding Reduction:
	  Wound
	Fluid Monitoring
	Hemodynamic
	  Regulation
	Hemorrhage Control
	Hypovolemia
	  Management
	Laboratory Data
	  Interpretation
	Shock Management
	Shock Prevention
		Autotransfusion
		Bedside Laboratory
		  Testing
		Blood Products
		  Administration
		Circulatory Precautions
		Fluid Resuscitation
		Intravenous (IV)
		  Insertion
		Intravenous (IV)
		  Therapy
		Invasive Hemodynamic
		  Monitoring
		Pneumatic Tourniquet
		  Precautions
		Shock Management:
		  Vasogenic
		Shock Management:
		  Volume

Continued

Outcome: Tissue Perfusion: Abdominal Organs

MAJOR INTERVENTIONS	SUGGESTED INTERVENTIONS	OPTIONAL INTERVENTIONS
Circulatory Care: Arterial Insufficiency Circulatory Care: Venous Insufficiency Intravenous (IV) Therapy Shock Management: Cardiac	Acid-Base Management Acid-Base Monitoring Bedside Laboratory Testing Bleeding Precautions Bleeding Reduction Electrolyte Management Electrolyte Monitoring Fluid Management Hemorrhage Control Hypovolemia Management Laboratory Data Interpretation Shock Management Shock Prevention Surveillance Vital Signs Monitoring	Autotransfusion Bleeding Reduction: Antepartum Uterus Bleeding Reduction: Gastrointestinal Bleeding Reduction: Postpartum Uterus Blood Products Administration Emergency Care Fluid Resuscitation Intravenous (IV) Insertion Intravenous (IV) Therapy

Outcome: Tissue Perfusion: Peripheral

MAJOR INTERVENTIONS	SUGGESTED INTERVENTIONS	OPTIONAL INTERVENTIONS
Circulatory Care: Arterial Insufficiency Circulatory Care: Venous Insufficiency Embolus Care: Peripheral	Bleeding Precautions Bleeding Reduction Blood Products Administration Cardiac Care: Acute Circulatory Care: Mechanical Assist Device Circulatory Precautions Fluid Management Hemodynamic Regulation Hypovolemia Management Pneumatic Tourniquet Precautions Shock Management: Cardiac Shock Prevention	Autotransfusion Fluid Resuscitation Intravenous (IV) Insertion Intravenous (IV) Therapy Resuscitation Resuscitation: Fetus Resuscitation: Neonate

Outcome: VITAL SIGNS STATUS

MAJOR INTERVENTIONS	SUGGESTED INTERVENTIONS	OPTIONAL INTERVENTIONS
Hemodynamic Regulation Vital Signs Monitoring	Acid-Base Management Anxiety Reduction Cardiac Care Dysrhythmia Management Electrolyte Management Fluid Management Hemorrhage Control Hypovolemia Management Intravenous (IV) Therapy Medication Administration Medication Management Medication Prescribing Shock Management Shock Prevention	Blood Products Administration Emergency Care Fluid Resuscitation Postanesthesia Care Postpartal Care Resuscitation Surveillance

Nursing Diagnosis: CAREGIVER ROLE STRAIN

DEFINITION: A caregiver's felt or exhibited difficulty in performing the family caregiver role.

Outcome: CAREGIVER LIFESTYLE DISRUPTION

MAJOR INTERVENTIONS	SUGGESTED INTERVENTIONS	OPTIONAL INTERVENTIONS

Caregiver Support
Coping Enhancement
Respite Care
	Assertiveness Training
	Decision-Making
	  Support
	Emotional Support
	Family Support
	Health System Guidance
	Mutual Goal Setting
	Support Group
	Support System
	  Enhancement
	Telephone Consultation
		Case Management
		Family Integrity
		  Promotion
		Family Involvement
		  Promotion
		Family Process
		  Maintenance
		Insurance Authorization

Outcome: CAREGIVER WELL-BEING

MAJOR INTERVENTIONS	SUGGESTED INTERVENTIONS	OPTIONAL INTERVENTIONS

Caregiver Support
Respite Care
Teaching: Individual
	Coping Enhancement
	Family Involvement
	  Promotion
	Family Mobilization
	Family Support
	Home Maintenance
	  Assistance
	Hope Instillation
	Support Group
	Support System
	  Enhancement
		Active Listening
		Anticipatory Guidance
		Counseling
		Emotional Support
		Family Integrity
		  Promotion
		Normalization
		  Promotion
		Presence

Outcome: ROLE PERFORMANCE

MAJOR INTERVENTIONS	SUGGESTED INTERVENTIONS	OPTIONAL INTERVENTIONS
Role Enhancement Parenting Promotion	Abuse Protection Support: Child Abuse Protection Support: Domestic Partner Abuse Protection Support: Elder Anticipatory Guidance Behavior Modification Caregiver Support Cognitive Restructuring Counseling Emotional Support Family Involvement Promotion Parent Education: Adolescent Parent Education: Childrearing Family Parent Education: Infant Values Clarification	Active Listening Attachment Promotion Childbirth Preparation Decision-Making Support Family Integrity Promotion Kangaroo Care Support Group Support System Enhancement Teaching: Individual Teaching: Infant Nutrition Teaching: Infant Safety Teaching: Sexuality Teaching: Toddler Safety

Nursing Diagnosis: COMMUNICATION, IMPAIRED VERBAL

Definition: The state in which an individual experiences a decreased, delayed, or absent ability to receive, process, transmit, and use a system of symbols; anything that has meaning, i.e., transmits meaning.

Outcome: COMMUNICATION ABILITY

MAJOR INTERVENTIONS	SUGGESTED INTERVENTIONS	OPTIONAL INTERVENTIONS
Active Listening Communication Enhancement: Hearing Deficit Communication Enhancement: Speech Deficit	Anxiety Reduction Communication Enhancement: Visual Deficit Presence Touch	Art Therapy Bibliotherapy Culture Brokerage Environmental Management Socialization Enhancement

Outcome: COMMUNICATION: EXPRESSIVE ABILITY

MAJOR INTERVENTIONS	SUGGESTED INTERVENTIONS	OPTIONAL INTERVENTIONS
Communication Enhancement: Speech Deficit	Active Listening Assertiveness Training Communication Enhancement: Hearing Deficit Communication Enhancement: Visual Deficit	Anxiety Reduction Bibliotherapy Socialization Enhancement

Outcome: COMMUNICATION: RECEPTIVE ABILITY

MAJOR INTERVENTIONS	SUGGESTED INTERVENTIONS	OPTIONAL INTERVENTIONS
Communication Enhancement: Hearing Deficit Communication Enhancement: Visual Deficit	Active Listening Communication Enhancement: Speech Deficit Learning Readiness Enhancement	Cognitive Stimulation Culture Brokerage Ear Care Environmental Management Eye Care Reality Orientation

Nursing Diagnosis: COMMUNITY COPING, INEFFECTIVE

DEFINITION: A pattern of community activities for adaptation and problem solving that is unsatisfactory for meeting the demands or needs of the community.

Outcome: COMMUNITY COMPETENCE

MAJOR INTERVENTIONS	SUGGESTED INTERVENTIONS	OPTIONAL INTERVENTIONS
Community Disaster Preparedness Environmental Management: Community	Conflict Mediation Environmental Management: Safety Environmental Management: Violence Prevention Environmental Risk Protection Fiscal Resource Management Health Policy Monitoring Program Development Risk Identification Surveillance: Community	Consultation Documentation Resiliency Promotion Triage: Disaster Vehicle Safety Promotion

Outcome: COMMUNITY HEALTH STATUS

MAJOR INTERVENTIONS	SUGGESTED INTERVENTIONS	OPTIONAL INTERVENTIONS
Communicable Disease Management Community Health Development Health Screening	Environmental Management: Safety Environmental Management: Violence Prevention Environmental Risk Protection Health Education Immunization/ Vaccination Management Infection Control Risk Identification Surveillance: Community	Documentation Health Policy Monitoring Risk Identification: Genetic Sports-Injury Prevention: Youth Vehicle Safety Promotion

Continued

Outcome: COMMUNITY HEALTH: IMMUNITY

MAJOR INTERVENTIONS	SUGGESTED INTERVENTIONS	OPTIONAL INTERVENTIONS
Immunization/ Vaccination Management	Communicable Disease Management Community Health Development Environmental Risk Protection Health Education Health Screening Infection Control Risk Identification Surveillance: Community	Documentation Health Policy Monitoring Program Development

Outcome: COMMUNITY RISK CONTROL: CHRONIC DISEASE

MAJOR INTERVENTIONS	SUGGESTED INTERVENTIONS	OPTIONAL INTERVENTIONS
Health Education Program Development	Community Health Development Environmental Risk Protection Health Policy Monitoring Health Screening Surveillance: Community	Documentation Environmental Management: Community Risk Identification

Outcome: COMMUNITY RISK CONTROL: COMMUNICABLE DISEASE

MAJOR INTERVENTIONS	SUGGESTED INTERVENTIONS	OPTIONAL INTERVENTIONS
Communicable Disease Management Immunization/ Vaccination Management	Health Education Health Policy Monitoring Health Screening Program Development Risk Identification Surveillance: Community	Documentation Infection Control

Outcome: COMMUNITY RISK CONTROL: LEAD EXPOSURE

MAJOR INTERVENTIONS	SUGGESTED INTERVENTIONS	OPTIONAL INTERVENTIONS
Environmental Management: Community Environmental Risk Protection	Community Health Development Environmental Management: Worker Safety Health Education Program Development Risk Identification Surveillance: Community	Documentation Health Screening Referral

Nursing Diagnosis: COMMUNITY COPING, POTENTIAL FOR ENHANCED

DEFINITION: A pattern of community activities for adaptation and problem solving that is satisfactory for meeting the demands or needs of the community but can be improved for management of current and future problems/stressors.

Outcome: COMMUNITY COMPETENCE

MAJOR INTERVENTIONS	SUGGESTED INTERVENTIONS	OPTIONAL INTERVENTIONS
Environmental Risk Protection Health Policy Monitoring Program Development	Environmental Management: Community Environmental Management: Worker Safety Environmental Management: Violence Management Community Health Development	Communicable Disease Management Community Disaster Preparedness Health Screening Immunization/ Vaccination Management Resiliency Promotion

Outcome: COMMUNITY HEALTH STATUS

MAJOR INTERVENTIONS	SUGGESTED INTERVENTIONS	OPTIONAL INTERVENTIONS
Communicable Disease Management Community Health Development	Environmental Management: Safety Environmental Management: Violence Prevention Environmental Risk Protection Health Education Health Screening Immunization/ Vaccination Management Infection Control Risk Identification Surveillance: Community	Documentation Health Policy Monitoring Risk Identification: Genetic Sports-Injury Prevention: Youth Vehicle Safety Promotion

Outcome: COMMUNITY HEALTH: IMMUNITY

MAJOR INTERVENTIONS	SUGGESTED INTERVENTIONS	OPTIONAL INTERVENTIONS
Immunization/ Vaccination Management	Community Health Development Health Education Health Policy Monitoring Health Screening Program Development Risk Identification Surveillance: Community	Communicable Disease Management Documentation Environmental Risk Protection Infection Control

Outcome: COMMUNITY RISK CONTROL: CHRONIC DISEASE

MAJOR INTERVENTIONS	SUGGESTED INTERVENTIONS	OPTIONAL INTERVENTIONS
Health Education Program Development	Community Health Development Health Policy Monitoring Health Screening Risk Identification Surveillance: Community	Documentation Environmental Management: Community Environmental Risk Protection

Outcome: COMMUNITY RISK CONTROL: COMMUNICABLE DISEASE

MAJOR INTERVENTIONS	SUGGESTED INTERVENTIONS	OPTIONAL INTERVENTIONS
Communicable Disease Management Program Development	Health Education Health Policy Monitoring Risk Identification Health Screening Immunization/ Vaccination Management Surveillance: Community	Documentation Infection Control

Continued

Outcome: **COMMUNITY RISK CONTROL: LEAD EXPOSURE**

MAJOR INTERVENTIONS	SUGGESTED INTERVENTIONS	OPTIONAL INTERVENTIONS
Environmental Management: Community Environmental Risk Protection	Community Health Development Environmental Management: Worker Safety Health Education Program Development Risk Identification Surveillance: Community	Documentation Health Screening Referral

Nursing Diagnosis: COMMUNITY MANAGEMENT OF THERAPEUTIC REGIMEN, INEFFECTIVE

DEFINITION: A pattern of regulating and integrating into community processes programs for treatment of illness and the sequelae of illness that are unsatisfactory for meeting health-related goals.

Outcome: COMMUNITY COMPETENCE

MAJOR INTERVENTIONS	SUGGESTED INTERVENTIONS	OPTIONAL INTERVENTIONS
Community Health Development Health Policy Monitoring Program Development	Communicable Disease Management Environmental Management: Community Environmental Management: Safety Environmental Risk Protection Health Education Health Screening Immunization/ Vaccination Management Risk Identification Surveillance: Community	Community Disaster Preparedness Conflict Mediation Documentation Environmental Management: Worker Safety Fiscal Resource Management Resiliency Promotion Sports-Injury Prevention: Youth Surveillance: Safety Vehicle Safety Promotion

Continued

Outcome: COMMUNITY HEALTH STATUS

MAJOR INTERVENTIONS	SUGGESTED INTERVENTIONS	OPTIONAL INTERVENTIONS
Community Health Development	Communicable Disease Management	Documentation
Environmental Management: Community	Environmental Management	Risk Identification: Genetic
	Environmental Management: Safety	Sports-Injury Prevention: Youth
	Environmental Management: Violence Prevention	Vehicle Safety Promotion
	Environmental Risk Protection	
	Health Education	
	Health Policy Monitoring	
	Health Screening	
	Immunization/ Vaccination Management	
	Infection Control	
	Program Development	
	Risk Identification	
	Surveillance: Community	

Nursing Diagnosis: CONFUSION, ACUTE

DEFINITION: The abrupt onset of a cluster of global, transient changes and disturbances in attention, cognition, psychomotor activity, level of consciousness, and/or sleep/wake cycle.

Outcome: COGNITIVE ORIENTATION

MAJOR INTERVENTIONS	SUGGESTED INTERVENTIONS	OPTIONAL INTERVENTIONS

Delirium Management
Delusion Management
Reality Orientation
	Acid-Base Management
	Environmental
	  Management: Safety
	Fall Prevention
	Hallucination
	  Management
	Medication
	  Administration
	Medication Management
	Pain Management
	Sleep Enhancement
	Surveillance: Safety
		Calming Technique
		Presence
		Self-Care Assistance
		Touch

Outcome: DISTORTED THOUGHT CONTROL

MAJOR INTERVENTIONS	SUGGESTED INTERVENTIONS	OPTIONAL INTERVENTIONS

Delirium Management
Delusion Management
Hallucination
  Management
	Anxiety Reduction
	Medication Management
	Reality Orientation
		Calming Technique
		Environmental
		  Management

Outcome: INFORMATION PROCESSING

MAJOR INTERVENTIONS	SUGGESTED INTERVENTIONS	OPTIONAL INTERVENTIONS

Cognitive Stimulation	Calming Technique
	Delirium Management
	Delusion Management
	Medication Management
	Reality Orientation
		Anxiety Reduction
		Environmental
		  Management
		Fluid/Electrolyte
		  Management
		Hallucination
		  Management
		Oxygen Therapy
		Pain Management
		Sleep Enhancement

Continued

Outcome: **Neurological Status: Consciousness**

MAJOR INTERVENTIONS	SUGGESTED INTERVENTIONS	OPTIONAL INTERVENTIONS
Cerebral Perfusion Promotion Neurologic Monitoring Reality Orientation	Airway Management Cerebral Edema Management Cognitive Stimulation Delirium Management Hyperglycemia Management Hypoglycemia Management Medication Administration Medication Administration: Intramuscular Medication Administration: Intravenous Medication Management Seizure Precautions Surveillance Vital Signs Monitoring	Environmental Management Fluid Resuscitation Intracranial Pressure (ICP) Monitoring Mechanical Ventilation Patient Rights Protection Shock Management Substance Use Treatment Substance Use Treatment: Alcohol Withdrawal Substance Use Treatment: Drug Withdrawal Substance Use Treatment: Overdose

Outcome: **Safety Behavior: Personal**

MAJOR INTERVENTIONS	SUGGESTED INTERVENTIONS	OPTIONAL INTERVENTIONS
Environmental Management: Safety Fall Prevention	Area Restriction Home Maintenance Assistance Physical Restraint Seclusion Surveillance: Safety	Behavior Management: Overactivity/Inattention Behavior Management: Self-Harm Security Enhancement Sleep Enhancement

Outcome: **SLEEP**		
MAJOR INTERVENTIONS	**SUGGESTED INTERVENTIONS**	**OPTIONAL INTERVENTIONS**
Sleep Enhancement	Analgesic Administration Calming Technique Energy Management Environmental Management Environmental Management: Comfort Music Therapy Simple Massage Simple Relaxation Therapy	Anxiety Reduction Distraction Emotional Support Exercise Promotion Presence

Nursing Diagnosis: CONFUSION, CHRONIC

DEFINITION: An irreversible, long-standing and/or progressive deterioration of intellect and personality characterized by decreased ability to interpret environmental stimuli, decreased capacity for intellectual thought processes and manifested by disturbances of memory, orientation, and behavior.

Outcome: COGNITIVE ABILITY

MAJOR INTERVENTIONS	SUGGESTED INTERVENTIONS	OPTIONAL INTERVENTIONS

Cognitive Stimulation
Dementia Management
Mood Management
	Anxiety Reduction
	Area Restriction
	Decision-Making
	  Support
	Family Involvement
	  Promotion
	Family Support
	Memory Training
	Milieu Therapy
	Reality Orientation
	Reminiscence Therapy
	Surveillance: Safety
		Environmental
		  Management
		Fall Prevention
		Patient Rights Protection
		Recreation Therapy

Outcome: COGNITIVE ORIENTATION

MAJOR INTERVENTIONS	SUGGESTED INTERVENTIONS	OPTIONAL INTERVENTIONS

Dementia Management
Reality Orientation
	Area Restriction
	Cognitive Stimulation
	Calming Technique
	Hallucination
	  Management
	Medication Management
	Memory Training
	Surveillance: Safety
		Animal-Assisted
		  Therapy
		Art Therapy
		Environmental
		  Management: Safety
		Milieu Therapy
		Neurologic Monitoring
		Patient Rights Protection
		Physical Restraint
		Presence
		Recreation Therapy
		Reminiscence Therapy
		Substance Use Treatment
		Visitation Facilitation

Outcome: CONCENTRATION

MAJOR INTERVENTIONS	SUGGESTED INTERVENTIONS	OPTIONAL INTERVENTIONS

Anxiety Reduction
Cognitive Stimulation
Dementia Management
	Hallucination
	  Management
	Medication Management
	Presence
	Substance Use Treatment
	Touch
		Calming Technique
		Cognitive Restructuring
		Environmental
		  Management
		Meditation Facilitation
		Simple Relaxation
		  Therapy

Outcome: DECISION MAKING

MAJOR INTERVENTIONS	SUGGESTED INTERVENTIONS	OPTIONAL INTERVENTIONS

Decision-Making
  Support
Family Involvement
  Promotion
	Emotional Support
	Health System Guidance
	Learning Facilitation
	Patient Rights Protection
	Support System
	  Enhancement
	Teaching: Individual
		Case Management
		Family Support
		Health Care Information
		  Exchange
		Multidisciplinary Care
		  Conference

Outcome: DISTORTED THOUGHT CONTROL

MAJOR INTERVENTIONS	SUGGESTED INTERVENTIONS	OPTIONAL INTERVENTIONS

Dementia Management
Delusion Management
	Anxiety Reduction
	Cognitive Stimulation
	Hallucination
	  Management
	Medication Management
	Milieu Therapy
	Reality Orientation
	Therapy Group
		Activity Therapy
		Animal-Assisted
		  Therapy
		Art Therapy
		Environmental
		  Management
		Memory Training
		Music Therapy
		Recreation Therapy

Continued

Outcome: IDENTITY

MAJOR INTERVENTIONS	SUGGESTED INTERVENTIONS	OPTIONAL INTERVENTIONS
Cognitive Restructuring Reality Orientation	Body Image Enhancement Medication Management Self-Awareness Enhancement Self-Esteem Enhancement Socialization Enhancement Spiritual Support Values Clarification	Dementia Management Environmental Management: Violence Prevention Family Mobilization Hallucination Management Milieu Therapy Therapy Group

Outcome: INFORMATION PROCESSING

MAJOR INTERVENTIONS	SUGGESTED INTERVENTIONS	OPTIONAL INTERVENTIONS
Cognitive Stimulation Decision-Making Support	Active Listening Calming Technique Dementia Management Learning Facilitation Learning Readiness Enhancement Medication Management Memory Training Reality Orientation	Anxiety Reduction Cerebral Perfusion Promotion Cognitive Restructuring Environmental Management Fluid/Electrolyte Management Hallucination Management Oxygen Therapy Pain Management Reminiscence Therapy Sleep Enhancement

Outcome: MEMORY

MAJOR INTERVENTIONS	SUGGESTED INTERVENTIONS	OPTIONAL INTERVENTIONS
Memory Training	Active Listening Cognitive Stimulation Learning Facilitation Milieu Therapy Reality Orientation Reminiscence Therapy	Bibliotherapy Cognitive Restructuring Coping Enhancement Medication Management Patient Rights Protection

Outcome: NEUROLOGICAL STATUS: CONSCIOUSNESS

MAJOR INTERVENTIONS	SUGGESTED INTERVENTIONS	OPTIONAL INTERVENTIONS
Cerebral Perfusion Promotion Neurologic Monitoring Reality Orientation	Cognitive Stimulation Dementia Management Environmental Management Environmental Management: Safety Laboratory Data Interpretation Medication Administration Medication Administration: Intramuscular Medication Management Patient Rights Protection Substance Use Treatment Surveillance Vital Signs Monitoring	Family Involvement Promotion Family Support Humor Seizure Precautions

Nursing Diagnosis: CONSTIPATION

DEFINITION: A decrease in a person's normal frequency of defecation accompanied by difficult or incomplete passage of stool and/or passage of excessively hard, dry stool.

Outcome: BOWEL ELIMINATION

MAJOR INTERVENTIONS	SUGGESTED INTERVENTIONS	OPTIONAL INTERVENTIONS
Bowel Management Constipation/Impaction Management	Bowel Irrigation Bowel Training Exercise Promotion Fluid Management Fluid Monitoring Medication Management Medication Prescribing Nutrition Management Nutritional Monitoring Self-Care Assistance: Toileting	Diet Staging Flatulence Reduction Medication Administration Ostomy Care Pain Management Rectal Prolapse Management Skin Surveillance Specimen Management

Outcome: HYDRATION

MAJOR INTERVENTIONS	SUGGESTED INTERVENTIONS	OPTIONAL INTERVENTIONS
Fluid Management Fluid/Electrolyte Management	Fluid Monitoring Intravenous (IV) Insertion Intravenous (IV) Therapy Medication Management Nutrition Management	Bottle Feeding Enteral Tube Feeding Feeding Fever Treatment

Outcome: SYMPTOM CONTROL

MAJOR INTERVENTIONS	SUGGESTED INTERVENTIONS	OPTIONAL INTERVENTIONS
Bowel Management	Bowel Irrigation Constipation/Impaction Management Exercise Promotion Fluid Management Medication Management Nutrition Management Rectal Prolapse Management	Anxiety Reduction Flatulence Reduction Pain Management Simple Relaxation Therapy

Nursing Diagnosis: CONSTIPATION, PERCEIVED

DEFINITION: The state in which an individual makes a self-diagnosis of constipation and ensures a daily bowel movement through abuse of laxatives, enemas, and suppositories.

Outcome: BOWEL ELIMINATION

MAJOR INTERVENTIONS	SUGGESTED INTERVENTIONS	OPTIONAL INTERVENTIONS

Bowel Management	Counseling
	Exercise Promotion
	Fluid Management
	Fluid Monitoring
	Medication Management
	Nutrition Management
	Teaching: Individual
		Distraction
		Simple Relaxation
		  Therapy
		Teaching: Prescribed
		  Diet

Outcome: HEALTH BELIEFS

MAJOR INTERVENTIONS	SUGGESTED INTERVENTIONS	OPTIONAL INTERVENTIONS

Health Education
Values Clarification
	Active Listening
	Behavior Modification
	Counseling
	Risk Identification
	Self-Modification
	  Assistance
		Culture Brokerage
		Learning Facilitation
		Learning Readiness
		  Enhancement
		Mutual Goal Setting
		Patient Contracting
		Teaching: Individual

Outcome: HEALTH BELIEFS: PERCEIVED THREAT

MAJOR INTERVENTIONS	SUGGESTED INTERVENTIONS	OPTIONAL INTERVENTIONS

Health Education
Teaching: Individual
	Active Listening
	Behavior Modification
	Counseling
	Learning Facilitation
	Learning Readiness
	  Enhancement
	Risk Identification
	Self-Modification
	  Assistance
	Self-Responsibility
	  Facilitation
	Truth Telling
	Values Clarification
		Anxiety Reduction
		Coping Enhancement
		Emotional Support
		Nutrition Management

Nursing Diagnosis: DEATH ANXIETY

DEFINITION: The apprehension, worry, or fear related to death or dying.

Outcome: ACCEPTANCE: HEALTH STATUS

MAJOR INTERVENTIONS	SUGGESTED INTERVENTIONS	OPTIONAL INTERVENTIONS

Coping Enhancement
Emotional Support
	Anticipatory Guidance
	Decision-Making
	  Support
	Grief Work Facilitation
	Hope Instillation
	Presence
	Spiritual Support
	Support System
	  Enhancement
	Values Clarification
		Active Listening
		Referral
		Truth Telling

Outcome: ANXIETY CONTROL

MAJOR INTERVENTIONS	SUGGESTED INTERVENTIONS	OPTIONAL INTERVENTIONS

Anxiety Reduction	Active Listening
	Calming Technique
	Coping Enhancement
	Music Therapy
	Presence
	Simple Massage
	Simple Relaxation
	  Therapy
	Spiritual Support
	Touch
		Animal-Assisted
		  Therapy
		Bibliotherapy
		Meditation Facilitation
		Sleep Enhancement

Outcome: DEPRESSION LEVEL

MAJOR INTERVENTIONS	SUGGESTED INTERVENTIONS	OPTIONAL INTERVENTIONS

Dying Care
Hope Instillation
Spiritual Support
	Bibliotherapy
	Emotional Support
	Grief Work Facilitation
	Medication Management
	Mood Management
	Sleep Enhancement
		Animal-Assisted
		  Therapy
		Music Therapy
		Reminiscence Therapy
		Support System
		  Enhancement

Outcome: DIGNIFIED DYING

MAJOR INTERVENTIONS	SUGGESTED INTERVENTIONS	OPTIONAL INTERVENTIONS

Dying Care
Spiritual Support
	Anticipatory Guidance
	Anxiety Reduction
	Decision-Making
	  Support
	Family Involvement
	  Promotion
	Family Mobilization
	Forgiveness Facilitation
	Grief Work Facilitation
	Medication Management
	Patient-Controlled
	  Analgesia (PCA)
	  Assistance
	Values Clarification
		Active Listening
		Anger Control
		  Assistance
		Animal-Assisted
		  Therapy
		Bibliotherapy
		Caregiver Support
		Coping Enhancement
		Culture Brokerage
		Emotional Support
		Family Integrity
		  Promotion
		Family Process
		  Maintenance
		Family Support
		Music Therapy
		Patient Rights Protection
		Presence
		Reminiscence Therapy
		Visitation Facilitation

Outcome: FEAR CONTROL

MAJOR INTERVENTIONS	SUGGESTED INTERVENTIONS	OPTIONAL INTERVENTIONS

Coping Enhancement
Dying Care
	Active Listening
	Anxiety Reduction
	Calming Technique
	Decision-Making
	  Support
	Emotional Support
	Family Mobilization
	Presence
	Spiritual Support
		Animal-Assisted
		  Therapy
		Caregiver Support
		Culture Brokerage
		Meditation Facilitation
		Pain Management
		Simple Guided Imagery
		Simple Relaxation
		  Therapy

Outcome: HOPE

MAJOR INTERVENTIONS	SUGGESTED INTERVENTIONS	OPTIONAL INTERVENTIONS
Hope Instillation Spiritual Support	Coping Enhancement Dying Care Emotional Support Grief Work Facilitation	Family Mobilization Mutual Goal Setting Presence Touch

Nursing Diagnosis: DECISIONAL CONFLICT (SPECIFY)

DEFINITION: The state of uncertainty about course of action to be taken when choice among competing actions involves risk, loss, or challenge to personal life values.

Outcome: DECISION MAKING

MAJOR INTERVENTIONS	SUGGESTED INTERVENTIONS	OPTIONAL INTERVENTIONS
Decision-Making Support Mutual Goal Setting	Coping Enhancement Counseling Emotional Support Genetic Counseling Preconception Counseling Self-Awareness Enhancement Support System Enhancement Teaching: Individual Telephone Consultation	Culture Brokerage Health Care Information Exchange Health Education Health System Guidance Patient Contracting Preparatory Sensory Information Simple Guided Imagery Teaching: Sexuality Values Clarification

Outcome: INFORMATION PROCESSING

MAJOR INTERVENTIONS	SUGGESTED INTERVENTIONS	OPTIONAL INTERVENTIONS
Learning Facilitation Decision-Making Support	Active Listening Coping Enhancement Counseling Teaching: Individual	Anxiety Reduction Culture Brokerage Dementia Management Developmental Enhancement: Adolescent Environmental Management Music Therapy Reminiscence Therapy Sleep Enhancement

Outcome: PARTICIPATION: HEALTH CARE DECISIONS

MAJOR INTERVENTIONS	SUGGESTED INTERVENTIONS	OPTIONAL INTERVENTIONS
Decision-Making Support Health System Guidance	Active Listening Admission Care Anticipatory Guidance Assertiveness Training Counseling Culture Brokerage Discharge Planning Patient Rights Protection Self-Responsibility Facilitation Telephone Consultation Values Clarification	Anxiety Reduction Behavior Modification Caregiver Support Coping Enhancement Family Involvement Promotion Health Care Information Exchange Insurance Authorization Referral Sustenance Support

Nursing Diagnosis: DEFENSIVE COPING

DEFINITION: The state in which an individual repeatedly projects falsely positive self-evaluation based on a self-protective pattern that defends against underlying perceived threats to positive self-regard.

Outcome: ACCEPTANCE: HEALTH STATUS

MAJOR INTERVENTIONS	SUGGESTED INTERVENTIONS	OPTIONAL INTERVENTIONS
Coping Enhancement Emotional Support Self-Awareness Enhancement	Body Image Enhancement Counseling Grief Work Facilitation Hope Instillation Presence Spiritual Support Support Group	Active Listening Cognitive Restructuring Normalization Promotion Support System Enhancement Truth Telling Values Clarification

Outcome: CHILD DEVELOPMENT: ADOLESCENCE (12-17 YEARS)

MAJOR INTERVENTIONS	SUGGESTED INTERVENTIONS	OPTIONAL INTERVENTIONS
Self-Esteem Enhancement Self-Responsibility Facilitation	Body Image Enhancement Environmental Management Exercise Promotion Nutrition Management Nutritional Counseling Patient Contracting Role Enhancement Self-Awareness Enhancement Self-Modification Assistance Socialization Enhancement Spiritual Support	Cognitive Restructuring Counseling Eating Disorders Management Family Support Family Therapy Sexual Counseling Sibling Support Support System Enhancement Truth Telling Values Clarification Weight Management

Outcome: COPING

MAJOR INTERVENTIONS	SUGGESTED INTERVENTIONS	OPTIONAL INTERVENTIONS
Coping Enhancement Counseling	Anxiety Reduction Calming Technique Complex Relationship Building Emotional Support Exercise Promotion Patient Contracting Self-Awareness Enhancement	Behavior Modification Mood Management Normalization Promotion Reminiscence Therapy

Outcome: SELF-ESTEEM

MAJOR INTERVENTIONS	SUGGESTED INTERVENTIONS	OPTIONAL INTERVENTIONS
Self-Esteem Enhancement	Active Listening Body Image Enhancement Cognitive Restructuring Counseling Developmental Enhancement: Adolescent Developmental Enhancement: Child Emotional Support Self-Awareness Enhancement Socialization Enhancement Support Group	Assertiveness Training Behavior Modification Behavior Modification: Social Skills Complex Relationship Building Coping Enhancement Eating Disorders Management Family Mobilization Milieu Therapy Security Enhancement Self-Modification Assistance Spiritual Support Weight Management

Continued

Outcome: **Social Interaction Skills**

MAJOR INTERVENTIONS	SUGGESTED INTERVENTIONS	OPTIONAL INTERVENTIONS
Behavior Modification: Social Skills Complex Relationship Building	Active Listening Assertiveness Training Counseling Developmental Enhancement: Adolescent Developmental Enhancement: Child Family Integrity Promotion Family Process Maintenance Recreation Therapy Role Enhancement Self-Awareness Enhancement Self-Esteem Enhancement Self-Responsibility Facilitation Socialization Enhancement Touch	Anger Control Assistance Anxiety Reduction Body Image Enhancement Coping Enhancement Culture Brokerage Family Therapy Guilt Work Facilitation Humor Reminiscence Therapy Therapy Group Visitation Facilitation

Nursing Diagnosis: DENIAL, INEFFECTIVE

DEFINITION: The state of a conscious or unconscious attempt to disavow the knowledge or meaning of an event to reduce anxiety/fear to the detriment of health.

Outcome: ACCEPTANCE: HEALTH STATUS

MAJOR INTERVENTIONS	SUGGESTED INTERVENTIONS	OPTIONAL INTERVENTIONS

Coping Enhancement
Counseling
Emotional Support
	Body Image
	  Enhancement
	Crisis Intervention
	Decision-Making
	  Support
	Hope Instillation
	Reality Orientation
	Spiritual Support
	Support Group
	Support System
	  Enhancement
	Truth Telling
	Values Clarification
		Cognitive Restructuring
		Mutual Goal Setting
		Normalization
		  Promotion
		Self-Awareness
		  Enhancement
		Therapy Group

Outcome: ANXIETY CONTROL

MAJOR INTERVENTIONS	SUGGESTED INTERVENTIONS	OPTIONAL INTERVENTIONS

Anxiety Reduction	Active Listening
	Calming Technique
	Coping Enhancement
	Counseling
	Medication
	  Administration
	Medication Prescribing
	Presence
	Recreation Therapy
	Security Enhancement
	Spiritual Support
	Support System
	  Enhancement
		Childbirth Preparation
		Decision-Making
		  Support
		Environmental
		  Management
		Family Therapy
		Guilt Work Facilitation
		Humor
		Milieu Therapy
		Support Group
		Therapeutic Play
		Therapy Group
		Truth Telling

Continued

Outcome: FEAR CONTROL

MAJOR INTERVENTIONS	SUGGESTED INTERVENTIONS	OPTIONAL INTERVENTIONS

Calming Technique
Coping Enhancement
Security Enhancement
	Active Listening
	Anticipatory Guidance
	Anxiety Reduction
	Counseling
	Decision-Making
	  Support
	Emotional Support
	Family Support
	Support System
	  Enhancement
	Truth Telling
		Dying Care
		Support Group
		Therapy Group

Outcome: HEALTH BELIEFS: PERCEIVED THREAT

MAJOR INTERVENTIONS	SUGGESTED INTERVENTIONS	OPTIONAL INTERVENTIONS

Health Education
Self-Awareness
  Enhancement
Teaching: Disease
  Process
	Active Listening
	Counseling
	Self-Modification
	  Assistance
	Self-Responsibility
	  Facilitation
	Teaching: Individual
	Truth Telling
	Values Clarification
		Anxiety Reduction
		Coping Enhancement
		Emotional Support
		Genetic Counseling
		Smoking Cessation
		  Assistance
		Substance Use
		  Prevention
		Substance Use Treatment

Outcome: SYMPTOM CONTROL

MAJOR INTERVENTIONS	SUGGESTED INTERVENTIONS	OPTIONAL INTERVENTIONS

Self-Modification
  Assistance
Self-Responsibility
  Facilitation
	Anticipatory Guidance
	Behavior Modification
	Health Education
	Health System Guidance
	Learning Facilitation
	Learning Readiness
	  Enhancement
	Self-Awareness
	  Enhancement
	Teaching: Disease
	  Process
	Teaching: Individual
		Coping Enhancement
		Counseling
		Emotional Support
		Family Involvement
		  Promotion
		Mutual Goal Setting
		Patient Contracting

Nursing Diagnosis: DENTITION, ALTERED

DEFINITION: Disruption in tooth development/eruption patterns or structural integrity of individual teeth.

Outcome: ORAL HEALTH

MAJOR INTERVENTIONS	SUGGESTED INTERVENTIONS	OPTIONAL INTERVENTIONS
Oral Health Maintenance Oral Health Restoration	Medication Management Nutrition Management Pain Management Referral Teaching: Individual	Health System Guidance Insurance Authorization Teaching: Psychomotor Skill

Outcome: SELF-CARE: ORAL HYGIENE

MAJOR INTERVENTIONS	SUGGESTED INTERVENTIONS	OPTIONAL INTERVENTIONS

Oral Health Maintenance
Oral Health Restoration
	Oral Health Promotion
	Self-Care Assistance:
	  Bathing/Hygiene
	Teaching: Individual
		Nutrition Management
		Self-Care Assistance:
		  Feeding
		Teaching: Psychomotor Skill

Nursing Diagnosis: **DIARRHEA**

DEFINITION: Passage of loose, unformed stools.

Outcome: **BOWEL ELIMINATION**

MAJOR INTERVENTIONS	SUGGESTED INTERVENTIONS	OPTIONAL INTERVENTIONS

Bowel Management
Diarrhea Management
	Fluid Management
	Fluid/Electrolyte
	  Management
	Medication Management
	Medication Prescribing
	Nutrition Management
	Perineal Care
	Skin Surveillance
		Anxiety Reduction
		Bowel Incontinence Care
		Bowel Incontinence
		  Care: Encopresis
		Fluid Monitoring
		Ostomy Care
		Self-Care Assistance:
		  Toileting
		Skin Care: Topical
		  Treatments
		Specimen Management

Outcome: **ELECTROLYTE & ACID/BASE BALANCE**

MAJOR INTERVENTIONS	SUGGESTED INTERVENTIONS	OPTIONAL INTERVENTIONS

Electrolyte Management
Fluid/Electrolyte
  Management
	Acid-Base Management
	Acid-Base Monitoring
	Diarrhea Management
	Electrolyte Monitoring
	Intravenous (IV)
	  Insertion
	Intravenous (IV)
	  Therapy
	Laboratory Data
	  Interpretation
	Vital Signs Monitoring
		Electrolyte Management:
		  Hypokalemia
		Electrolyte Management:
		  Hyponatremia
		Specimen Management
		Total Parenteral
		  Nutrition (TPN)
		  Administration

Outcome: FLUID BALANCE

MAJOR INTERVENTIONS	SUGGESTED INTERVENTIONS	OPTIONAL INTERVENTIONS

Fluid Management
Fluid/Electrolyte
  Management
	Diarrhea Management
	Electrolyte Management
	Electrolyte Monitoring
	Fluid Monitoring
	Fluid Resuscitation
	Intravenous (IV)
	  Insertion
	Intravenous (IV)
	  Therapy
	Nutrition Management
	Nutrition Therapy
	Nutritional Monitoring
	Vital Signs Monitoring
		Enteral Tube Feeding
		Peripherally Inserted
		  Central (PIC)
		  Catheter Care
		Total Parenteral
		  Nutrition (TPN)
		  Administration
		Venous Access Device
		  (VAD) Maintenance

Outcome: HYDRATION

MAJOR INTERVENTIONS	SUGGESTED INTERVENTIONS	OPTIONAL INTERVENTIONS

Fluid Management
Fluid/Electrolyte
  Management
	Bottle Feeding
	Diarrhea Management
	Electrolyte Management
	Electrolyte Monitoring
	Feeding
	Fluid Monitoring
	Fluid Resuscitation
	Nutrition Management
	Nutritional Monitoring
		Intravenous (IV)
		  Insertion
		Intravenous (IV)
		  Therapy
		Temperature Regulation
		Vital Signs Monitoring

Outcome: SYMPTOM SEVERITY

MAJOR INTERVENTIONS	SUGGESTED INTERVENTIONS	OPTIONAL INTERVENTIONS

Diarrhea Management	Anxiety Reduction
	Bowel Management
	Coping Enhancement
	Emotional Support
	Energy Management
	Medication
	  Administration
	Medication Management
	Medication Prescribing
	Pain Management
		Flatulence Reduction
		Perineal Care
		Skin Care: Topical
		  Treatments
		Surveillance
		Weight Management

Nursing Diagnosis: DIVERSIONAL ACTIVITY DEFICIT

DEFINITION: The state in which an individual experiences a decreased stimulation from or interest or engagement in recreational or leisure activities.

Outcome: LEISURE PARTICIPATION

MAJOR INTERVENTIONS	SUGGESTED INTERVENTIONS	OPTIONAL INTERVENTIONS
Recreation Therapy Self-Responsibility Facilitation	Activity Therapy Exercise Promotion Socialization Enhancement Therapeutic Play	Animal-Assisted Therapy Art Therapy Bibliotherapy Family Mobilization Humor Music Therapy Reminiscence Therapy

Outcome: PLAY PARTICIPATION

MAJOR INTERVENTIONS	SUGGESTED INTERVENTIONS	OPTIONAL INTERVENTIONS
Therapeutic Play	Exercise Promotion Recreation Therapy Socialization Enhancement	Activity Therapy Animal-Assisted Therapy Art Therapy Music Therapy Surveillance: Safety

Outcome: SOCIAL INVOLVEMENT

MAJOR INTERVENTIONS	SUGGESTED INTERVENTIONS	OPTIONAL INTERVENTIONS
Socialization Enhancement	Activity Therapy Animal-Assisted Therapy Art Therapy Developmental Enhancement: Adolescent Developmental Enhancement: Child Milieu Therapy Mutual Goal Setting Recreation Therapy Role Enhancement Self-Awareness Enhancement Self-Esteem Enhancement Self-Responsibility Facilitation Therapeutic Play Visitation Facilitation	Active Listening Assertiveness Training Behavior Management Body Image Enhancement Communication Enhancement: Hearing Deficit Communication Enhancement: Speech Deficit Communication Enhancement: Visual Deficit Complex Relationship Building Counseling Culture Brokerage Emotional Support Family Mobilization Family Therapy Humor Presence Support Group Support System Enhancement

Nursing Diagnosis: DYSREFLEXIA

DEFINITION: The state in which an individual with a spinal cord injury at T7 or above experiences a life threatening uninhibited sympathetic response of the nervous system to a noxious stimulus.

Outcome: NEUROLOGICAL STATUS

MAJOR INTERVENTIONS	SUGGESTED INTERVENTIONS	OPTIONAL INTERVENTIONS

Dysreflexia Management
Vital Signs Monitoring
	Emergency Care
	Medication
	  Administration
	Neurologic Monitoring
	Respiratory Monitoring
	Seizure Management
	Seizure Precautions
	Temperature Regulation
		Code Management
		Teaching: Disease
		  Process
		Teaching: Prescribed
		  Medication

Outcome: NEUROLOGICAL STATUS: AUTONOMIC

MAJOR INTERVENTIONS	SUGGESTED INTERVENTIONS	OPTIONAL INTERVENTIONS

Dysreflexia Management
Vital Signs Monitoring
	Bowel Management
	Emergency Care
	Medication
	  Administration
	Medication Management
	Neurologic Monitoring
	Positioning
	Respiratory Monitoring
	Surveillance
	Urinary Elimination
	  Management
		Code Management
		Fever Treatment
		Infection Control
		Intravenous (IV)
		  Therapy
		Phlebotomy: Arterial
		  Blood Sample
		Phlebotomy: Venous
		  Blood Sample
		Technology Management
		Temperature Regulation
		Urinary Catheterization
		Urinary Catheterization:
		  Intermittent

Outcome: VITAL SIGNS STATUS

MAJOR INTERVENTIONS	SUGGESTED INTERVENTIONS	OPTIONAL INTERVENTIONS

Vital Signs Monitoring	Airway Management
	Anxiety Reduction
	Dysreflexia Management
	Environmental
	  Management
	Fluid Management
	Medication
	  Administration
	Medication Management
	Medication Prescribing
	Shock Prevention
		Cough Enhancement
		Emergency Care
		Infection Protection
		Pain Management
		Teaching: Individual
		Teaching: Prescribed
		  Medication

Nursing Diagnosis: ENERGY FIELD DISTURBANCE

DEFINITION: A disruption of the flow of energy surrounding a person's being that results in disharmony of the body, mind and/or spirit.

Outcome: SPIRITUAL WELL-BEING

MAJOR INTERVENTIONS	SUGGESTED INTERVENTIONS	OPTIONAL INTERVENTIONS

Hope Instillation
Spiritual Growth
  Facilitation
	Forgiveness Facilitation
	Meditation Facilitation
	Self-Awareness
	  Enhancement
	Spiritual Support
	Support Group
	Therapeutic Touch
	Values Clarification
		Bibliotherapy
		Counseling
		Family Support
		Grief Work Facilitation
		Guilt Work Facilitation
		Self-Esteem
		  Enhancement
		Socialization
		  Enhancement
		Support System
		  Enhancement
		Touch

Outcome: WELL-BEING

MAJOR INTERVENTIONS	SUGGESTED INTERVENTIONS	OPTIONAL INTERVENTIONS

Self-Awareness
  Enhancement
Therapeutic Touch
	Acupressure
	Emotional Support
	Energy Management
	Hope Instillation
	Meditation Facilitation
	Pain Management
	Self-Esteem
	  Enhancement
	Simple Guided Imagery
	Spiritual Support
	Temperature Regulation
	Values Clarification
		Communication
		  Enhancement: Hearing
		  Deficit
		Communication
		  Enhancement: Speech
		  Deficit
		Communication
		  Enhancement: Visual
		  Deficit
		Counseling
		Environmental
		  Management
		Risk Identification
		Security Enhancement
		Support System
		  Enhancement

Nursing Diagnosis: ENVIRONMENTAL INTERPRETATION SYNDROME, IMPAIRED

DEFINITION: Consistent lack of orientation to person, place, time or circumstances over more than three to six months necessitating a protective environment.

Outcome: COGNITIVE ORIENTATION

MAJOR INTERVENTIONS	SUGGESTED INTERVENTIONS	OPTIONAL INTERVENTIONS
Dementia Management Reality Orientation	Anxiety Reduction Cognitive Stimulation Emotional Support Environmental Management Memory Training Milieu Therapy	Area Restriction Behavior Management Mood Management Patient Rights Protection Presence

Outcome: CONCENTRATION

MAJOR INTERVENTIONS	SUGGESTED INTERVENTIONS	OPTIONAL INTERVENTIONS

Anxiety Reduction
Cognitive Stimulation
	Cerebral Perfusion
	  Promotion
	Dementia Management
	Environmental
	  Management
	Medication Management
	Reality Orientation
		Active Listening
		Calming Technique
		Communication
		  Enhancement: Hearing
		  Deficit
		Communication
		  Enhancement: Speech
		  Deficit
		Communication
		  Enhancement: Visual
		  Deficit
		Touch

Continued

Outcome: INFORMATION PROCESSING

MAJOR INTERVENTIONS	SUGGESTED INTERVENTIONS	OPTIONAL INTERVENTIONS
Cognitive Stimulation Learning Facilitation Reality Orientation	Anxiety Reduction Calming Technique Communication Enhancement: Hearing Deficit Communication Enhancement: Speech Deficit Communication Enhancement: Visual Deficit Dementia Management Learning Readiness Enhancement Medication Management	Environmental Management Milieu Therapy Music Therapy Reminiscence Therapy Sleep Enhancement

Outcome: MEMORY

MAJOR INTERVENTIONS	SUGGESTED INTERVENTIONS	OPTIONAL INTERVENTIONS
Dementia Management Memory Training	Cognitive Stimulation Learning Facilitation Milieu Therapy Reality Orientation Reminiscence Therapy	Coping Enhancement Medication Management Patient Rights Protection Sleep Enhancement

Outcome: NEUROLOGICAL STATUS: CONSCIOUSNESS

MAJOR INTERVENTIONS	SUGGESTED INTERVENTIONS	OPTIONAL INTERVENTIONS
Cerebral Perfusion Promotion Environmental Management: Safety Neurologic Monitoring	Cognitive Stimulation Dementia Management Environmental Management Medication Administration Medication Management	Aspiration Precautions Patient Rights Protection Security Enhancement Seizure Precautions Surveillance Vital Signs Monitoring

Outcome: SAFETY BEHAVIOR: HOME PHYSICAL ENVIRONMENT

MAJOR INTERVENTIONS	SUGGESTED INTERVENTIONS	OPTIONAL INTERVENTIONS
Environmental Management: Safety Surveillance: Safety	Area Restriction Environmental Management: Violence Prevention Fire-Setting Precautions Home Maintenance Assistance Limit Setting Risk Identification Security Enhancement	Dementia Management Hallucination Management Incident Reporting Risk Identification Self-Care Assistance

Nursing Diagnosis: FAILURE TO THRIVE, ADULT

DEFINITION: A progressive functional deterioration of a physical and cognitive nature; the individual's ability to live with multisystem diseases, cope with ensuing problems, and manage his/her care are remarkably diminished.

Outcome: NUTRITIONAL STATUS

MAJOR INTERVENTIONS	SUGGESTED INTERVENTIONS	OPTIONAL INTERVENTIONS

Nutrition Management
Nutrition Therapy
	Energy Management
	Feeding
	Fluid/Electrolyte
	  Management
	Nutritional Monitoring
	Teaching:
	  Prescribed Diet
	Weight Gain Assistance
		Eating Disorders
		  Management
		Enteral Tube Feeding
		Self-Care Assistance:
		  Feeding
		Sustenance Support
		Total Parenteral
		  Nutrition (TPN)
		  Administration

Outcome: PHYSICAL AGING STATUS

MAJOR INTERVENTIONS	SUGGESTED INTERVENTIONS	OPTIONAL INTERVENTIONS

Environmental
  Management
Home Maintenance
  Assistance
Risk Identification
	Body Mechanics
	  Promotion
	Case Management
	Coping Enhancement
	Diet Staging
	Emotional Support
	Energy Management
	Family Mobilization
	Medication Management
	Nutrition Management
	Nutrition Therapy
	Nutritional Monitoring
		Bathing
		Bowel Management
		Dressing
		Family Support
		Feeding
		Foot Care
		Hair Care
		Nail Care
		Skin Surveillance
		Urinary Elimination
		  Management

Outcome: PSYCHOSOCIAL ADJUSTMENT: LIFE CHANGES

MAJOR INTERVENTIONS	SUGGESTED INTERVENTIONS	OPTIONAL INTERVENTIONS
Coping Enhancement	Emotional Support Family Involvement Promotion Family Mobilization Family Process Maintenance Financial Resource Assistance Spiritual Support	Animal-Assisted Therapy Dying Care Mood Management Sustenance Support

Outcome: SELF-CARE: ACTIVITIES OF DAILY LIVING (ADL)

MAJOR INTERVENTIONS	SUGGESTED INTERVENTIONS	OPTIONAL INTERVENTIONS
Self-Care Assistance	Caregiver Support Case Management Environmental Management: Comfort Self-Care Assistance: Bathing/Hygiene Self-Care Assistance: Dressing/Grooming Self-Care Assistance: Feeding Self-Care Assistance: Toileting	Energy Management Environmental Management: Safety Exercise Promotion Fall Prevention Home Maintenance Assistance

Outcome: WILL TO LIVE

MAJOR INTERVENTIONS	SUGGESTED INTERVENTIONS	OPTIONAL INTERVENTIONS
Hope Instillation Spiritual Support	Emotional Support Family Support Patient Rights Protection Support System Enhancement	Animal-Assisted Therapy Coping Enhancement

Nursing Diagnosis: FAMILIES MANAGEMENT OF THERAPEUTIC REGIMEN, INEFFECTIVE

DEFINITION: A pattern of regulating and integrating into family processes a program for treatment of illness and the sequelae of illness that is unsatisfactory for meeting specific health goals.

Outcome: FAMILY COPING

MAJOR INTERVENTIONS	SUGGESTED INTERVENTIONS	OPTIONAL INTERVENTIONS

Coping Enhancement
Family Process
    Maintenance
	Counseling
	Decision-Making
	    Support
	Emotional Support
	Family Integrity
	    Promotion
	Family Mobilization
	Family Support
	Family Therapy
	Financial Resource
	    Assistance
	Normalization
	    Promotion
	Support System
	    Enhancement
		Family Involvement
		    Promotion
		Home Maintenance
		    Assistance
		Respite Care
		Role Enhancement
		Support Group

Outcome: FAMILY FUNCTIONING

MAJOR INTERVENTIONS	SUGGESTED INTERVENTIONS	OPTIONAL INTERVENTIONS

Family Integrity
    Promotion
Family Involvement
    Promotion
Family Process
    Maintenance
	Counseling
	Family Mobilization
	Family Support
	Family Therapy
	Financial Resource
	    Assistance
	Normalization
	    Promotion
	Role Enhancement
	Sibling Support
		Abuse Protection
		    Support
		Caregiver Support
		Health System Guidance
		Home Maintenance
		    Assistance
		Referral
		Respite Care
		Support System
		    Enhancement

Outcome: FAMILY NORMALIZATION

MAJOR INTERVENTIONS	SUGGESTED INTERVENTIONS	OPTIONAL INTERVENTIONS
Family Involvement Promotion Family Mobilization Normalization Promotion	Case Management Coping Enhancement Counseling Family Integrity Promotion Family Process Maintenance Family Support Family Therapy Health System Guidance Home Maintenance Assistance Respite Care Role Enhancement Sibling Support Support System Enhancement Sustenance Support	Caregiver Support Culture Brokerage Referral Respite Care Risk Identification Support Group

Outcome: FAMILY PARTICIPATION IN PROFESSIONAL CARE

MAJOR INTERVENTIONS	SUGGESTED INTERVENTIONS	OPTIONAL INTERVENTIONS
Decision-Making Support Health System Guidance	Active Listening Anticipatory Guidance Assertiveness Training Counseling Culture Brokerage Discharge Planning Patient Rights Protection Self-Responsibility Facilitation Telephone Consultation	Anxiety Reduction Behavior Modification Caregiver Support Coping Enhancement Family Involvement Promotion Health Care Information Exchange Referral Sustenance Support

Continued

Outcome: KNOWLEDGE: TREATMENT REGIMEN

MAJOR INTERVENTIONS	SUGGESTED INTERVENTIONS	OPTIONAL INTERVENTIONS
Teaching: Disease Process Teaching: Procedure/ Treatment	Anticipatory Guidance Learning Facilitation Learning Readiness Enhancement Medication Management Nutrition Management Teaching: Group Teaching: Individual Teaching: Prescribed Activity/Exercise Teaching: Prescribed Diet Teaching: Prescribed Medication Teaching: Psychomotor Skill	Family Involvement Promotion Health System Guidance Prenatal Care Weight Management

Nursing Diagnosis: FAMILY COPING: COMPROMISED, INEFFECTIVE

DEFINITION: A usually supportive primary person (family member or close friend) is providing insufficient, ineffective, or compromised support, comfort assistance, or encouragement that may be needed by the client to manage or master adaptive tasks related to his/her health challenge.

Outcome: CAREGIVER EMOTIONAL HEALTH

MAJOR INTERVENTIONS	SUGGESTED INTERVENTIONS	OPTIONAL INTERVENTIONS

Emotional Support
Respite Care
	Anger Control
	  Assistance
	Anticipatory Guidance
	Caregiver Support
	Decision-Making
	  Support
	Family Involvement
	  Promotion
	Grief Work Facilitation
	Guilt Work Facilitation
	Resiliency Promotion
	Spiritual Support
	Support Group
	Support System
	  Enhancement
		Abuse Protection
		  Support
		Coping Enhancement
		Family Integrity
		  Promotion
		Family Mobilization
		Family Process
		  Maintenance
		Family Support
		Forgiveness Facilitation
		Health System Guidance
		Referral
		Role Enhancement
		Simple Relaxation
		  Therapy

Outcome: CAREGIVER-PATIENT RELATIONSHIP

MAJOR INTERVENTIONS	SUGGESTED INTERVENTIONS	OPTIONAL INTERVENTIONS

Caregiver Support	Conflict Mediation
	Emotional Support
	Family Integrity
	  Promotion
	Family Involvement
	  Promotion
	Family Mobilization
	Family Support
	Home Maintenance
	  Assistance
	Respite Care
	Support Group
	Support System
	  Enhancement
		Abuse Protection
		  Support
		Anxiety Reduction
		Complex Relationship
		  Building
		Environmental
		  Management:
		  Attachment Process
		Environmental
		  Management: Violence
		  Prevention
		Mutual Goal Setting

Continued

Outcome: CAREGIVER STRESSORS

MAJOR INTERVENTIONS	SUGGESTED INTERVENTIONS	OPTIONAL INTERVENTIONS

Caregiver Support
Coping Enhancement
	Decision-Making
	  Support
	Emotional Support
	Family Involvement
	  Promotion
	Family Mobilization
	Family Support
	Mediation Facilitation
	Role Enhancement
	Simple Relaxation
	  Therapy
	Support Group
	Support System
	  Enhancement
		Active Listening
		Anticipatory Guidance
		Energy Management
		Family Integrity
		  Promotion
		Financial Resource
		  Assistance
		Grief Work Facilitation
		Spiritual Support

Outcome: FAMILY COPING

MAJOR INTERVENTIONS	SUGGESTED INTERVENTIONS	OPTIONAL INTERVENTIONS

Coping Enhancement
Family Involvement
  Promotion
Family Mobilization
	Caregiver Support
	Complex Relationship
	  Building
	Conflict Mediation
	Counseling
	Family Integrity
	  Promotion
	Family Process
	  Maintenance
	Family Support
	Normalization
	  Promotion
	Resiliency Promotion
	Spiritual Support
		Abuse Protection
		  Support: Child
		Abuse Protection
		  Support: Domestic
		  Partner
		Abuse Protection
		  Support: Elder
		Anger Control
		  Assistance
		Case Management
		Consultation
		Crisis Intervention
		Decision-Making
		  Support
		Family Therapy
		Financial Resource
		  Assistance
		Grief Work Facilitation
		Mutual Goal Setting
		Respite Care
		Sibling Support

Outcome: FAMILY NORMALIZATION

MAJOR INTERVENTIONS	SUGGESTED INTERVENTIONS	OPTIONAL INTERVENTIONS
Family Process Maintenance Family Support Normalization Promotion	Caregiver Support Coping Enhancement Counseling Decision-Making Support Family Integrity Promotion Family Involvement Promotion Family Mobilization Respite Care Sibling Support Spiritual Support	Complex Relationship Building Consultation Mutual Goal Setting Reminiscence Therapy Role Enhancement Sustenance Support

Nursing Diagnosis: FAMILY COPING: DISABLING, INEFFECTIVE

DEFINITION: Behavior of significant person (family member or other primary person) that disables his/her capacities and the client's capacities to effectively address tasks essential to either person's adaptation to the health challenge.

Outcome: CAREGIVER EMOTIONAL HEALTH

MAJOR INTERVENTIONS	SUGGESTED INTERVENTIONS	OPTIONAL INTERVENTIONS
Caregiver Support	Anger Control	Abuse Protection
Emotional Support	Assistance	Support
Respite Care	Decision-Making	Assertiveness Training
	Support	Coping Enhancement
	Family Involvement	Family Integrity
	Promotion	Promotion
	Grief Work Facilitation	Family Mobilization
	Guilt Work Facilitation	Family Process
	Hope Instillation	Maintenance
	Self-Esteem	Family Support
	Enhancement	Referral
	Socialization	Role Enhancement
	Enhancement	Simple Relaxation
	Spiritual Support	Therapy
		Support Group
		Support System
		Enhancement

Outcome: CAREGIVER-PATIENT RELATIONSHIP

MAJOR INTERVENTIONS	SUGGESTED INTERVENTIONS	OPTIONAL INTERVENTIONS
Caregiver Support	Abuse Protection Support: Child Abuse Protection Support: Domestic Partner Abuse Protection Support: Elder Emotional Support Family Integrity Promotion Family Involvement Promotion Family Mobilization Family Support Home Maintenance Assistance Respite Care Support Group Support System Enhancement	Abuse Protection Support Anger Control Assistance Complex Relationship Building Counseling Environmental Management: Violence Prevention Mutual Goal Setting Self-Modification Assistance

Outcome: CAREGIVING ENDURANCE POTENTIAL

MAJOR INTERVENTIONS	SUGGESTED INTERVENTIONS	OPTIONAL INTERVENTIONS
Caregiver Support Coping Enhancement	Decision-Making Support Energy Management Exercise Promotion Family Involvement Promotion Respite Care Spiritual Support Support Group Support System Enhancement	Assertiveness Training Emotional Support Family Mobilization Family Support Mutual Goal Setting Recreation Therapy Simple Relaxation Therapy

Continued

Outcome: FAMILY COPING

MAJOR INTERVENTIONS	SUGGESTED INTERVENTIONS	OPTIONAL INTERVENTIONS

Coping Enhancement
Family Support
Family Therapy
	Abuse Protection
	  Support: Child
	Abuse Protection
	  Support: Domestic
	  Partner
	Abuse Protection
	  Support: Elder
	Complex Relationship
	  Building
	Conflict Mediation
	Counseling
	Family Integrity
	  Promotion
	Normalization
	  Promotion
	Resiliency Promotion
	Spiritual Support
	Sustenance Support
		Abuse Protection
		  Support
		Anger Control
		  Assistance
		Case Management
		Consultation
		Environmental
		  Management: Violence
		  Prevention
		Family Involvement
		  Promotion
		Family Process
		  Maintenance
		Financial Resource
		  Assistance

Outcome: FAMILY NORMALIZATION

MAJOR INTERVENTIONS	SUGGESTED INTERVENTIONS	OPTIONAL INTERVENTIONS

Family Support
Family Therapy
Normalization
  Promotion
	Coping Enhancement
	Counseling
	Family Integrity
	  Promotion
	Family Involvement
	  Promotion
	Family Mobilization
	Family Process
	  Maintenance
	Spiritual Support
		Abuse Protection
		  Support
		Anxiety Reduction
		Case Management
		Consultation
		Decision-Making
		  Support
		Environmental
		  Management: Home
		  Preparation
		Mutual Goal Setting

Nursing Diagnosis: FAMILY COPING: POTENTIAL FOR GROWTH

DEFINITION: Effective managing of adaptive tasks by family member involved with the client's health challenge, who now is exhibiting desire and readiness for enhanced health and growth in regard to self and in relation to the client.

Outcome: CAREGIVER WELL-BEING

MAJOR INTERVENTIONS	SUGGESTED INTERVENTIONS	OPTIONAL INTERVENTIONS

Caregiver Support
Respite Care
	Coping Enhancement
	Emotional Support
	Family Involvement
	   Promotion
	Family Mobilization
	Family Support
	Hope Instillation
	Support Group
	Support System
	   Enhancement
		Counseling
		Family Integrity
		   Promotion
		Home Maintenance
		   Assistance
		Normalization
		   Promotion
		Role Enhancement

Outcome: FAMILY COPING

MAJOR INTERVENTIONS	SUGGESTED INTERVENTIONS	OPTIONAL INTERVENTIONS

Family Involvement
   Promotion
Family Support
	Consultation
	Counseling
	Family Integrity
	   Promotion
	Family Mobilization
	Normalization
	   Promotion
	Parent Education: Infant
	Resiliency Promotion
		Coping Enhancement
		High-Risk
		   Pregnancy Care
		Mutual Goal Setting
		Preconception
		   Counseling
		Role Enhancement

Continued

Outcome: FAMILY NORMALIZATION

MAJOR INTERVENTIONS	SUGGESTED INTERVENTIONS	OPTIONAL INTERVENTIONS

Family Support
Normalization
  Promotion
	Anticipatory Guidance
	Consultation
	Developmental
	  Enhancement:
	  Adolescent
	Developmental
	  Enhancement: Child
	Family Integrity
	  Promotion
	Family Involvement
	  Promotion
	Role Enhancement
	Sibling Support
		Complex Relationship
		  Building
		Counseling
		Genetic Counseling
		Pass Facilitation
		Respite Care

Outcome: HEALTH PROMOTING BEHAVIOR

MAJOR INTERVENTIONS	SUGGESTED INTERVENTIONS	OPTIONAL INTERVENTIONS

Health Education
Self-Modification
  Assistance
	Behavior Modification
	Counseling
	Emotional Support
	Exercise Promotion
	Health Screening
	Mutual Goal Setting
	Self-Awareness
	  Enhancement
	Support Group
	Support System
	  Enhancement
		Developmental
		  Enhancement:
		  Adolescent
		Developmental
		  Enhancement: Child
		Family Mobilization
		Family Planning:
		  Contraception
		Nutrition Management
		Prenatal Care
		Smoking Cessation
		  Assistance
		Substance Use
		  Prevention
		Teaching: Safe Sex
		Weight Management

Outcome: HEALTH SEEKING BEHAVIOR

MAJOR INTERVENTIONS	SUGGESTED INTERVENTIONS	OPTIONAL INTERVENTIONS
Decision-Making Support Health Education	Anticipatory Guidance Counseling Developmental Enhancement: Adolescent Developmental Enhancement: Child Family Integrity Promotion Health Screening Health System Guidance Learning Facilitation Self-Awareness Enhancement Self-Modification Assistance Support Group	Exercise Promotion Nutrition Management Parenting Promotion Smoking Cessation Assistance Substance Use Prevention Weight Management

Outcome: PARTICIPATION: HEALTH CARE DECISIONS

MAJOR INTERVENTIONS	SUGGESTED INTERVENTIONS	OPTIONAL INTERVENTIONS
Decision-Making Support Health System Guidance	Active Listening Anticipatory Guidance Assertiveness Training Counseling Culture Brokerage Patient Rights Protection Self-Responsibility Facilitation	Behavior Modification Caregiver Support Coping Enhancement Family Involvement Promotion Health Care Information Exchange Referral

Nursing Diagnosis: FAMILY PROCESSES, ALTERED

DEFINITION: A change in family relationships and/or functioning.

Outcome: FAMILY COPING

MAJOR INTERVENTIONS	SUGGESTED INTERVENTIONS	OPTIONAL INTERVENTIONS

Coping Enhancement
Family Support
	Conflict Mediation
	Counseling
	Decision-Making
	  Support
	Emotional Support
	Family Mobilization
	Family Process
	  Maintenance
	Family Therapy
	Financial Resource
	  Assistance
	Grief Work Facilitation
	Respite Care
	Support Group
	Support System
	  Enhancement
		Behavior Management
		Behavior Modification
		Caregiver Support
		Dementia Management
		Family Integrity
		  Promotion
		Guilt Work Facilitation
		Home Maintenance
		  Assistance
		Newborn Care
		Parent Education:
		  Adolescent
		Parent Education:
		  Childrearing Family
		Reproductive
		  Technology
		  Management

Outcome: FAMILY ENVIRONMENT: INTERNAL

MAJOR INTERVENTIONS	SUGGESTED INTERVENTIONS	OPTIONAL INTERVENTIONS

Family Integrity
  Promotion
Family Process
  Maintenance
	Behavior Management
	Conflict Mediation
	Counseling
	Decision-Making
	  Support
	Family Involvement
	  Promotion
	Family Support
	Home Maintenance
	  Assistance
	Mutual Goal Setting
	Role Enhancement
		Behavior Modification
		Caregiver Support
		Developmental
		  Enhancement:
		  Adolescent
		Developmental
		  Enhancement: Child
		Family Therapy
		Financial Resource
		  Assistance

Outcome: FAMILY FUNCTIONING

MAJOR INTERVENTIONS	SUGGESTED INTERVENTIONS	OPTIONAL INTERVENTIONS
Family Integrity Promotion Family Process Maintenance	Conflict Mediation Counseling Developmental Enhancement: Adolescent Developmental Enhancement: Child Family Involvement Promotion Family Mobilization Family Support Family Therapy Financial Resource Assistance Normalization Promotion Role Enhancement Support System Enhancement	Attachment Promotion Behavior Management Coping Enhancement Decision-Making Support Family Integrity Promotion: Childbearing Family Family Planning: Contraception Family Planning: Infertility Family Planning: Unplanned Pregnancy Parent Education: Adolescent Parent Education: Childrearing Family Spiritual Support Support Group

Outcome: FAMILY NORMALIZATION

MAJOR INTERVENTIONS	SUGGESTED INTERVENTIONS	OPTIONAL INTERVENTIONS
Family Process Maintenance Normalization Promotion	Caregiver Support Coping Enhancement Counseling Emotional Support Family Mobilization Family Support Financial Resource Assistance Home Maintenance Assistance Respite Care Role Enhancement Support System Enhancement	Behavior Management Behavior Modification Dementia Management Developmental Enhancement: Adolescent Developmental Enhancement: Child Family Integrity Promotion Family Therapy Grief Work Facilitation Guilt Work Facilitation

Continued

Outcome: PARENTING

MAJOR INTERVENTIONS	SUGGESTED INTERVENTIONS	OPTIONAL INTERVENTIONS
Parent Education: Adolescent	Abuse Protection Support: Child	Breastfeeding Assistance
Parent Education: Childrearing Family	Anticipatory Guidance	Emotional Support
Parenting Promotion	Coping Enhancement	Family Integrity Promotion
	Counseling	Family Therapy
	Developmental Enhancement: Adolescent	Guilt Work Facilitation
	Developmental Enhancement: Child	Health System Guidance
	Family Integrity Promotion: Childbearing Family	Home Maintenance Assistance
	Family Involvement Promotion	Prenatal Care
	Family Process Maintenance	Security Enhancement
	Family Support	Self-Esteem Enhancement
	Normalization Promotion	Socialization Enhancement
	Respite Care	Support Group
	Role Enhancement	Sustenance Support
	Sibling Support	Telephone Consultation
	Support System Enhancement	

Nursing Diagnosis: FAMILY PROCESSES, ALTERED: ALCOHOLISM

DEFINITION: The state in which the psychosocial, spiritual, and physiological functions of the family unit are chronically disorganized, leading to conflict, denial of problems, resistance to change, ineffective problem-solving, and a series of self-perpetuating crises.

Outcome: FAMILY COPING

MAJOR INTERVENTIONS	SUGGESTED INTERVENTIONS	OPTIONAL INTERVENTIONS

Coping Enhancement
Family Process
  Maintenance
Substance Use Treatment
	Abuse Protection
	  Support
	Abuse Protection
	  Support: Child
	Abuse Protection
	  Support: Domestic
	  Partner
	Abuse Protection
	  Support: Elder
	Crisis Intervention
	Counseling
	Family Integrity
	  Promotion
	Family Support
	Family Therapy
	Normalization
	  Promotion
	Spiritual Support
	Support Group
		Anger Control
		  Assistance
		Behavior Management
		Impulse Control Training
		Referral
		Self-Awareness
		  Enhancement
		Self-Responsibility
		  Facilitation

Outcome: FAMILY FUNCTIONING

MAJOR INTERVENTIONS	SUGGESTED INTERVENTIONS	OPTIONAL INTERVENTIONS

Family Integrity
  Promotion
Family Process
  Maintenance
Substance Use Treatment
	Behavior Management
	Counseling
	Family Mobilization
	Family Support
	Family Therapy
	Mutual Goal Setting
	Normalization
	  Promotion
	Substance Use
	  Prevention
	Support System
	  Enhancement
		Abuse Protection
		  Support
		Anger Control
		  Assistance
		Coping Enhancement
		Decision-Making
		  Support
		Impulse Control Training
		Referral
		Self-Responsibility
		  Facilitation
		Spiritual Support
		Support Group

Continued

Outcome: SUBSTANCE ADDICTION CONSEQUENCES

MAJOR INTERVENTIONS	SUGGESTED INTERVENTIONS	OPTIONAL INTERVENTIONS
Substance Use Prevention Substance Use Treatment	Anxiety Reduction Behavior Management Behavior Management: Self-Harm Behavior Modification Behavior Modification: Social Skills Coping Enhancement Counseling Crisis Intervention Emotional Support Family Involvement Promotion Family Mobilization Family Support Impulse Control Training Limit Setting Mutual Goal Setting Patient Contracting Self-Awareness Enhancement Self-Esteem Enhancement Self-Modification Assistance Self-Responsibility Facilitation Spiritual Support Support Group Support System Enhancement Teaching: Disease Process Therapy Group	Active Listening Anger Control Assistance Body Image Enhancement Complex Relationship Building Decision-Making Support Environmental Management Family Therapy Mood Management Progressive Muscle Relaxation Socialization Enhancement

Nursing Diagnosis: FATIGUE

DEFINITION: An overwhelming sustained sense of exhaustion and decreased capacity for physical and mental work at usual level.

Outcome: ACTIVITY TOLERANCE

MAJOR INTERVENTIONS	SUGGESTED INTERVENTIONS	OPTIONAL INTERVENTIONS
Energy Management	Environmental Management Exercise Promotion Exercise Promotion: Strength Training Teaching: Prescribed Activity/Exercise	Exercise Promotion: Stretching Self-Care Assistance

Outcome: ENDURANCE

MAJOR INTERVENTIONS	SUGGESTED INTERVENTIONS	OPTIONAL INTERVENTIONS
Activity Therapy Energy Management	Exercise Promotion Health Screening Mutual Goal Setting Nutrition Management Risk Identification Sleep Enhancement Teaching: Prescribed Activity/Exercise Teaching: Prescribed Diet	Exercise Promotion: Strength Training Exercise Therapy: Ambulation Exercise Therapy: Balance Exercise Therapy: Joint Mobility Exercise Therapy: Muscle Control Mood Management Self-Care Assistance Support System Enhancement Weight Management

Continued

Outcome: ENERGY CONSERVATION

MAJOR INTERVENTIONS	SUGGESTED INTERVENTIONS	OPTIONAL INTERVENTIONS

Energy Management
Environmental
   Management
	Body Mechanics
	   Promotion
	Exercise Promotion
	Nutrition Management
	Nutrition Therapy
	Nutritional Monitoring
	Sleep Enhancement
	Teaching: Prescribed
	   Activity/Exercise
		Dying Care
		Exercise Therapy:
		   Ambulation
		Exercise Therapy:
		   Balance
		Exercise Therapy: Joint
		   Mobility
		Exercise Therapy:
		   Muscle Control
		Simple Guided Imagery
		Simple Relaxation
		   Therapy
		Weight Management

Outcome: NUTRITIONAL STATUS: ENERGY

MAJOR INTERVENTIONS	SUGGESTED INTERVENTIONS	OPTIONAL INTERVENTIONS

Energy Management
Nutrition Management
	Feeding
	Nutrition Therapy
	Nutritional Counseling
	Nutritional Monitoring
	Self-Care Assistance:
	   Feeding
	Teaching:
	   Prescribed Diet
		Diet Staging
		Eating Disorders
		   Management
		Enteral Tube Feeding
		Sustenance Support
		Total Parenteral
		   Nutrition (TPN)
		   Administration
		Weight Management

Outcome: PSYCHOMOTOR ENERGY

MAJOR INTERVENTIONS	SUGGESTED INTERVENTIONS	OPTIONAL INTERVENTIONS

Energy Management
Mood Management
	Coping Enhancement
	Counseling
	Crisis Intervention
	Grief Work Facilitation
	Guilt Work Facilitation
	Medication Management
	Self-Esteem
	  Enhancement
		Animal-Assisted
		  Therapy
		Art Therapy
		Bibliotherapy
		Exercise Promotion
		Music Therapy
		Pain Management
		Progressive Muscle
		  Relaxation
		Simple Guided Imagery
		Simple Massage
		Simple Relaxation
		  Therapy
		Sleep Enhancement

Nursing Diagnosis: FEAR

DEFINITION: Fear is anxiety caused by consciously recognized and realistic danger. It is a perceived threat, real or imagined. Operationally, fear is the presence of immediate feeling of apprehension and fright; source known and specific; subjective responses that act as energizers but cannot be observed; and objective signs that are the result of the transformation of energy into relief behaviors and responses.

Outcome: ANXIETY CONTROL

MAJOR INTERVENTIONS	SUGGESTED INTERVENTIONS	OPTIONAL INTERVENTIONS
Anxiety Reduction	Active Listening	Abuse Protection
	Calming Technique	Support
	Coping Enhancement	Biofeedback
	Counseling	Childbirth Preparation
	Distraction	Environmental
	Meditation Facilitation	Management
	Music Therapy	Examination Assistance
	Preparatory Sensory	Sleep Enhancement
	Information	Support Group
	Presence	Therapy Group
	Security Enhancement	
	Simple Relaxation	
	Therapy	
	Support System	
	Enhancement	
	Therapeutic Play	

Outcome: FEAR CONTROL

MAJOR INTERVENTIONS	SUGGESTED INTERVENTIONS	OPTIONAL INTERVENTIONS
Coping Enhancement Security Enhancement	Active Listening Anticipatory Guidance Anxiety Reduction Calming Technique Counseling Crisis Intervention Decision-Making Support Emotional Support Environmental Management Examination Assistance Family Involvement Promotion Preparatory Sensory Information Presence Support System Enhancement Teaching: Preoperative Teaching: Procedure/ Treatment Therapeutic Touch Truth Telling	Abuse Protection Support Abuse Protection Support: Child Abuse Protection Support: Elder Autogenic Training Biofeedback Childbirth Preparation Culture Brokerage Dying Care Hypnosis Meditation Facilitation Pain Management Progressive Muscle Relaxation Rape-Trauma Treatment Self-Esteem Enhancement Simple Guided Imagery Simple Relaxation Therapy Support Group Therapy Group

Nursing Diagnosis: FLUID VOLUME DEFICIT

DEFINITION: The state in which an individual experiences decreased intravascular, interstitial and/or intracellular fluid. This refers to dehydration, water loss alone without change in sodium.

Outcome: ELECTROLYTE & ACID/BASE BALANCE

MAJOR INTERVENTIONS	SUGGESTED INTERVENTIONS	OPTIONAL INTERVENTIONS
Acid-Base Management Electrolyte Management Fluid/Electrolyte Management	Acid-Base Monitoring Electrolyte Monitoring Fluid Management Fluid Monitoring Hemodynamic Regulation Intravenous (IV) Insertion Intravenous (IV) Therapy Laboratory Data Interpretation Neurologic Monitoring Surveillance Vital Signs Monitoring	Electrolyte Management: Hypercalcemia Electrolyte Management: Hyperkalemia Electrolyte Management: Hypermagnesemia Electrolyte Management: Hypernatremia Electrolyte Management: Hyperphosphatemia Electrolyte Management: Hypocalcemia Electrolyte Management: Hypokalemia Electrolyte Management: Hypomagnesemia Electrolyte Management: Hyponatremia Electrolyte Management: Hypophosphatemia Phlebotomy: Arterial Blood Sample Phlebotomy: Venous Blood Sample Total Parenteral Nutrition (TPN) Administration

Outcome: FLUID BALANCE

MAJOR INTERVENTIONS	SUGGESTED INTERVENTIONS	OPTIONAL INTERVENTIONS

Fluid Management
Fluid Monitoring
Hypovolemia
  Management
	Cardiac Care: Acute
	Diarrhea Management
	Electrolyte Management
	Electrolyte Monitoring
	Fluid Resuscitation
	Intravenous (IV)
	  Insertion
	Intravenous (IV)
	  Therapy
	Laboratory Data
	  Interpretation
	Medication
	  Administration
	Medication Management
	Medication Prescribing
	Nutrition Management
	Shock Management:
	  Volume
	Total Parenteral
	  Nutrition (TPN)
	  Administration
	Urinary Elimination
	  Management
	Vital Signs Monitoring
		Bleeding Reduction
		Blood Products
		  Administration
		Hemodynamic
		  Regulation
		Hemorrhage Control
		Invasive Hemodynamic
		  Monitoring
		Peripherally Inserted
		  Central (PIC)
		  Catheter Care
		Resuscitation: Fetus
		Shock Management
		Shock Prevention
		Venous Access Devices
		  (VAD) Maintenance

Continued

Outcome: HYDRATION

MAJOR INTERVENTIONS	SUGGESTED INTERVENTIONS	OPTIONAL INTERVENTIONS

Fluid Management
Fluid/Electrolyte
  Management
Hypovolemia
  Management
Intravenous (IV)
  Therapy
	Bottle Feeding
	Diarrhea Management
	Electrolyte Management
	Electrolyte Monitoring
	Feeding
	Fever Treatment
	Fluid Monitoring
	Fluid Resuscitation
	Intravenous (IV)
	  Insertion
	Intravenous (IV)
	  Therapy
	Nutrition Management
	Shock Management:
	  Volume
	Urinary Elimination
	  Management
	Vital Signs Monitoring
		Bleeding Precautions
		Bleeding Reduction
		Bleeding Reduction:
		  Antepartum Uterus
		Bleeding Reduction:
		  Gastrointestinal
		Bleeding Reduction:
		  Postpartum Uterus
		Hemorrhage Control
		Gastrointestinal
		  Intubation
		Temperature Regulation

Outcome: NUTRITIONAL STATUS: FOOD & FLUID INTAKE

MAJOR INTERVENTIONS	SUGGESTED INTERVENTIONS	OPTIONAL INTERVENTIONS

Fluid Management
Fluid Monitoring
Nutrition Management
Nutritional Monitoring
	Enteral Tube Feeding
	Feeding
	Nutrition Therapy
	Self-Care Assistance:
	  Feeding
	Total Parenteral
	  Nutrition (TPN)
	  Administration
		Bottle Feeding
		Intravenous (IV)
		  Therapy
		Oral Health Restoration
		Swallowing Therapy
		Teaching:
		  Prescribed Diet

Nursing Diagnosis: **FLUID VOLUME EXCESS**

DEFINITION: The state in which an individual experiences increased isotonic fluid retention.

Outcome: **ELECTROLYTE & ACID/BASE BALANCE**

MAJOR INTERVENTIONS	SUGGESTED INTERVENTIONS	OPTIONAL INTERVENTIONS
Fluid Management Fluid Monitoring Fluid/Electrolyte Management	Acid-Base Management Electrolyte Management Electrolyte Monitoring Hemodialysis Therapy Hemodynamic Regulation Invasive Hemodynamic Monitoring Laboratory Data Interpretation Neurologic Monitoring Vital Signs Monitoring	Electrolyte Management: Hypocalcemia Electrolyte Management: Hypokalemia Electrolyte Management: Hypomagnesemia Electrolyte Management: Hyponatremia Electrolyte Management: Hypophosphatemia Phlebotomy: Arterial Blood Sample Phlebotomy: Venous Blood Sample

Outcome: **FLUID BALANCE**

MAJOR INTERVENTIONS	SUGGESTED INTERVENTIONS	OPTIONAL INTERVENTIONS
Fluid Management Fluid Monitoring Fluid/Electrolyte Management	Bedside Laboratory Testing Cerebral Edema Management Electrolyte Management Electrolyte Monitoring Hypervolemia Management Intravenous (IV) Insertion Intravenous (IV) Therapy Laboratory Data Interpretation Medication Administration Medication Management Nutrition Management Urinary Elimination Management Vital Signs Monitoring	Cardiac Care: Acute Hemodialysis Therapy Hemodynamic Regulation Intracranial Pressure (ICP) Monitoring Invasive Hemodynamic Monitoring Neurologic Monitoring Peritoneal Dialysis Therapy Respiratory Monitoring Weight Management

Continued

Outcome: **HYDRATION**		
MAJOR INTERVENTIONS	**SUGGESTED INTERVENTIONS**	**OPTIONAL INTERVENTIONS**
Fluid/Electrolyte Management Hypervolemia Management	Electrolyte Management Electrolyte Monitoring Fluid Management Fluid Monitoring Urinary Elimination Management Vital Signs Monitoring	Nutrition Management Nutritional Monitoring Temperature Regulation

Nursing Diagnosis: GAS EXCHANGE, IMPAIRED

DEFINITION: Excess or deficit in oxygenation and/or carbon dioxide elimination at the alveolar-capillary membrane.

Outcome: ELECTROLYTE & ACID/BASE BALANCE

MAJOR INTERVENTIONS	SUGGESTED INTERVENTIONS	OPTIONAL INTERVENTIONS
Acid-Base Management Electrolyte Management Laboratory Data Interpretation	Acid-Base Management: Respiratory Acidosis Acid-Base Management: Respiratory Alkalosis Acid-Base Monitoring Electrolyte Monitoring Fluid Management Fluid/Electrolyte Management Hemodynamic Regulation Intravenous (IV) Therapy Peripherally Inserted Central (PIC) Catheter Care Respiratory Monitoring Vital Signs Monitoring	Electrolyte Management: Hypercalcemia Electrolyte Management: Hyperkalemia Electrolyte Management: Hypermagnesemia Electrolyte Management: Hypernatremia Electrolyte Management: Hypocalcemia Electrolyte Management: Hypomagnesemia Electrolyte Management: Hyponatremia Specimen Management

Outcome: RESPIRATORY STATUS: GAS EXCHANGE

MAJOR INTERVENTIONS	SUGGESTED INTERVENTIONS	OPTIONAL INTERVENTIONS
Acid-Base Management Oxygen Therapy Ventilation Assistance	Acid-Base Management: Respiratory Acidosis Acid-Base Management: Respiratory Alkalosis Acid-Base Monitoring Airway Management Anxiety Reduction Bedside Laboratory Testing Chest Physiotherapy Energy Management Positioning Respiratory Monitoring	Airway Insertion and Stabilization Airway Suctioning Artificial Airway Management Aspiration Precautions Cough Enhancement Embolus Care: Pulmonary Laboratory Data Interpretation Mechanical Ventilation Phlebotomy: Arterial Blood Sample

Continued

Outcome: RESPIRATORY STATUS: VENTILATION

MAJOR INTERVENTIONS	SUGGESTED INTERVENTIONS	OPTIONAL INTERVENTIONS
Airway Management Respiratory Monitoring Ventilation Assistance	Airway Insertion and Stabilization Airway Suctioning Artificial Airway Management Aspiration Precautions Chest Physiotherapy Cough Enhancement Mechanical Ventilation Positioning	Acid-Base Monitoring Anxiety Reduction Embolus Care: Pulmonary Energy Management Mechanical Ventilatory Weaning Oxygen Therapy Pain Management Postanesthesia Care Resuscitation Resuscitation: Neonate Smoking Cessation Assistance

Outcome: TISSUE PERFUSION: PULMONARY

MAJOR INTERVENTIONS	SUGGESTED INTERVENTIONS	OPTIONAL INTERVENTIONS
Acid-Base Management: Respiratory Acidosis Acid-Base Management: Respiratory Alkalosis Embolus Care: Pulmonary Hemodynamic Regulation	Acid-Base Monitoring Bedside Laboratory Testing Fluid Management Fluid Monitoring Intravenous (IV) Insertion Intravenous (IV) Therapy Invasive Hemodynamic Monitoring Laboratory Data Interpretation Medication Administration Medication Management Oxygen Therapy Respiratory Monitoring Surveillance Vital Signs Monitoring	Chest Physiotherapy Cough Enhancement Emergency Care Mechanical Ventilation Resuscitation Resuscitation: Fetus Specimen Management Tube Care: Chest Ventilation Assistance

Outcome: VITAL SIGNS STATUS

MAJOR INTERVENTIONS	SUGGESTED INTERVENTIONS	OPTIONAL INTERVENTIONS
Airway Management Respiratory Monitoring Vital Signs Monitoring	Acid-Base Management Acid-Base Monitoring Anxiety Reduction Electrolyte Management Fluid Management Hemodynamic Regulation Intravenous (IV) Insertion Intravenous (IV) Therapy Medication Administration Medication Management Medication Prescribing Oxygen Therapy Ventilation Assistance	Biofeedback Emergency Care Pain Management Resuscitation

Nursing Diagnosis: GRIEVING, ANTICIPATORY

DEFINITION: Intellectual and emotional responses and behaviors by which individuals, families, communities work through the process of modifying self-concept based on the perception of loss.

Outcome: COPING

MAJOR INTERVENTIONS	SUGGESTED INTERVENTIONS	OPTIONAL INTERVENTIONS
Coping Enhancement Grief Work Facilitation Grief Work Facilitation: Perinatal Death	Anticipatory Guidance Anxiety Reduction Caregiver Support Counseling Dying Care Emotional Support Family Integrity Promotion Family Support Forgiveness Facilitation Hope Instillation Meditation Facilitation Presence Resiliency Promotion Spiritual Support Support Group Support System Enhancement Touch	Body Image Enhancement Mood Management Normalization Promotion Reminiscence Therapy Sibling Support Therapeutic Play Therapy Group Truth Telling

Outcome: FAMILY COPING

MAJOR INTERVENTIONS	SUGGESTED INTERVENTIONS	OPTIONAL INTERVENTIONS
Family Support Grief Work Facilitation	Coping Enhancement Counseling Family Integrity Promotion Family Process Maintenance Family Therapy Resiliency Promotion Spiritual Support Support System Enhancement	Caregiver Support Support Group

Outcome: FAMILY ENVIRONMENT: INTERNAL

MAJOR INTERVENTIONS	SUGGESTED INTERVENTIONS	OPTIONAL INTERVENTIONS
Family Integrity Promotion Family Support Grief Work Facilitation	Emotional Support Family Therapy Support Group Support System Enhancement	Counseling Spiritual Support

Outcome: GRIEF RESOLUTION

MAJOR INTERVENTIONS	SUGGESTED INTERVENTIONS	OPTIONAL INTERVENTIONS
Grief Work Facilitation Grief Work Facilitation: Perinatal Death	Active Listening Anger Control Assistance Anticipatory Guidance Coping Enhancement Counseling Dying Care Emotional Support Hope Instillation Spiritual Support Support Group Support System Enhancement	Animal-Assisted Therapy Bibliotherapy Guilt Work Facilitation Music Therapy Pregnancy Termination Care Presence Sibling Support Touch Visitation Facilitation

Outcome: PSYCHOSOCIAL ADJUSTMENT: LIFE CHANGE

MAJOR INTERVENTIONS	SUGGESTED INTERVENTIONS	OPTIONAL INTERVENTIONS
Anticipatory Guidance Coping Enhancement	Counseling Dying Care Emotional Support Truth Telling	Decision-Making Support Family Integrity Promotion Family Mobilization Family Process Maintenance Humor Spiritual Support

Nursing Diagnosis: GRIEVING, DYSFUNCTIONAL

DEFINITION: Extended, unsuccessful use of intellectual and emotional responses by which individuals, families, and communities attempt to work through the process of modifying self-concept based upon the perception of loss.

Outcome: COPING

MAJOR INTERVENTIONS	SUGGESTED INTERVENTIONS	OPTIONAL INTERVENTIONS
Coping Enhancement	Anxiety Reduction	Art Therapy
Counseling	Calming Technique	Behavior Management:
Grief Work Facilitation	Caregiver Support	Self-Harm
Grief Work Facilitation:	Conflict Mediation	Body Image
Perinatal Death	Crisis Intervention	Enhancement
	Decision-Making	Cognitive Restructuring
	Support	Family Therapy
	Emotional Support	Normalization
	Family Support	Promotion
	Forgiveness Facilitation	Reminiscence Therapy
	Guilt Work Facilitation	Sibling Support
	Hope Instillation	Simple Relaxation
	Presence	Therapy
	Support Group	Spiritual Growth
		Facilitation
		Spiritual Support
		Support System
		Enhancement
		Therapeutic Play
		Therapy Group
		Touch
		Truth Telling
		Values Clarification
		Visitation Facilitation

Outcome: FAMILY COPING

MAJOR INTERVENTIONS	SUGGESTED INTERVENTIONS	OPTIONAL INTERVENTIONS

Coping Enhancement
Family Integrity
  Promotion
Family Therapy
	Active Listening
	Counseling
	Crisis Intervention
	Emotional Support
	Family Process
	  Maintenance
	Family Support
	Grief Work Facilitation
	Grief Work Facilitation:
	  Perinatal Death
	Sibling Support
		Decision-Making
		  Support
		Normalization
		  Promotion
		Support Group
		Support System
		  Enhancement
		Values Clarification

Outcome: GRIEF RESOLUTION

MAJOR INTERVENTIONS	SUGGESTED INTERVENTIONS	OPTIONAL INTERVENTIONS

Grief Work Facilitation
Grief Work Facilitation:
  Perinatal Death
	Active Listening
	Anger Control
	  Assistance
	Coping Enhancement
	Counseling
	Culture Brokerage
	Emotional Support
	Family Integrity
	  Promotion
	Spiritual Support
	Support Group
	Support System
	  Enhancement
		Guilt Work Facilitation
		Hope Instillation
		Mutual Goal Setting
		Presence
		Sibling Support
		Suicide Prevention
		Touch
		Visitation Facilitation

Continued

Outcome: **Psychosocial Adjustment: Life Change**

MAJOR INTERVENTIONS	SUGGESTED INTERVENTIONS	OPTIONAL INTERVENTIONS
Coping Enhancement	Conflict Mediation Counseling Crisis Intervention Emotional Support Grief Work Facilitation Role Enhancement	Decision-Making Support Family Integrity Promotion Family Mobilization Family Process Maintenance Spiritual Growth Facilitation Spiritual Support Values Clarification

Nursing Diagnosis: GROWTH AND DEVELOPMENT, ALTERED

DEFINITION: The state in which an individual demonstrates deviations in norms from his/her age group.

Outcome: CHILD DEVELOPMENT: 2 MONTHS

MAJOR INTERVENTIONS	SUGGESTED INTERVENTIONS	OPTIONAL INTERVENTIONS
Developmental Enhancement: Child Infant Care Parenting Promotion	Attachment Promotion Family Integrity Promotion: Childbearing Family Family Support Parent Education: Infant Teaching: Infant Nutrition	Abuse Protection Support: Child Caregiver Support Health System Guidance Lactation Counseling Nutrition Management Nutritional Monitoring Respite Care Support System Enhancement Sustenance Support

Outcome: CHILD DEVELOPMENT: 4 MONTHS

MAJOR INTERVENTIONS	SUGGESTED INTERVENTIONS	OPTIONAL INTERVENTIONS
Developmental Enhancement: Child Infant Care Parenting Promotion	Family Integrity Promotion: Childbearing Family Family Process Maintenance Family Support Parent Education: Infant Teaching: Infant Nutrition Teaching: Infant Safety	Abuse Protection Support: Child Attachment Promotion Caregiver Support Health Screening Health System Guidance Lactation Counseling Nonnutritive Sucking Nutrition Management Nutritional Counseling Nutritional Monitoring Respite Care Support System Enhancement Sustenance Support

Continued

Outcome: CHILD DEVELOPMENT: 6 MONTHS

MAJOR INTERVENTIONS	SUGGESTED INTERVENTIONS	OPTIONAL INTERVENTIONS
Developmental Enhancement: Child Health Screening Parenting Promotion	Family Integrity Promotion: Childbearing Family Family Process Maintenance Family Support Infant Care Nutritional Counseling Parent Education: Infant Security Enhancement Teaching: Infant Nutrition Teaching: Infant Safety	Abuse Protection Support: Child Attachment Promotion Caregiver Support Environmental Management: Safety Health System Guidance Nutrition Management Nutritional Monitoring Support System Enhancement Surveillance: Safety Sustenance Support

Outcome: CHILD DEVELOPMENT: 12 MONTHS

MAJOR INTERVENTIONS	SUGGESTED INTERVENTIONS	OPTIONAL INTERVENTIONS
Developmental Enhancement: Child Health Screening Parenting Promotion	Anticipatory Guidance Bottle Feeding Family Integrity Promotion: Childbearing Family Family Process Maintenance Family Support Nutritional Counseling Parent Education: Childrearing Family Security Enhancement Socialization Enhancement Teaching: Toddler Nutrition Teaching: Toddler Safety	Abuse Protection Support: Child Attachment Promotion Caregiver Support Environmental Management: Safety Health System Guidance Nutrition Management Nutritional Monitoring Support System Enhancement Surveillance: Safety Sustenance Support Therapeutic Play

Outcome: **Child Development: 2 Years**

MAJOR INTERVENTIONS	SUGGESTED INTERVENTIONS	OPTIONAL INTERVENTIONS
Developmental Enhancement: Child Health Screening Parent Education: Childrearing Family	Family Integrity Promotion Family Support Family Therapy Nutrition Management Parenting Promotion Security Enhancement Socialization Enhancement Teaching: Toddler Nutrition Teaching: Toddler Safety	Abuse Protection Support: Child Activity Therapy Behavior Management Behavior Management: Overactivity/ Inattention Bowel Training Family Process Maintenance Health System Guidance Nutrition Counseling Support System Enhancement Surveillance: Safety Therapeutic Play Urinary Habit Training

Continued

Outcome: **CHILD DEVELOPMENT: 3 YEARS**

MAJOR INTERVENTIONS	SUGGESTED INTERVENTIONS	OPTIONAL INTERVENTIONS
Developmental Enhancement: Child Health Screening Parent Education: Childrearing Family	Behavior Management Behavior Management: Overactivity/ Inattention Bowel Incontinence Care: Encopresis Bowel Management Bowel Training Family Integrity Promotion Family Support Family Therapy Nutrition Management Parenting Promotion Security Enhancement Socialization Enhancement Support System Enhancement Teaching: Toddler Nutrition Teaching: Toddler Safety Urinary Habit Training Urinary Incontinence Care: Enuresis	Abuse Protection Support: Child Activity Therapy Behavior Modification Family Process Maintenance Health System Guidance Nutritional Counseling Nutritional Monitoring Sleep Enhancement Surveillance: Safety Sustenance Support Therapeutic Play

Outcome: CHILD DEVELOPMENT: 4 YEARS

MAJOR INTERVENTIONS	SUGGESTED INTERVENTIONS	OPTIONAL INTERVENTIONS
Developmental Enhancement: Child Health Screening Parent Education: Childrearing Family	Activity Therapy Behavior Management Behavior Management: Overactivity/ Inattention Behavior Modification Nutrition Management Nutrition Therapy Parenting Promotion Security Enhancement Socialization Enhancement Support System Enhancement Teaching: Psychomotor Skill Urinary Incontinence Care: Enuresis	Abuse Protection Support: Child Family Integrity Promotion Family Process Maintenance Family Support Family Therapy Health System Guidance Nutritional Counseling Nutritional Monitoring Sleep Enhancement Sustenance Support Therapeutic Play Urinary Habit Training

Outcome: CHILD DEVELOPMENT: 5 YEARS

MAJOR INTERVENTIONS	SUGGESTED INTERVENTIONS	OPTIONAL INTERVENTIONS
Developmental Enhancement: Child Health Screening	Activity Therapy Behavior Management: Overactivity/ Inattention Behavior Modification Learning Facilitation Nutrition Management Nutrition Therapy Parent Education: Childrearing Family Parenting Promotion Security Enhancement Socialization Enhancement Support System Enhancement Teaching: Psychomotor Skill Therapeutic Play Urinary Incontinence Care: Enuresis	Abuse Protection Support: Child Behavior Management Family Integrity Promotion Family Support Family Therapy Health System Guidance Nutritional Monitoring Sleep Enhancement Sustenance Support Urinary Habit Training

Continued

Outcome: Child Development: Middle Childhood (6-11 Years)

MAJOR INTERVENTIONS	SUGGESTED INTERVENTIONS	OPTIONAL INTERVENTIONS
Developmental Enhancement: Child Health Screening	Behavior Management Behavior Management: Sexual Behavior Modification Behavior Modification: Social Skills Exercise Promotion Learning Facilitation Mutual Goal Setting Nutrition Management Nutrition Therapy Parent Education: Childrearing Family Parenting Promotion Patient Contracting Self-Responsibility Facilitation Socialization Enhancement Weight Management	Abuse Protection Support: Child Body Image Enhancement Counseling Family Integrity Promotion Family Support Family Therapy Health System Guidance Nutritional Counseling Nutritional Monitoring Self-Awareness Enhancement Self-Esteem Enhancement Spiritual Support Substance Use Prevention Teaching: Individual Teaching: Safe Sex Teaching: Sexuality Values Clarification

Outcome: CHILD DEVELOPMENT: ADOLESCENCE (12-17 YEARS)

MAJOR INTERVENTIONS	SUGGESTED INTERVENTIONS	OPTIONAL INTERVENTIONS
Developmental Enhancement: Adolescent Health Screening Risk Identification Self-Responsibility Facilitation	Behavior Management Behavior Management: Sexual Behavior Modification Behavior Modification: Social Skills Eating Disorders Management Exercise Promotion Health System Guidance Learning Readiness Enhancement Mutual Goal Setting Nutrition Therapy Nutritional Monitoring Parent Education: Adolescent Parenting Promotion Self-Esteem Enhancement Socialization Enhancement Substance Use Prevention	Abuse Protection Support Bibliotherapy Body Image Enhancement Counseling Environmental Management: Violence Prevention Family Integrity Promotion Family Support Family Therapy Nutrition Management Nutritional Counseling Role Enhancement Self-Awareness Enhancement Self-Modification Assistance Sexual Counseling Spiritual Support Sports Injury Prevention: Youth Support System Enhancement Sustenance Support Teaching: Safe Sex Teaching: Sexuality Values Clarification Weight Management

Outcome: GROWTH

MAJOR INTERVENTIONS	SUGGESTED INTERVENTIONS	OPTIONAL INTERVENTIONS
Health Screening Nutrition Management Nutrition Therapy	Eating Disorders Management Nutritional Counseling Nutritional Monitoring Teaching: Prescribed Diet Weight Gain Assistance Weight Management	Bottle Feeding Breastfeeding Assistance Feeding Lactation Counseling Referral Sustenance Support

Continued

Outcome: PHYSICAL AGING STATUS

MAJOR INTERVENTIONS	SUGGESTED INTERVENTIONS	OPTIONAL INTERVENTIONS
Health Screening Risk Identification	Anticipatory Guidance Behavior Modification Cognitive Restructuring Communication Enhancement: Hearing Deficit Communication Enhancement: Visual Deficit Nutrition Management Nutrition Therapy Patient Contracting Self-Modification Assistance Self-Responsibility Facilitation Teaching: Prescribed Activity/Exercise Teaching: Prescribed Diet Teaching: Prescribed Medication	Body Mechanics Promotion Bowel Management Coping Enhancement Emotional Support Energy Management Exercise Promotion Family Support Medication Management Medication Prescribing Mutual Goal Setting Nutritional Counseling Nutritional Monitoring Sexual Counseling Teaching: Sexuality Urinary Elimination Management Vital Signs Monitoring Weight Management

Outcome: PHYSICAL MATURATION: FEMALE

MAJOR INTERVENTIONS	SUGGESTED INTERVENTIONS	OPTIONAL INTERVENTIONS
Developmental Enhancement: Adolescent Health Screening	Behavior Management: Sexual Impulse Control Training Nutrition Management Risk Identification Self-Awareness Enhancement Teaching: Sexuality	Eating Disorders Management Health System Guidance Nutrition Therapy Nutritional Counseling Nutritional Monitoring Parent Education: Adolescent

Outcome: **PHYSICAL MATURATION: MALE**

MAJOR INTERVENTIONS	SUGGESTED INTERVENTIONS	OPTIONAL INTERVENTIONS
Developmental Enhancement: Adolescent Health Screening	Behavior Management: Sexual Impulse Control Training Nutrition Management Parent Education: Adolescent Risk Identification Self-Awareness Enhancement Teaching: Sexuality	Eating Disorders Management Health System Guidance Nutrition Therapy Nutritional Counseling Nutritional Monitoring

Nursing Diagnosis: HEALTH MAINTENANCE, ALTERED

DEFINITION: Inability to identify, manage, and/or seek out help to maintain health.

Outcome: HEALTH BELIEFS: PERCEIVED RESOURCES

MAJOR INTERVENTIONS	SUGGESTED INTERVENTIONS	OPTIONAL INTERVENTIONS
Health System Guidance Support System Enhancement	Family Mobilization Family Support Insurance Authorization Sustenance Support	Energy Management Referral Self-Care Assistance

Outcome: HEALTH PROMOTING BEHAVIOR

MAJOR INTERVENTIONS	SUGGESTED INTERVENTIONS	OPTIONAL INTERVENTIONS

Health Education
Self-Modification
    Assistance
	Behavior Modification
	Cognitive Restructuring
	Coping Enhancement
	Counseling
	Exercise Promotion
	Health Screening
	Risk Identification
	Self-Awareness
	    Enhancement
	Self-Responsibility
	    Facilitation
	Support System
	    Enhancement
		Family Mobilization
		Nutrition Management
		Oral Health Promotion
		Referral
		Sleep Enhancement
		Smoking Cessation
		    Assistance
		Sports Injury Prevention:
		    Youth
		Substance Use
		    Prevention
		Teaching: Safe Sex
		Values Clarification
		Weight Management

Outcome: HEALTH SEEKING BEHAVIOR

MAJOR INTERVENTIONS	SUGGESTED INTERVENTIONS	OPTIONAL INTERVENTIONS
Decision-Making Support Self-Responsibility Facilitation	Anticipatory Guidance Counseling Health Education Health Screening Health System Guidance Learning Facilitation Mutual Goal Setting Patient Contracting Self-Modification Assistance	Culture Brokerage Exercise Promotion Nutrition Management Referral Self-Awareness Enhancement Smoking Cessation Assistance Substance Use Prevention Support Group Teaching: Safe Sex Values Clarification Weight Management

Outcome: KNOWLEDGE: HEALTH BEHAVIORS

MAJOR INTERVENTIONS	SUGGESTED INTERVENTIONS	OPTIONAL INTERVENTIONS
Health Education	Anticipatory Guidance Learning Facilitation Teaching: Group Teaching: Individual Teaching: Infant Nutrition Teaching: Prescribed Activity/Exercise Teaching: Prescribed Diet Teaching: Prescribed Medication Teaching: Toddler Nutrition Teaching: Toddler Safety	Health System Guidance Learning Readiness Enhancement Parent Education: Adolescent Parent Education: Childrearing Family Parent Education: Infant Preconception Counseling Risk Identification Self-Awareness Enhancement Teaching: Psychomotor Skill Teaching: Safe Sex Teaching: Sexuality Telephone Consultation Values Clarification

Continued

Outcome: KNOWLEDGE: HEALTH PROMOTION

MAJOR INTERVENTIONS	SUGGESTED INTERVENTIONS	OPTIONAL INTERVENTIONS

Health Education
Teaching: Individual
	Learning Facilitation
	Nutritional Counseling
	Oral Health Promotion
	Preconception
	  Counseling
	Risk Identification
	Teaching: Safe Sex
		Childbirth Preparation
		Health System Guidance
		Learning Readiness
		  Facilitation
		Parent Education:
		  Childrearing Family

Outcome: KNOWLEDGE: HEALTH RESOURCES

MAJOR INTERVENTIONS	SUGGESTED INTERVENTIONS	OPTIONAL INTERVENTIONS

Health System Guidance	Discharge Planning
	Health Education
	Learning Facilitation
	Teaching: Individual
		Health Care Information
		  Exchange
		Learning Readiness
		  Enhancement
		Teaching: Group
		Telephone Consultation

Outcome: KNOWLEDGE: TREATMENT REGIMEN

MAJOR INTERVENTIONS	SUGGESTED INTERVENTIONS	OPTIONAL INTERVENTIONS

Teaching: Procedure/
  Treatment
	Chemotherapy
	  Management
	Learning Facilitation
	Medication Management
	Nutrition Management
	Radiation Therapy
	  Management
	Surgical Preparation
	Teaching: Disease
	  Process
	Teaching: Individual
	Teaching: Preoperative
	Teaching: Prescribed
	  Activity/Exercise
	Teaching:
	  Prescribed Diet
	Teaching: Prescribed
	  Medication
		Family Involvement
		  Promotion
		Health System Guidance
		Learning Readiness
		  Enhancement
		Prenatal Care
		Teaching: Group
		Weight Gain Assistance
		Weight Management
		Weight Reduction
		  Assistance

Outcome: PARTICIPATION: HEALTH CARE DECISIONS

MAJOR INTERVENTIONS	SUGGESTED INTERVENTIONS	OPTIONAL INTERVENTIONS
Decision-Making Support Health System Guidance	Active Listening Admission Care Anticipatory Guidance Assertiveness Training Counseling Culture Brokerage Discharge Planning Patient Rights Protection Self-Responsibility Facilitation Values Clarification	Anxiety Reduction Behavior Modification Coping Enhancement Family Involvement Promotion Health Care Information Exchange Referral Telephone Consultation

Outcome: RISK DETECTION

MAJOR INTERVENTIONS	SUGGESTED INTERVENTIONS	OPTIONAL INTERVENTIONS
Health Screening Risk Identification Risk Identification: Childbearing Family Self-Responsibility Facilitation	Anticipatory Guidance Environmental Management: Safety Health System Guidance Learning Facilitation Self-Modification Assistance Surveillance: Safety Teaching: Disease Process Teaching: Group Teaching: Individual Values Clarification	Abuse Protection Support Abuse Protection Support: Child Abuse Protection Support: Elder Health Education Learning Readiness Enhancement Self-Awareness Enhancement

Continued

Outcome: SELF-DIRECTION OF CARE

MAJOR INTERVENTIONS	SUGGESTED INTERVENTIONS	OPTIONAL INTERVENTIONS
Self-Responsibility Facilitation	Assertiveness Training Coping Enhancement Culture Brokerage Decision-Making Support	Family Support Health System Guidance Medication Management Nutrition Management Role Enhancement Self-Awareness Enhancement Self-Esteem Enhancement

Outcome: SOCIAL SUPPORT

MAJOR INTERVENTIONS	SUGGESTED INTERVENTIONS	OPTIONAL INTERVENTIONS
Family Involvement Promotion Support Group Support System Enhancement	Financial Resource Assistance Referral Socialization Enhancement Telephone Consultation	Caregiver Support Coping Enhancement Emotional Support Family Support Role Enhancement Spiritual Support Sustenance Support Therapy Group

Outcome: Treatment Behavior: Illness or Injury

MAJOR INTERVENTIONS	SUGGESTED INTERVENTIONS	OPTIONAL INTERVENTIONS
Self-Responsibility Facilitation Teaching: Disease Process	Behavior Management Behavior Modification Health System Guidance Mutual Goal Setting Patient Contracting Self-Modification Assistance Support System Enhancement Teaching: Prescribed Activity/Exercise Teaching: Prescribed Diet Teaching: Prescribed Medication Teaching: Procedure/ Treatment Teaching: Psychomotor Skill	Coping Enhancement Self-Awareness Enhancement Self-Care Assistance Smoking Cessation Assistance Substance Use Treatment Support Group Telephone Consultation Weight Gain Assistance Weight Reduction Assistance

Nursing Diagnosis: HEALTH-SEEKING BEHAVIORS (SPECIFY)

DEFINITION: A state in which an individual in stable health is actively seeking ways to alter personal health habits, and/or the environment in order to move toward a higher level of health.

Outcome: ADHERENCE BEHAVIOR

MAJOR INTERVENTIONS	SUGGESTED INTERVENTIONS	OPTIONAL INTERVENTIONS
Health Education Self-Modification Assistance	Coping Enhancement Decision-Making Support Emotional Support Health System Guidance Self-Awareness Enhancement Support System Enhancement Telephone Consultation Values Clarification	Assertiveness Training Counseling Health Screening Risk Identification Teaching: Individual

Outcome: HEALTH BELIEFS

MAJOR INTERVENTIONS	SUGGESTED INTERVENTIONS	OPTIONAL INTERVENTIONS
Self-Awareness Enhancement Values Clarification	Counseling Culture Brokerage Health Education Risk Identification Self-Esteem Enhancement	Bibliotherapy Health System Guidance Teaching: Individual Truth Telling

Outcome: HEALTH ORIENTATION

MAJOR INTERVENTIONS	SUGGESTED INTERVENTIONS	OPTIONAL INTERVENTIONS
Health Education Values Clarification	Counseling Culture Brokerage Decision-Making Support Self-Awareness Enhancement Self-Modification Assistance Self-Responsibility Facilitation	Active Listening Bibliotherapy Teaching: Group Teaching: Individual

Outcome: HEALTH PROMOTING BEHAVIOR

MAJOR INTERVENTIONS	SUGGESTED INTERVENTIONS	OPTIONAL INTERVENTIONS

Health Education
Self-Modification
  Assistance
	Behavior Modification
	Breast Examination
	Coping Enhancement
	Emotional Support
	Exercise Promotion
	Exercise Promotion:
	  Strength Training
	Exercise Promotion:
	  Stretching
	Health Screening
	Immunization/
	  Vaccination
	  Management
	Preconception
	  Counseling
	Risk Identification
	Self-Responsibility
	  Facilitation
	Smoking Cessation
	  Assistance
	Spiritual Support
	Substance Use
	  Prevention
	Weight Management
		Nutrition Management
		Oral Health Promotion
		Sexual Counseling
		Sleep Enhancement
		Spiritual Growth
		  Facilitation
		Support Group
		Support System
		  Enhancement
		Telephone Consultation

Continued

Outcome: HEALTH SEEKING BEHAVIOR

MAJOR INTERVENTIONS	SUGGESTED INTERVENTIONS	OPTIONAL INTERVENTIONS
Decision-Making Support Health Education Values Clarification	Activity Therapy Developmental Enhancement: Adolescent Developmental Enhancement: Child Emotional Support Family Integrity Promotion Health System Guidance Learning Facilitation Self-Modification Assistance Self-Responsibility Facilitation Support Group	Bibliotherapy Culture Brokerage Exercise Promotion Mutual Goal Setting Nutrition Management Patient Contracting Self-Awareness Enhancement Smoking Cessation Assistance Substance Use Prevention Teaching: Safe Sex Weight Management

Outcome: KNOWLEDGE: HEALTH PROMOTION

MAJOR INTERVENTIONS	SUGGESTED INTERVENTIONS	OPTIONAL INTERVENTIONS
Health Education Teaching: Individual	Learning Facilitation Nutritional Counseling Oral Health Promotion Preconception Counseling Risk Identification Teaching: Safe Sex	Childbirth Preparation Genetic Counseling Health System Guidance Learning Readiness Enhancement Parent Education: Childrearing Family Sexual Counseling

Outcome: KNOWLEDGE: HEALTH RESOURCES

MAJOR INTERVENTIONS	SUGGESTED INTERVENTIONS	OPTIONAL INTERVENTIONS
Health System Guidance	Discharge Planning Health Education Learning Facilitation Learning Readiness Enhancement Teaching: Individual	Financial Resource Assistance Health Care Information Exchange Teaching: Group Telephone Consultation

Outcome: **WELL-BEING**		
MAJOR INTERVENTIONS	**SUGGESTED INTERVENTIONS**	**OPTIONAL INTERVENTIONS**
Health System Guidance Risk Identification	Coping Enhancement Counseling Decision-Making Support Developmental Enhancement: Child Emotional Support Family Integrity Promotion Family Support Health Education Health Screening Meditation Facilitation Role Enhancement Security Enhancement Self-Awareness Enhancement Self-Esteem Enhancement Self-Modification Assistance Self-Responsibility Facilitation Socialization Enhancement Spiritual Growth Facilitation Support System Enhancement	Communication Enhancement: Hearing Deficit Communication Enhancement: Speech Deficit Communication Enhancement: Visual Deficit Exercise Promotion Pain Management Substance Use Prevention Surveillance: Safety

Nursing Diagnosis: HOME MAINTENANCE MANAGEMENT, IMPAIRED

DEFINITION: Inability to independently maintain a safe growth-promoting immediate environment.

Outcome: FAMILY FUNCTIONING

MAJOR INTERVENTIONS	SUGGESTED INTERVENTIONS	OPTIONAL INTERVENTIONS
Family Integrity Promotion Family Integrity Promotion: Childbearing Family	Family Mobilization Family Support Parenting Promotion	Case Management Financial Resource Assistance Mutual Goal Setting Resiliency Promotion Role Enhancement

Outcome: OUTCOME: PARENTING

MAJOR INTERVENTIONS	SUGGESTED INTERVENTIONS	OPTIONAL INTERVENTIONS
Home Maintenance Assistance	Abuse Protection Support: Child Environmental Management: Safety Family Support Respite Care Support System Enhancement Surveillance Sustenance Support	Parent Education: Childrearing Family Security Enhancement Support Group Telephone Consultation

Outcome: PARENTING: SOCIAL SAFETY

MAJOR INTERVENTIONS	SUGGESTED INTERVENTIONS	OPTIONAL INTERVENTIONS
Parent Education: Adolescent Parent Education: Childrearing Family Risk Identification: Childbearing Family	Abuse Protection Support: Child Anticipatory Guidance Developmental Enhancement: Child Family Integrity Promotion: Childbearing Family Surveillance: Safety	Counseling Family Support Family Therapy Mutual Goal Setting Self-Modification Assistance Support Group Teaching: Individual

Outcome: ROLE PERFORMANCE

MAJOR INTERVENTIONS	SUGGESTED INTERVENTIONS	OPTIONAL INTERVENTIONS

Role Enhancement	Anticipatory Guidance
	Behavior Modification
	Caregiver Support
	Counseling
	Emotional Support
	Self-Awareness
	  Enhancement
	Values Clarification
		Decision-Making
		  Support
		Family Therapy
		Health Education
		Mutual Goal Setting
		Respite Care
		Self-Esteem
		  Enhancement
		Support Group
		Support System
		  Enhancement
		Sustenance Support

Outcome: SELF-CARE: INSTRUMENTAL ACTIVITIES OF DAILY LIVING (IADL)

MAJOR INTERVENTIONS	SUGGESTED INTERVENTIONS	OPTIONAL INTERVENTIONS

Home Maintenance
  Assistance
	Energy Management
	Environmental
	  Management
	Environmental
	  Management: Home
	  Preparation
	Family Mobilization
	Role Enhancement
	Support System
	  Enhancement
	Surveillance: Safety
		Body Mechanics
		  Promotion
		Family Support
		Referral
		Self-Care Assistance
		Teaching: Individual
		Teaching: Prescribed
		  Activity/Exercise
		Telephone Consultation

Nursing Diagnosis: HOPELESSNESS

DEFINITION: A subjective state in which an individual sees limited or no alternatives or personal choices available and is unable to mobilize energy on own behalf.

Outcome: DECISION MAKING

MAJOR INTERVENTIONS	SUGGESTED INTERVENTIONS	OPTIONAL INTERVENTIONS
Decision-Making Support	Counseling Emotional Support Self-Awareness Enhancement Support System Enhancement Values Clarification	Family Support Mutual Goal Setting

Outcome: DEPRESSION CONTROL

MAJOR INTERVENTIONS	SUGGESTED INTERVENTIONS	OPTIONAL INTERVENTIONS
Mood Management Resiliency Promotion Self-Modification Assistance	Behavior Modification Coping Enhancement Emotional Support Energy Management Grief Work Facilitation Grief Work Facilitation: Perinatal Death Guilt Work Facilitation Hope Instillation Mutual Goal Setting Patient Contracting Self-Awareness Enhancement Therapy Group	Animal-Assisted Therapy Art Therapy Exercise Promotion Music Therapy Presence Recreation Therapy Socialization Enhancement Therapeutic Play

Outcome: DEPRESSION LEVEL

MAJOR INTERVENTIONS	SUGGESTED INTERVENTIONS	OPTIONAL INTERVENTIONS

Hope Instillation
Mood Management
	Coping Enhancement
	Counseling
	Crisis Intervention
	Emotional Support
	Grief Work Facilitation
	Grief Work Facilitation:
	  Perinatal Death
	Self-Esteem
	  Enhancement
	Support Group
	Therapy Group
		Activity Therapy
		Behavior Management:
		  Self-Harm
		Cognitive Stimulation
		Dying Care
		Recreation Therapy
		Security Enhancement

Outcome: HOPE

MAJOR INTERVENTIONS	SUGGESTED INTERVENTIONS	OPTIONAL INTERVENTIONS

Hope Instillation
Spiritual Growth
  Facilitation
	Active Listening
	Complex Relationship
	  Building
	Coping Enhancement
	Emotional Support
	Energy Management
	Reminiscence Therapy
	Resiliency Promotion
	Sleep Enhancement
	Spiritual Support
	Support Group
	Support System
	  Enhancement
	Values Clarification
		Counseling
		Family Mobilization
		Grief Work Facilitation
		Mutual Goal Setting
		Presence
		Socialization
		  Enhancement
		Suicide Prevention
		Touch

Continued

Outcome: **Mood Equilibrium**		
MAJOR INTERVENTIONS	**SUGGESTED INTERVENTIONS**	**OPTIONAL INTERVENTIONS**
Mood Management	Anger Control Assistance Counseling Crisis Intervention Emotional Support Grief Work Facilitation Grief Work Facilitation: Perinatal Death Hope Instillation Presence Resiliency Promotion Spiritual Support Suicide Prevention Support Group Touch	Animal-Assisted Therapy Anxiety Reduction Exercise Promotion Music Therapy Pain Management Self-Care Assistance Sleep Enhancement Support System Enhancement Therapeutic Play Therapy Group

Outcome: **Quality of Life**		
MAJOR INTERVENTIONS	**SUGGESTED INTERVENTIONS**	**OPTIONAL INTERVENTIONS**
Hope Instillation Values Clarification	Coping Enhancement Decision-Making Support Emotional Support Family Support Grief Work Facilitation Resiliency Promotion Role Enhancement Security Enhancement Self-Awareness Enhancement Socialization Enhancement Spiritual Support Support System Enhancement	Body Image Enhancement Guilt Work Facilitation Mood Management Reminiscence Therapy Support Group Sustenance Support

Nursing Diagnosis: HYPERTHERMIA

DEFINITION: A state in which an individual's body temperature is elevated above normal range.

Outcome: THERMOREGULATION

MAJOR INTERVENTIONS	SUGGESTED INTERVENTIONS	OPTIONAL INTERVENTIONS

Fever Treatment
Malignant Hyperthermia
  Precautions
Temperature Regulation
Temperature Regulation:
  Intraoperative
Vital Signs Monitoring
	Bathing
	Environmental
	  Management
	Fluid Management
	Heat Exposure
	  Treatment
	Infection Control
	Medication
	  Administration
		Emergency Care
		Heat/Cold Application
		Shock Management
		Skin Surveillance

Outcome: THERMOREGULATION: NEONATE

MAJOR INTERVENTIONS	SUGGESTED INTERVENTIONS	OPTIONAL INTERVENTIONS

Fever Treatment
Newborn Care
Temperature Regulation
	Bathing
	Environmental
	  Management
	Fluid Management
	Infection Control
	Newborn Monitoring
	Vital Signs Monitoring
		Heat Exposure
		  Treatment
		Parent Education: Infant
		Seizure Management
		Seizure Precautions
		Skin Surveillance

Nursing Diagnosis: HYPOTHERMIA

DEFINITION: The state in which an individual's body temperature is reduced below normal range.

Outcome: THERMOREGULATION

MAJOR INTERVENTIONS	SUGGESTED INTERVENTIONS	OPTIONAL INTERVENTIONS

Hypothermia Treatment
Temperature Regulation
Temperature Regulation:
  Intraoperative
Vital Signs Monitoring
	Circulatory Precautions
	Environmental
	  Management
	Fluid Management
	Hemodynamic
	  Regulation
		Heat/Cold Application
		Shock Management
		Shock Prevention

Outcome: THERMOREGULATION: NEONATE

MAJOR INTERVENTIONS	SUGGESTED INTERVENTIONS	OPTIONAL INTERVENTIONS
Hypothermia Treatment Newborn Care Temperature Regulation Vital Signs Monitoring	Environmental Management Fluid Management Newborn Monitoring Technology Management	Acid-Base Management Heat/Cold Application Parent Education: Infant Shock Prevention

Nursing Diagnosis: INCONTINENCE: BOWEL

DEFINITION: Change in normal bowel habits characterized by involuntary passage of stool.

Outcome: BOWEL CONTINENCE

MAJOR INTERVENTIONS	SUGGESTED INTERVENTIONS	OPTIONAL INTERVENTIONS

Bowel Incontinence Care
Bowel Training
	Bowel Incontinence
	  Care: Encopresis
	Bowel Irrigation
	Bowel Management
	Diarrhea Management
	Fluid Management
	Medication Management
	Rectal Prolapse
	  Management
	Self-Care Assistance:
	  Toileting
		Emotional Support
		Environmental
		  Management
		Exercise Promotion
		Exercise Therapy:
		  Ambulation
		Flatulence Reduction
		Nutrition Management
		Teaching: Prescribed
		  Activity/Exercise
		Teaching:
		  Prescribed Diet
		Teaching: Prescribed
		  Medication
		Teaching: Procedure/
		  Treatment

Outcome: BOWEL ELIMINATION

MAJOR INTERVENTIONS	SUGGESTED INTERVENTIONS	OPTIONAL INTERVENTIONS

Bowel Incontinence Care
Bowel Management
	Bowel Incontinence
	  Care: Encopresis
	Bowel Training
	Diarrhea Management
	Nutrition Management
	Nutritional Monitoring
	Rectal Prolapse
	  Management
		Exercise Promotion
		Fluid Monitoring
		Ostomy Care

Outcome: TISSUE INTEGRITY: SKIN & MUCOUS MEMBRANES

MAJOR INTERVENTIONS	SUGGESTED INTERVENTIONS	OPTIONAL INTERVENTIONS
Bowel Incontinence Care Perineal Care	Bathing Diarrhea Management Skin Surveillance	Ostomy Care

Nursing Diagnosis: Individual Coping, Ineffective

Definition: Inability to form a valid appraisal of the stressors, inadequate choices of practiced responses, and/or inability to use available resources.

Outcome: Aggression Control

MAJOR INTERVENTIONS	SUGGESTED INTERVENTIONS	OPTIONAL INTERVENTIONS
Anger Control Assistance	Area Restriction	Art Therapy
Environmental Management: Violence Prevention	Behavior Management: Self-Harm	Behavior Management: Overactivity/ Inattention
Impulse Control Training	Behavior Management: Sexual	Behavior Modification
	Behavior Modification: Social Skills	Delusion Management
	Calming Technique	Environmental Management
	Coping Enhancement	Environmental Management: Safety
	Counseling	Hallucination Management
	Crisis Intervention	Presence
	Fire-Setting Precautions	Self-Awareness Enhancement
	Limit Setting	Self-Modification Assistance
	Patient Contracting	Self-Responsibility Facilitation
	Physical Restraint	Substance Use Treatment
	Seclusion	
	Suicide Prevention	
	Surveillance Safety	

Outcome: COPING

MAJOR INTERVENTIONS	SUGGESTED INTERVENTIONS	OPTIONAL INTERVENTIONS
Coping Enhancement Decision-Making Support	Anxiety Reduction Calming Technique Caregiver Support Complex Relationship Building Counseling Crisis Intervention Distraction Emotional Support Meditation Facilitation Mood Management Pass Facilitation Presence Progressive Muscle Relaxation Reminiscence Therapy Resiliency Promotion Sleep Enhancement Support Group Support System Enhancement Therapy Group Touch	Abuse Protection Support Abuse Protection Support: Child Abuse Protection Support: Domestic Partner Abuse Protection Support: Elder Abuse Protection Support: Religious Activity Therapy Animal-Assisted Therapy Art Therapy Autogenic Training Behavior Management: Self-Harm Behavior Modification Biofeedback Cognitive Restructuring Family Therapy Grief Work Facilitation Grief Work Facilitation: Perinatal Death Hypnosis Mutual Goal Setting Rape-Trauma Treatment Self-Awareness Enhancement Self-Esteem Enhancement Sibling Support Simple Relaxation Therapy Spiritual Support Sustenance Support Weight Management

Continued

Outcome: DECISION MAKING

MAJOR INTERVENTIONS	SUGGESTED INTERVENTIONS	OPTIONAL INTERVENTIONS
Decision-Making Support	Counseling Emotional Support Genetic Counseling Learning Facilitation Patient Rights Protection Support System Enhancement Teaching: Individual Values Clarification	Culture Brokerage Family Involvement Promotion Family Support Health Care Information Exchange Parent Education: Adolescent Parent Education: Childrearing Family Parent Education: Infant Teaching: Prescribed Medication Teaching: Safe Sex

Outcome: IMPULSE CONTROL

MAJOR INTERVENTIONS	SUGGESTED INTERVENTIONS	OPTIONAL INTERVENTIONS

Coping Enhancement
Impulse Control Training
	Anger Control
	  Assistance
	Anxiety Reduction
	Area Restriction
	Behavior Management
	Behavior Management:
	  Self-Harm
	Behavior Management:
	  Sexual
	Behavior Modification:
	  Social Skills
	Elopement Precautions
	Environmental
	  Management: Safety
	Environmental
	  Management: Violence
	  Prevention
	Fire-Setting Precautions
	Limit Setting
	Mutual Goal Setting
	Patient Contracting
	Seclusion
	Self-Modification
	  Assistance
	Self-Responsibility
	  Facilitation
	Substance Use
	  Prevention
		Emotional Support
		Medication
		  Administration
		Mood Management
		Presence
		Risk Identification
		Security Enhancement
		Substance Use Treatment
		Support Group
		Support System
		  Enhancement
		Surveillance: Safety
		Teaching: Safe Sex
		Therapy Group

Continued

Outcome: INFORMATION PROCESSING

MAJOR INTERVENTIONS	SUGGESTED INTERVENTIONS	OPTIONAL INTERVENTIONS
Learning Facilitation Learning Readiness Enhancement	Cognitive Restructuring Delusion Management Dementia Management Medication Management Memory Training Reality Orientation	Activity Therapy Anxiety Reduction Art Therapy Counseling Delirium Management Environmental Management Hallucination Management Reminiscence Therapy Sleep Enhancement

Outcome: ROLE PERFORMANCE

MAJOR INTERVENTIONS	SUGGESTED INTERVENTIONS	OPTIONAL INTERVENTIONS
Role Enhancement	Anticipatory Guidance Behavior Modification Caregiver Support Cognitive Restructuring Counseling Emotional Support Parenting Promotion Self-Awareness Enhancement	Childbirth Preparation Decision-Making Support Health Education Parent Education: Adolescent Parent Education: Childrearing Family Parent Education: Infant Self-Esteem Enhancement Substance Use Treatment Support Group Support System Enhancement Sustenance Support

Outcome: SOCIAL SUPPORT

MAJOR INTERVENTIONS	SUGGESTED INTERVENTIONS	OPTIONAL INTERVENTIONS
Family Involvement Promotion Support Group Support System Enhancement	Coping Enhancement Emotional Support Referral Socialization Enhancement Telephone Consultation	Caregiver Support Family Support Role Enhancement Spiritual Support Sustenance Support Therapy Group

Nursing Diagnosis: INDIVIDUAL MANAGEMENT OF THERAPEUTIC REGIMEN, EFFECTIVE

DEFINITION: A pattern of regulating and integrating into daily living a program for treatment of illness and its sequelae that are satisfactory for meeting specific health goals.

Outcome: ADHERENCE BEHAVIOR

MAJOR INTERVENTIONS	SUGGESTED INTERVENTIONS	OPTIONAL INTERVENTIONS

Anticipatory Guidance
Health Education
Health System Guidance
	Decision-Making
	  Support
	Health Screening
	Learning Facilitation
	Learning Readiness
	  Enhancement
	Risk Identification
	Self-Modification
	  Assistance
		Culture Brokerage
		Referral
		Teaching: Individual
		Telephone Consultation
		Telephone Follow-up

Outcome: COMPLIANCE BEHAVIOR

MAJOR INTERVENTIONS	SUGGESTED INTERVENTIONS	OPTIONAL INTERVENTIONS

Behavior Modification
Mutual Goal Setting
Patient Contracting
	Health System Guidance
	Learning Facilitation
	Learning Readiness
	  Enhancement
	Self-Modification
	  Assistance
	Self-Responsibility
	  Facilitation
	Support System
	  Enhancement
	Surveillance
	Teaching: Individual
	Teaching: Prescribed
	  Activity/Exercise
	Teaching:
	  Prescribed Diet
	Teaching: Prescribed
	  Medication
	Teaching: Procedure/
	  Treatment
	Teaching: Psychomotor
	  Skill
	Teaching: Safe Sex
	Telephone Consultation
	Telephone Follow-up
	Values Clarification
		Culture Brokerage
		Patient Rights Protection
		Smoking Cessation
		  Assistance
		Substance Use
		  Prevention

Continued

Outcome: FAMILY PARTICIPATION IN PROFESSIONAL CARE

MAJOR INTERVENTIONS	SUGGESTED INTERVENTIONS	OPTIONAL INTERVENTIONS
Family Involvement Promotion	Family Mobilization Health Education Health System Guidance	Caregiver Support Culture Brokerage Family Process Maintenance Family Support Fiscal Resource Management

Outcome: KNOWLEDGE: TREATMENT REGIMEN

MAJOR INTERVENTIONS	SUGGESTED INTERVENTIONS	OPTIONAL INTERVENTIONS
Teaching: Procedure/ Treatment	Anticipatory Guidance Chemotherapy Management Learning Facilitation Learning Readiness Enhancement Medication Management Nutrition Management Radiation Therapy Management Teaching: Group Teaching: Individual Teaching: Prescribed Activity/Exercise Teaching: Prescribed Diet Teaching: Prescribed Medication Teaching: Psychomotor Skill	Health System Guidance Nausea Management Teaching: Disease Process Vomiting Management Weight Gain Assistance Weight Management Weight Reduction Assistance

Outcome: PARTICIPATION: HEALTH CARE DECISIONS

MAJOR INTERVENTIONS	SUGGESTED INTERVENTIONS	OPTIONAL INTERVENTIONS
Decision-Making Support Health System Guidance	Anticipatory Guidance Assertiveness Training Culture Brokerage Discharge Planning Patient Rights Protection Self-Responsibility Facilitation Telephone Consultation Values Clarification	Caregiver Support Family Involvement Promotion Health Care Information Exchange Referral

Outcome: RISK CONTROL

MAJOR INTERVENTIONS	SUGGESTED INTERVENTIONS	OPTIONAL INTERVENTIONS
Health Education Risk Identification Self-Modification Assistance	Health Screening Health System Guidance Learning Facilitation Learning Readiness Enhancement Surveillance	Environmental Management: Safety Environmental Management: Worker Safety Immunization/ Vaccination Management Infection Control Laser Precautions Latex Precautions Surgical Precautions

Outcome: SYMPTOM CONTROL

MAJOR INTERVENTIONS	SUGGESTED INTERVENTIONS	OPTIONAL INTERVENTIONS
Anticipatory Guidance Self-Modification Assistance	Health Education Health Screening Health System Guidance Learning Facilitation Learning Readiness Enhancement Teaching: Disease Process Teaching: Individual	Coping Enhancement Emotional Support Family Involvement Promotion Nausea Management Vomiting Management

Nursing Diagnosis: INDIVIDUAL MANAGEMENT OF THERAPEUTIC REGIMEN, INEFFECTIVE

DEFINITION: A pattern of regulating and integrating into daily living a program for treatment of illness and the sequelae of illness that is unsatisfactory for meeting specific health goals.

Outcome: COMPLIANCE BEHAVIOR

MAJOR INTERVENTIONS	SUGGESTED INTERVENTIONS	OPTIONAL INTERVENTIONS
Behavior Modification	Case Management	Bibliotherapy
Mutual Goal Setting	Cognitive Restructuring	Consultation
Patient Contracting	Coping Enhancement	Exercise Promotion
Self-Modification	Counseling	Family Involvement
Assistance	Culture Brokerage	Promotion
	Emotional Support	Family Mobilization
	Family Support	Patient Rights Protection
	Health System Guidance	Self-Awareness
	Learning Facilitation	Enhancement
	Learning Readiness	Self-Esteem
	Enhancement	Enhancement
	Risk Identification	Smoking Cessation
	Self-Responsibility	Assistance
	Facilitation	Support Group
	Support System	Surveillance
	Enhancement	Teaching: Prescribed
	Teaching: Disease	Activity/Exercise
	Process	Teaching:
	Teaching: Procedure/	Prescribed Diet
	Treatment	Teaching: Prescribed
	Teaching: Psychomotor	Medication
	Skill	Teaching: Safe Sex
	Telephone Consultation	
	Telephone Follow-up	
	Values Clarification	

Outcome: KNOWLEDGE: TREATMENT REGIMEN

MAJOR INTERVENTIONS	SUGGESTED INTERVENTIONS	OPTIONAL INTERVENTIONS
Teaching: Procedure/ Treatment	Active Listening Chemotherapy Management Learning Facilitation Learning Readiness Enhancement Medication Management Nutrition Management Radiation Therapy Management Teaching: Disease Process Teaching: Group Teaching: Individual Teaching: Prescribed Activity/Exercise Teaching: Prescribed Diet Teaching: Prescribed Medication Teaching: Psychomotor Skill	Family Involvement Promotion Health System Guidance High-Risk Pregnancy Care Prenatal Care Weight Gain Assistance Weight Management Weight Reduction Assistance

Outcome: PARTICIPATION: HEALTH CARE DECISIONS

MAJOR INTERVENTIONS	SUGGESTED INTERVENTIONS	OPTIONAL INTERVENTIONS
Decision-Making Support Health System Guidance	Active Listening Assertiveness Training Counseling Culture Brokerage Discharge Planning Patient Rights Protection Self-Responsibility Facilitation Telephone Consultation Values Clarification	Behavior Modification Bibliotherapy Coping Enhancement Family Involvement Promotion Health Care Information Exchange Referral Sustenance Support

Continued

Outcome: **TREATMENT BEHAVIOR: ILLNESS OR INJURY**

MAJOR INTERVENTIONS	SUGGESTED INTERVENTIONS	OPTIONAL INTERVENTIONS

Behavior Modification
Self-Responsibility
  Facilitation
Teaching: Disease
  Process
	Cognitive Restructuring
	Coping Enhancement
	Counseling
	Emotional Support
	Learning Facilitation
	Learning Readiness
	  Enhancement
	Mutual Goal Setting
	Patient Contracting
	Self-Modification
	  Assistance
	Support Group
	Support System
	  Enhancement
	Teaching: Individual
	Teaching: Prescribed
	  Activity/Exercise
	Teaching:
	  Prescribed Diet
	Teaching: Prescribed
	  Medication
	Teaching: Procedure/
	  Treatment
	Teaching: Psychomotor
	  Skill
	Telephone Consultation
	Telephone Follow-up
	Values Clarification
		Active Listening
		Family Involvement
		  Promotion
		Family Mobilization
		Self-Awareness
		  Enhancement
		Self-Care Assistance
		Smoking Cessation
		  Assistance
		Substance Use Treatment
		Surveillance
		Weight Gain Assistance
		Weight Reduction
		  Assistance

Nursing Diagnosis: **INFANT BEHAVIOR, DISORGANIZED**

DEFINITION: Disintegrated physiological and neurobehavioral responses to the environment.

Outcome: **NEUROLOGICAL STATUS**

MAJOR INTERVENTIONS	SUGGESTED INTERVENTIONS	OPTIONAL INTERVENTIONS

Neurologic Monitoring	Fluid Management
	Nutritional Monitoring
	Positioning
	Respiratory Monitoring
	Surveillance
	Temperature Regulation
	Vital Signs Monitoring
		Laboratory Data
		  Interpretation
		Medication
		  Administration
		Medication Management
		Newborn Monitoring
		Sleep Enhancement

Outcome: **PRETERM INFANT ORGANIZATION**

MAJOR INTERVENTIONS	SUGGESTED INTERVENTIONS	OPTIONAL INTERVENTIONS

Environmental
  Management
Newborn Care
	Attachment Promotion
	Breastfeeding Assistance
	Developmental Care
	Environmental
	  Management:
	    Attachment Process
	Kangaroo Care
	Lactation Counseling
	Newborn Monitoring
	Nonnutritive Sucking
	Nutritional Monitoring
	Pain Management
	Respiratory Monitoring
	Sleep Enhancement
		Bottle Feeding
		Cutaneous Stimulation
		Parent Education: Infant
		Positioning
		Surveillance
		Sustenance Support

Outcome: **SLEEP**

MAJOR INTERVENTIONS	SUGGESTED INTERVENTIONS	OPTIONAL INTERVENTIONS

Sleep Enhancement	Energy Management
	Environmental
	  Management
	Environmental
	  Management: Comfort
	Pain Management
		Presence

Continued

Outcome: THERMOREGULATION: NEONATE

MAJOR INTERVENTIONS	SUGGESTED INTERVENTIONS	OPTIONAL INTERVENTIONS
Newborn Care Temperature Regulation	Environmental Management Fluid Management Newborn Monitoring Vital Signs Monitoring	Parent Education: Infant

Nursing Diagnosis: INFANT BEHAVIOR, ORGANIZED, POTENTIAL FOR ENHANCED

DEFINITION: A pattern of modulation of the physiologic and behavioral systems of functioning (i.e. autonomic, motor, state, organizational, self-regulators, and attentional-interactional systems) in an infant that is satisfactory but that can be improved resulting in higher levels of integration in response to environmental stimuli.

Outcome: CHILD DEVELOPMENT: 2 MONTHS

MAJOR INTERVENTIONS	SUGGESTED INTERVENTIONS	OPTIONAL INTERVENTIONS
Developmental Care Infant Care	Attachment Promotion Environmental Management Environmental Management: Attachment Process Family Integrity Promotion: Childbearing Family Family Mobilization Kangaroo Care Nonnutritive Sucking Sleep Enhancement Touch	Lactation Counseling Newborn Care Newborn Monitoring Parent Education: Infant Surveillance

Outcome: CHILD DEVELOPMENT: 4 MONTHS

MAJOR INTERVENTIONS	SUGGESTED INTERVENTIONS	OPTIONAL INTERVENTIONS
Developmental Care Health Screening	Bottle Feeding Infant Care Lactation Counseling Parent Education: Infant Sleep Enhancement	Attachment Promotion Caregiver Support Environmental Management Health System Guidance Nonnutritive Sucking Support System Enhancement Surveillance

Continued

Outcome: SLEEP

MAJOR INTERVENTIONS	SUGGESTED INTERVENTIONS	OPTIONAL INTERVENTIONS
Sleep Enhancement	Calming Technique Energy Management Environmental Management Environmental Management: Comfort Music Therapy	Newborn Care Newborn Monitoring Vital Signs Monitoring

Nursing Diagnosis: **INFANT FEEDING PATTERN, INEFFECTIVE**

DEFINITION: A state in which an infant demonstrates an impaired ability to suck or coordinate the suck swallow response.

Outcome: **BREASTFEEDING ESTABLISHMENT: INFANT**

MAJOR INTERVENTIONS	SUGGESTED INTERVENTIONS	OPTIONAL INTERVENTIONS
Breastfeeding Assistance Lactation Counseling	Calming Technique Environmental Management: Attachment Process Environmental Management: Comfort Infant Care Newborn Monitoring	Nonnutritive Sucking Nutritional Monitoring Parent Education: Infant

Outcome: **BREASTFEEDING MAINTENANCE**

MAJOR INTERVENTIONS	SUGGESTED INTERVENTIONS	OPTIONAL INTERVENTIONS
Breastfeeding Assistance Lactation Counseling	Attachment Promotion Environmental Management Environmental Management: Comfort Kangaroo Care Newborn Care Newborn Monitoring Nutrition Management	Caregiver Support Parent Education: Infant

Outcome: **MUSCLE FUNCTION**

MAJOR INTERVENTIONS	SUGGESTED INTERVENTIONS	OPTIONAL INTERVENTIONS
Nonnutritive Sucking	Aspiration Precautions Energy Management	Referral

Continued

Outcome: **NUTRITIONAL STATUS: FOOD & FLUID INTAKE**		
MAJOR INTERVENTIONS	**SUGGESTED INTERVENTIONS**	**OPTIONAL INTERVENTIONS**
Enteral Tube Feeding Tube Care: Umbilical 　Line	Bottle Feeding Fluid Management Fluid Monitoring Lactation Counseling Nutrition Management Nutritional Monitoring Weight Management	Gastrointestinal 　Intubation Sustenance Support

Outcome: **SWALLOWING STATUS**		
MAJOR INTERVENTIONS	**SUGGESTED INTERVENTIONS**	**OPTIONAL INTERVENTIONS**
Nonnutritive Sucking Swallowing Therapy	Aspiration Precautions Calming Technique Surveillance	Bottle Feeding Breastfeeding Assistance Nutrition Management Referral

Nursing Diagnosis: INTRACRANIAL ADAPTIVE CAPACITY, DECREASED

DEFINITION: A clinical state in which intracranial fluid dynamic mechanisms that normally compensate for increases in intracranial volumes are compromised, resulting in repeated disproportionate increases in intracranial pressure in response to a variety of noxious and non-noxious stimuli.

Outcome: ELECTROLYTE & ACID/BASE BALANCE

MAJOR INTERVENTIONS	SUGGESTED INTERVENTIONS	OPTIONAL INTERVENTIONS

Electrolyte Management
Fluid/Electrolyte
  Management
	Acid-Base Management
	Acid-Base Monitoring
	Electrolyte Monitoring
	Fluid Management
	Fluid Monitoring
	Intravenous (IV)
	  Insertion
	Intravenous (IV)
	  Therapy
	Laboratory Data
	  Interpretation
	Neurologic Monitoring
	Vital Signs Monitoring
		Respiratory Monitoring
		Specimen Management

Outcome: FLUID BALANCE

MAJOR INTERVENTIONS	SUGGESTED INTERVENTIONS	OPTIONAL INTERVENTIONS

Fluid Management
Fluid/Electrolyte
  Management
	Bedside Laboratory
	  Testing
	Electrolyte Management
	Electrolyte Monitoring
	Fluid Monitoring
	Intracranial Pressure
	  (ICP) Monitoring
	Intravenous (IV)
	  Insertion
	Intravenous (IV)
	  Therapy
	Laboratory Data
	  Interpretation
	Medication
	  Administration
	Medication Management
	Vital Signs Monitoring
		Respiratory Monitoring
		Urinary Elimination
		  Management
		Venous Access Devices
		  (VAD) Maintenance

Continued

Outcome: NEUROLOGICAL STATUS

MAJOR INTERVENTIONS	SUGGESTED INTERVENTIONS	OPTIONAL INTERVENTIONS
Cerebral Edema Management Cerebral Perfusion Promotion Intracranial Pressure (ICP) Monitoring Neurologic Monitoring	Fluid Management Fluid Monitoring Fluid/Electrolyte Management Laboratory Data Interpretation Medication Administration Medication Management Peripheral Sensation Management Positioning: Neurologic Surveillance Surveillance: Safety Tube Care: Ventriculostomy/ Lumbar Drain Vital Signs Monitoring	Acid-Base Management Acid-Base Monitoring Airway Management Code Management Emergency Care Positioning Respiratory Monitoring Seizure Management Seizure Precautions

Outcome: NEUROLOGICAL STATUS: CONSCIOUSNESS

MAJOR INTERVENTIONS	SUGGESTED INTERVENTIONS	OPTIONAL INTERVENTIONS
Cerebral Edema Management Cerebral Perfusion Promotion Neurologic Monitoring	Airway Management Aspiration Precautions Emergency Care Intracranial Pressure (ICP) Monitoring Intravenous (IV) Insertion Intravenous (IV) Therapy Laboratory Data Interpretation Medication Administration Medication Management Respiratory Monitoring Surveillance Vital Signs Monitoring	Anxiety Reduction Environmental Management: Safety Patient Rights Protection Presence Seizure Precautions Skin Surveillance Touch

Nursing Diagnosis: KNOWLEDGE DEFICIT (SPECIFY)

DEFINITION: Absence or deficiency of cognitive information related to a specific topic.

Outcome: KNOWLEDGE: BREASTFEEDING

MAJOR INTERVENTIONS	SUGGESTED INTERVENTIONS	OPTIONAL INTERVENTIONS

Breastfeeding Assistance
Lactation Counseling
	Childbirth Preparation
	Learning Facilitation
	Learning Readiness
	  Enhancement
	Teaching: Infant
	  Nutrition
		Health System Guidance
		Infant Care
		Lactation Suppression
		Nonnutritive Sucking
		Parent Education: Infant

Outcome: KNOWLEDGE: CHILD SAFETY

MAJOR INTERVENTIONS	SUGGESTED INTERVENTIONS	OPTIONAL INTERVENTIONS

Teaching: Infant Safety
Teaching: Toddler Safety
	Health Education
	Learning Facilitation
	Learning Readiness
	  Enhancement
	Parent Education: Infant
	Risk Identification
	Surveillance: Safety
	Teaching: Individual
		Counseling
		Family Support
		Health Screening
		Parenting Promotion
		Risk Identification:
		  Childbearing Family
		Teaching: Group
		Vehicle Safety Promotion

Outcome: KNOWLEDGE: CONCEPTION PREVENTION

MAJOR INTERVENTIONS	SUGGESTED INTERVENTIONS	OPTIONAL INTERVENTIONS

Family Planning:
  Contraception
Teaching: Safe Sex
	Health Education
	Parent Education:
	  Adolescent
	Parenting Promotion
	Learning Facilitation
	Learning Readiness
	  Enhancement
	Self-Responsibility
	  Facilitation
	Teaching: Individual
		Behavior Management:
		  Sexual
		Behavior Modification
		Family Planning:
		  Unplanned Pregnancy
		Impulse Control Training
		Pregnancy Termination
		  Care

Continued

Outcome: KNOWLEDGE: DIABETES MANAGEMENT

MAJOR INTERVENTIONS	SUGGESTED INTERVENTIONS	OPTIONAL INTERVENTIONS
Teaching: Disease Process Teaching: Prescribed Diet Teaching: Prescribed Medication	Hyperglycemia Management Hypoglycemia Management Medication Administration: Subcutaneous Teaching: Prescribed Activity/Exercise Teaching: Psychomotor Skill	Behavior Modification Health Education Medication Management Nutrition Management Referral

Outcome: KNOWLEDGE: DIET

MAJOR INTERVENTIONS	SUGGESTED INTERVENTIONS	OPTIONAL INTERVENTIONS
Teaching: Prescribed Diet Teaching: Infant Nutrition Teaching: Toddler Nutrition	Breastfeeding Assistance Health Education Lactation Counseling Learning Facilitation Learning Readiness Enhancement Nutritional Counseling Preconception Counseling Teaching: Individual	Behavior Management Chemotherapy Management Eating Disorders Management Nutrition Management Nutritional Monitoring Patient Contracting Prenatal Care Self-Modification Assistance Teaching: Group Weight Management

Outcome: KNOWLEDGE: DISEASE PROCESS

MAJOR INTERVENTIONS	SUGGESTED INTERVENTIONS	OPTIONAL INTERVENTIONS
Teaching: Disease Process	Health System Guidance Learning Facilitation Learning Readiness Enhancement Teaching: Individual	Admission Care Allergy Management Anxiety Reduction Discharge Planning Risk Identification Teaching: Group Truth Telling

Outcome: KNOWLEDGE: ENERGY CONSERVATION

MAJOR INTERVENTIONS	SUGGESTED INTERVENTIONS	OPTIONAL INTERVENTIONS
Teaching: Prescribed Activity/Exercise	Health Education Learning Facilitation Learning Readiness Enhancement Teaching: Disease Process Teaching: Individual	Body Mechanics Promotion Energy Management Exercise Promotion Progressive Muscle Relaxation Recreation Therapy Simple Relaxation Therapy Teaching: Group

Outcome: KNOWLEDGE: FERTILITY PROMOTION

MAJOR INTERVENTIONS	SUGGESTED INTERVENTIONS	OPTIONAL INTERVENTIONS
Family Planning: Infertility Fertility Preservation Reproductive Technology Management	Patients Rights Protection Preconception Counseling Teaching: Procedure/ Treatment	Counseling Decision-Making Support Genetic Counseling Specimen Management

Outcome: KNOWLEDGE: HEALTH BEHAVIORS

MAJOR INTERVENTIONS	SUGGESTED INTERVENTIONS	OPTIONAL INTERVENTIONS
Health Education	Active Listening Anticipatory Guidance Breast Examination Health System Guidance Learning Facilitation Learning Readiness Enhancement Parent Education: Adolescent Parent Education: Childrearing Family Parent Education: Infant Self-Awareness Enhancement Teaching: Group Teaching: Individual Teaching: Safe Sex Values Clarification	Behavior Modification Genetic Counseling Health Screening Infection Protection Oral Health Promotion Preconception Counseling Risk Identification Substance Use Prevention

Continued

Outcome: Knowledge: Health Resources

MAJOR INTERVENTIONS	SUGGESTED INTERVENTIONS	OPTIONAL INTERVENTIONS
Health System Guidance	Discharge Planning Health Education Learning Facilitation Learning Readiness Enhancement Support System Enhancement Teaching: Individual	Health Care Information Exchange Teaching: Group Telephone Consultation

Outcome: Knowledge: Illness Care

MAJOR INTERVENTIONS	SUGGESTED INTERVENTIONS	OPTIONAL INTERVENTIONS
Teaching: Individual Teaching: Procedure/Treatment	Teaching: Disease Process Teaching: Prescribed Activity/Exercise Teaching: Prescribed Diet Teaching: Prescribed Medication	Energy Management Health System Guidance Infection Control

Outcome: Knowledge: Infant Care

MAJOR INTERVENTIONS	SUGGESTED INTERVENTIONS	OPTIONAL INTERVENTIONS
Parent Education: Infant	Breastfeeding Assistance Lactation Counseling Teaching: Individual Teaching: Infant Nutrition Teaching: Infant Safety	Newborn Care Parenting Promotion

Outcome: KNOWLEDGE: INFECTION CONTROL

MAJOR INTERVENTIONS	SUGGESTED INTERVENTIONS	OPTIONAL INTERVENTIONS

Infection Protection
Risk Identification
Teaching: Safe Sex
	Health Education
	Incision Site Care
	Infection Control
	Learning Facilitation
	Learning Readiness
	  Enhancement
	Teaching: Disease
	  Process
	Teaching: Individual
	Teaching: Procedure/
	  Treatment
	Teaching: Psychomotor
	  Skill
		Home Maintenance
		  Assistance
		Immunization/
		  Vaccination
		  Management
		Medication Management
		Teaching: Group
		Teaching: Preoperative
		Teaching: Prescribed
		  Medication
		Urinary Elimination
		  Management
		Wound Care

Outcome: KNOWLEDGE: LABOR & DELIVERY

MAJOR INTERVENTIONS	SUGGESTED INTERVENTIONS	OPTIONAL INTERVENTIONS
Childbirth Preparation	Anticipatory Guidance Teaching: Individual	Intrapartal Care Labor Induction Labor Suppression Teaching: Group

Outcome: KNOWLEDGE: MATERNAL-CHILD HEALTH

MAJOR INTERVENTIONS	SUGGESTED INTERVENTIONS	OPTIONAL INTERVENTIONS

Health Education
Teaching: Individual
	Childbirth Preparation
	Genetic Counseling
	Lactation Counseling
	Parent Education: Infant
	Reproductive
	  Technology
	  Management
	Teaching: Infant Safety
	Teaching: Prescribed
	  Activity/Exercise
	Teaching:
	  Prescribed Diet
	Teaching: Safe Sex
	Teaching: Sexuality
		Energy Management
		Fertility Preservation
		Health System Guidance
		Nutrition Management
		Parenting Promotion
		Sexual Counseling
		Substance Use
		  Prevention
		Teaching: Toddler Safety
		Weight Management

Continued

Outcome: KNOWLEDGE: MEDICATION

MAJOR INTERVENTIONS	SUGGESTED INTERVENTIONS	OPTIONAL INTERVENTIONS
Teaching: Prescribed Medication	Allergy Management Analgesic Administration Chemotherapy Management Hyperglycemia Management Hypoglycemia Management Immunization/ Vaccination Management Learning Facilitation Learning Readiness Enhancement Medication Management Patient-Controlled Analgesia (PCA) Assistance Teaching: Individual	Constipation/Impaction Management Pain Management Preconception Counseling Prenatal Care Teaching: Disease Process Teaching: Group

Outcome: KNOWLEDGE: PERSONAL SAFETY

MAJOR INTERVENTIONS	SUGGESTED INTERVENTIONS	OPTIONAL INTERVENTIONS
Health Education Teaching: Infant Safety Teaching: Toddler Safety	Counseling Learning Facilitation Learning Readiness Enhancement Patient Rights Protection Risk Identification Teaching: Individual	Abuse Protection Support Abuse Protection Support: Child Abuse Protection Support: Domestic Partner Abuse Protection Support: Elder Fall Prevention Infection Protection Substance Use Prevention Teaching: Psychomotor Skill Vehicle Safety Promotion

Outcome: KNOWLEDGE: POSTPARTUM

MAJOR INTERVENTIONS	SUGGESTED INTERVENTIONS	OPTIONAL INTERVENTIONS

Lactation Counseling
Teaching: Prescribed
  Activity/Exercise
	Health Education
	Learning Facilitation
	Learning Readiness
	  Enhancement
	Nutritional Counseling
	Teaching: Individual
	Weight Reduction
	  Assistance
		Cesarean Section Care
		Health System Guidance
		Postpartal Care

Outcome: KNOWLEDGE: PRECONCEPTION

MAJOR INTERVENTIONS	SUGGESTED INTERVENTIONS	OPTIONAL INTERVENTIONS

Health Education
Preconception
  Counseling
	Counseling
	Genetic Counseling
	Learning Facilitation
	Learning Readiness
	  Enhancement
	Teaching: Individual
		Behavior Modification
		Sexual Counseling
		Substance Use
		  Prevention

Outcome: KNOWLEDGE: PREGNANCY

MAJOR INTERVENTIONS	SUGGESTED INTERVENTIONS	OPTIONAL INTERVENTIONS

Childbirth Preparation	Anticipatory Guidance
	Health Education
	Learning Facilitation
	Learning Readiness
	  Enhancement
	Prenatal Care
	Teaching: Individual
	Teaching: Prescribed
	  Medication
		Health System Guidance
		High-Risk
		  Pregnancy Care

Continued

Outcome: KNOWLEDGE: PRESCRIBED ACTIVITY

MAJOR INTERVENTIONS	SUGGESTED INTERVENTIONS	OPTIONAL INTERVENTIONS
Teaching: Prescribed Activity/Exercise	Energy Management Exercise Promotion Learning Facilitation Learning Readiness Enhancement Patient Contracting Teaching: Individual	Activity Therapy Behavior Modification Recreation Therapy Self-Modification Assistance Teaching: Group Therapeutic Play

Outcome: KNOWLEDGE: SEXUAL FUNCTIONING

MAJOR INTERVENTIONS	SUGGESTED INTERVENTIONS	OPTIONAL INTERVENTIONS
Teaching: Safe Sex Teaching: Sexuality	Behavior Management: Sexual Family Planning: Contraception Learning Facilitation Learning Readiness Enhancement Sexual Counseling Teaching: Individual	Genetic Counseling Patient Rights Protection Self-Awareness Enhancement

Outcome: Knowledge: Substance Use Control

MAJOR INTERVENTIONS	SUGGESTED INTERVENTIONS	OPTIONAL INTERVENTIONS
Substance Use Prevention	Behavior Management Health Education Learning Facilitation Learning Readiness Enhancement Medication Management Teaching: Group Teaching: Individual Teaching: Prescribed Medication	Analgesic Administration Controlled Substance Checking Health Screening Health System Guidance Mutual Goal Setting Nutritional Counseling Patient Contracting Preconception Counseling Smoking Cessation Assistance Substance Use Treatment Substance Use Treatment: Alcohol Withdrawal Substance Use Treatment: Drug Withdrawal

Outcome: Knowledge: Treatment Procedure(s)

MAJOR INTERVENTIONS	SUGGESTED INTERVENTIONS	OPTIONAL INTERVENTIONS
Preparatory Sensory Information Teaching: Procedure/Treatment Teaching: Psychomotor Skill	Anticipatory Guidance Learning Facilitation Learning Readiness Enhancement Parent Education: Adolescent Parent Education: Childrearing Family Parent Education: Infant Patients Rights Protection Presence Teaching: Disease Process Teaching: Individual	Anxiety Reduction Culture Brokerage Decision-Making Support Examination Assistance

Continued

Outcome: KNOWLEDGE: TREATMENT REGIMEN

MAJOR INTERVENTIONS	SUGGESTED INTERVENTIONS	OPTIONAL INTERVENTIONS
Teaching: Preoperative Teaching: Procedure/ Treatment	Anticipatory Guidance Chemotherapy Management Learning Facilitation Learning Readiness Enhancement Medication Management Nutrition Management Parent Education: Adolescent Parent Education: Childrearing Family Parent Education: Infant Radiation Therapy Management Teaching: Disease Process Teaching: Individual Teaching: Prescribed Activity/Exercise Teaching: Prescribed Diet Teaching: Prescribed Medication	Health System Guidance Labor Induction Prenatal Care Teaching: Group Weight Gain Assistance Weight Management Weight Reduction Assistance

Nursing Diagnosis: LATEX ALLERGY RESPONSE.

DEFINITION: An allergic response to natural latex rubber products.

Outcome: IMMUNE HYPERSENSITIVITY CONTROL

MAJOR INTERVENTIONS	SUGGESTED INTERVENTIONS	OPTIONAL INTERVENTIONS
Allergy Management Latex Precautions	Emergency Care Environmental Management Environmental Risk Protection Medication Administration Medication Administration: Skin Medication Management Respiratory Monitoring Risk Identification Surveillance Teaching: Individual Vital Signs Monitoring	Anaphylaxis Management Code Management Fluid Management Intravenous (IV) Insertion Intravenous (IV) Therapy Shock Prevention Skin Surveillance

Outcome: TISSUE INTEGRITY: SKIN & MUCOUS MEMBRANES

MAJOR INTERVENTIONS	SUGGESTED INTERVENTIONS	OPTIONAL INTERVENTIONS
Allergy Management Latex Precautions	Environmental Risk Protection Medication Administration Medication Administration: Skin Medication Management Skin Care: Topical Treatments Skin Surveillance Teaching: Individual	Fluid Management Pruritus Management Wound Care

Nursing Diagnosis: MEMORY, IMPAIRED

DEFINITION: The state in which an individual experiences the inability to remember or recall bits of information or behavioral skills. Impaired memory may be attributed to pathophysiological or situational causes that are either temporary or permanent.

Outcome: COGNITIVE ORIENTATION

MAJOR INTERVENTIONS	SUGGESTED INTERVENTIONS	OPTIONAL INTERVENTIONS
Reality Orientation	Cognitive Stimulation Delirium Management Dementia Management Environmental Management Environmental Management: Safety Medication Management Memory Training Surveillance: Safety	Animal-Assisted Therapy Area Restriction Calming Technique Milieu Therapy Neurologic Monitoring Patient Rights Protection Reminiscence Therapy Substance Use Treatment Surveillance Visitation Facilitation

Outcome: MEMORY

MAJOR INTERVENTIONS	SUGGESTED INTERVENTIONS	OPTIONAL INTERVENTIONS
Memory Training	Active Listening Anxiety Reduction Cognitive Stimulation Learning Facilitation Milieu Therapy Reminiscence Therapy	Coping Enhancement Emotional Support Family Support Medication Management Patient Rights Protection Reality Orientation

Outcome: NEUROLOGICAL STATUS

MAJOR INTERVENTIONS	SUGGESTED INTERVENTIONS	OPTIONAL INTERVENTIONS
Cerebral Perfusion Promotion Neurologic Monitoring	Electrolyte Management Electrolyte Monitoring Fluid Management Fluid Monitoring Fluid/Electrolyte Management Medication Administration Medication Management Reality Orientation Substance Use Treatment Surveillance	Oxygen Therapy Respiratory Monitoring

Nursing Diagnosis: MOBILITY, IMPAIRED BED

DEFINITION: Limitation of independent movement from one bed position to another.

Outcome: BODY POSITIONING: SELF-INITIATED

MAJOR INTERVENTIONS	SUGGESTED INTERVENTIONS	OPTIONAL INTERVENTIONS
Exercise Promotion: Strength Training Self-Care Assistance	Body Mechanics Promotion Exercise Promotion: Stretching Exercise Therapy: Joint Mobility Exercise Therapy: Muscle Control Positioning Teaching: Prescribed Activity/Exercise	Energy Management Fall Prevention Positioning: Neurologic Traction/Immobilization Care

Outcome: IMMOBILITY CONSEQUENCES: PHYSIOLOGICAL

MAJOR INTERVENTIONS	SUGGESTED INTERVENTIONS	OPTIONAL INTERVENTIONS
Bed Rest Care Positioning	Exercise Promotion Exercise Promotion: Strength Training Exercise Promotion: Stretching Exercise Therapy: Joint Mobility Exercise Therapy: Muscle Control	Pressure Management Simple Massage Teaching: Prescribed Activity/Exercise

Outcome: JOINT MOVEMENT: ACTIVE

MAJOR INTERVENTIONS	SUGGESTED INTERVENTIONS	OPTIONAL INTERVENTIONS
Exercise Therapy: Joint Mobility	Exercise Promotion: Strength Training Exercise Promotion: Stretching Exercise Therapy: Muscle Control Teaching: Prescribed Activity/Exercise	Body Mechanics Promotion Heat/Cold Application Pain Management

Outcome: MOBILITY LEVEL

MAJOR INTERVENTIONS	SUGGESTED INTERVENTIONS	OPTIONAL INTERVENTIONS

Bed Rest Care
Exercise Promotion:
  Strength Training
	Body Mechanics
	  Promotion
	Exercise Therapy: Joint
	  Mobility
	Exercise Therapy:
	  Muscle Control
	Teaching: Prescribed
	  Activity/Exercise
		Exercise Promotion
		Exercise Promotion:
		  Stretching
		Medication Management
		Pain Management
		Positioning
		Self-Care Assistance
		Self-Care Assistance:
		  Bathing/Hygiene
		Self-Care Assistance:
		  Dressing/Grooming
		Self-Care Assistance:
		  Toileting

Outcome: MUSCLE FUNCTION

MAJOR INTERVENTIONS	SUGGESTED INTERVENTIONS	OPTIONAL INTERVENTIONS

Exercise Promotion:
  Strength Training
	Body Mechanics
	  Promotion
	Exercise Promotion:
	  Stretching
	Exercise Therapy:
	  Joint Mobility
	Exercise Therapy:
	  Muscle Control
	Progressive Muscle
	  Relaxation
		Exercise Promotion
		Pain Management
		Simple Massage
		Simple Relaxation
		  Therapy
		Sleep Enhancement
		Teaching: Prescribed
		  Activity/Exercise

Nursing Diagnosis: NAUSEA

DEFINITION: An unpleasant, wave-like sensation in the back of the throat, epigastrium, or throughout the abdomen, that may or may not lead to vomiting.

Outcome: COMFORT LEVEL

MAJOR INTERVENTIONS	SUGGESTED INTERVENTIONS	OPTIONAL INTERVENTIONS
Medication Management Nausea Management	Calming Technique Environmental Management: Comfort Medication Administration Medication Prescribing Pain Management Simple Relaxation Therapy	Acupressure Aspiration Precautions Vomiting Management

Outcome: HYDRATION

MAJOR INTERVENTIONS	SUGGESTED INTERVENTIONS	OPTIONAL INTERVENTIONS
Fluid/Electrolyte Management	Electrolyte Management Electrolyte Monitoring Fluid Management Fluid Monitoring Fluid Resuscitation Intravenous (IV) Insertion Intravenous (IV) Therapy Vomiting Management	Temperature Regulation Venous Access Devices (VAD) Maintenance

Outcome: NUTRITIONAL STATUS: FOOD & FLUID INTAKE

MAJOR INTERVENTIONS	SUGGESTED INTERVENTIONS	OPTIONAL INTERVENTIONS
Fluid Monitoring	Diet Staging Nausea Management Nutritional Monitoring Vomiting Management	Intravenous (IV) Insertion Intravenous (IV) Therapy

Outcome: SYMPTOM SEVERITY

MAJOR INTERVENTIONS	SUGGESTED INTERVENTIONS	OPTIONAL INTERVENTIONS

Nausea Management
Vomiting Management
	Anxiety Reduction
	Calming Technique
	Distraction
	Medication
	  Administration
	Medication Management
	Pain Management
		Acupressure
		Flatulence Reduction
		Simple Relaxation
		  Therapy
		Temperature Regulation

Nursing Diagnosis: **NONCOMPLIANCE (SPECIFY)**

DEFINITION: The extent to which a person's and/or caregiver's behavior coincides or fails to coincide with a health-promoting or therapeutic plan agreed upon by the person (and/or family, and/or community) and health care professional. In the presence of an agreed-upon, health-promoting or therapeutic plan, person's or caregiver's behavior is fully or partially nonadherent and may lead to clinically effective, partially effective, or ineffective outcomes.

Outcome: **ADHERENCE BEHAVIOR**

MAJOR INTERVENTIONS	SUGGESTED INTERVENTIONS	OPTIONAL INTERVENTIONS
Health Education	Behavior Modification	Risk Identification
Self-Modification Assistance	Coping Enhancement	Teaching: Individual
Self-Responsibility Facilitation	Counseling	Truth Telling
	Decision-Making Support	
	Family Support	
	Health System Guidance	
	Mutual Goal Setting	
	Support System Enhancement	
	Telephone Consultation	
	Values Clarification	

Outcome: COMPLIANCE BEHAVIOR

MAJOR INTERVENTIONS	SUGGESTED INTERVENTIONS	OPTIONAL INTERVENTIONS

Health System Guidance
Mutual Goal Setting
Patient Contracting
Self-Modification
  Assistance
	Behavior Modification
	Counseling
	Culture Brokerage
	Decision-Making
	  Support
	Elopement Precautions
	Financial Resource
	  Assistance
	Learning Facilitation
	Learning Readiness
	  Enhancement
	Patient Rights Protection
	Self-Responsibility
	  Facilitation
	Support System
	  Enhancement
	Teaching: Disease
	  Process
	Teaching: Individual
	Teaching: Prescribed
	  Activity/Exercise
	Teaching:
	  Prescribed Diet
	Teaching: Prescribed
	  Medication
	Teaching: Procedure/
	  Treatment
	Teaching: Psychomotor
	  Skill
	Telephone Consultation
	Values Clarification
		Case Management
		Discharge Planning
		Family Involvement
		  Promotion
		Parent Education:
		  Adolescent
		Parent Education:
		  Childrearing Family
		Parent Education: Infant
		Smoking Cessation
		  Assistance
		Substance Use
		  Prevention
		Surveillance
		Teaching: Safe Sex
		Truth Telling

Continued

Outcome: SYMPTOM CONTROL

MAJOR INTERVENTIONS	SUGGESTED INTERVENTIONS	OPTIONAL INTERVENTIONS
Energy Management Nutrition Management Self-Modification Assistance Self-Responsibility Facilitation	Fever Treatment Health Education Health Screening Health System Guidance Learning Facilitation Learning Readiness Enhancement Nausea Management Pain Management Teaching: Disease Process Teaching: Individual Values Clarification	Coping Enhancement Counseling Emotional Support Family Involvement Promotion Medication Management Mutual Goal Setting Patient Contracting Teaching: Group Vomiting Management

Outcome: TREATMENT BEHAVIOR: ILLNESS OR INJURY		
MAJOR INTERVENTIONS	**SUGGESTED INTERVENTIONS**	**OPTIONAL INTERVENTIONS**
Self-Responsibility Facilitation Teaching: Disease Process Teaching: Individual	Behavior Modification Coping Enhancement Counseling Environmental Management Health Education Health System Guidance Learning Facilitation Learning Readiness Enhancement Mutual Goal Setting Patient Contracting Self-Modification Assistance Support System Enhancement Surveillance Teaching: Prescribed Activity/Exercise Teaching: Prescribed Diet Teaching: Prescribed Medication Teaching: Procedure/ Treatment Teaching: Psychomotor Skill Telephone Consultation Values Clarification	Home Maintenance Assistance Referral Self-Care Assistance Smoking Cessation Assistance Substance Use Treatment Support Group Weight Gain Assistance Weight Reduction Assistance

Nursing Diagnosis: NUTRITION, ALTERED: LESS THAN BODY REQUIREMENTS

Definition: The state in which an individual is experiencing an intake of nutrients insufficient to meet metabolic needs.

Outcome: NUTRITIONAL STATUS

MAJOR INTERVENTIONS	SUGGESTED INTERVENTIONS	OPTIONAL INTERVENTIONS
Diet Staging	Nutrition Therapy	Energy Management
Eating Disorders Management	Nutritional Counseling	Enteral Tube Feeding
Nutrition Management	Nutritional Monitoring	Fluid/Electrolyte Management
Weight Gain Assistance	Teaching: Prescribed Diet	Gastrointestinal Intubation
	Vital Signs Monitoring	Self-Care Assistance: Feeding
	Weight Management	Sustenance Support
		Total Parenteral Nutrition (TPN) Administration

Outcome: NUTRITIONAL STATUS: FOOD & FLUID INTAKE

MAJOR INTERVENTIONS	SUGGESTED INTERVENTIONS	OPTIONAL INTERVENTIONS
Fluid Monitoring	Enteral Tube Feeding	Bottle Feeding
Nutrition Monitoring	Feeding	Intravenous (IV) Therapy
	Fluid Management	Sustenance Support
	Lactation Counseling	Teaching: Prescribed Diet
	Nutrition Management	Weight Gain Assistance
	Nutrition Therapy	Weight Management
	Self-Care Assistance: Feeding	
	Swallowing Therapy	
	Total Parenteral Nutrition (TPN) Administration	

Outcome: NUTRITIONAL STATUS: NUTRIENT INTAKE

MAJOR INTERVENTIONS	SUGGESTED INTERVENTIONS	OPTIONAL INTERVENTIONS

Nutrition Management
Nutrition Monitoring
	Enteral Tube Feeding
	Medication Management
	Nutrition Therapy
	Nutritional Counseling
	Teaching:
	  Prescribed Diet
	Total Parenteral
	  Nutrition (TPN)
	  Administration
		Bottle Feeding
		Feeding
		Laboratory Data
		  Interpretation
		Lactation Counseling
		Self-Care Assistance:
		  Feeding
		Sustenance Support
		Swallowing Therapy
		Weight Gain Assistance
		Weight Management

Outcome: WEIGHT CONTROL

MAJOR INTERVENTIONS	SUGGESTED INTERVENTIONS	OPTIONAL INTERVENTIONS
Weight Gain Assistance Eating Disorders Management	Nutrition Management Nutrition Therapy Nutritional Counseling Nutritional Monitoring Weight Management	Behavior Modification Exercise Promotion Mutual Goal Setting Patient Contracting Teaching: Individual

Nursing Diagnosis: **Nutrition, Altered: More than Body Requirements**

Definition: The state in which an individual is experiencing an intake of nutrients that exceeds metabolic needs.

Outcome: **Nutritional Status**

MAJOR INTERVENTIONS	SUGGESTED INTERVENTIONS	OPTIONAL INTERVENTIONS

Nutrition Management
Weight Reduction
  Assistance
	Exercise Promotion
	Fluid Management
	Nutritional Counseling
	Nutritional Monitoring
	Weight Management
		Exercise Therapy:
		  Ambulation
		Fluid Management
		Lactation Counseling
		Teaching:
		  Prescribed Diet

Outcome: **Nutritional Status: Nutrient Intake**

MAJOR INTERVENTIONS	SUGGESTED INTERVENTIONS	OPTIONAL INTERVENTIONS

Nutrition Management
Nutritional Monitoring
	Nutritional Counseling
	Teaching:
	  Prescribed Diet
	Weight Management
	Weight Reduction
	  Assistance
		Bottle Feeding
		Enteral Tube Feeding
		Feeding
		Nutrition Therapy

Outcome: **Weight Control**

MAJOR INTERVENTIONS	SUGGESTED INTERVENTIONS	OPTIONAL INTERVENTIONS

Behavior Modification
Eating Disorders
  Management
Weight Reduction
  Assistance
	Behavior Management
	Mutual Goal Setting
	Nutrition Management
	Nutritional Counseling
	Nutritional Monitoring
	Patient Contracting
	Self-Responsibility
	  Facilitation
	Teaching:
	  Prescribed Diet
		Anxiety Reduction
		Coping Enhancement
		Limit Setting
		Referral

Nursing Diagnosis: ORAL MUCOUS MEMBRANE, ALTERED

DEFINITION: Disruptions of the lips and soft tissue of the oral cavity.

Outcome: ORAL HEALTH

MAJOR INTERVENTIONS	SUGGESTED INTERVENTIONS	OPTIONAL INTERVENTIONS
Oral Health Restoration	Chemotherapy Management Fluid/Electrolyte Management Fluid Management Nutrition Management Oral Health Maintenance	Airway Suctioning Artificial Airway Management Chemotherapy Management Dying Care Pain Management

Outcome: TISSUE INTEGRITY: SKIN & MUCOUS MEMBRANES

MAJOR INTERVENTIONS	SUGGESTED INTERVENTIONS	OPTIONAL INTERVENTIONS
Oral Health Restoration	Chemotherapy Management Infection Protection Medication Administration: Skin Medication Management Nutrition Management Oral Health Maintenance Radiation Therapy Management	Fluid Management Wound Care Wound Irrigation

Nursing Diagnosis: PAIN

DEFINITION: An unpleasant sensory and emotional experience arising from actual or potential tissue damage or described in terms of such damage (International Association for the Study of Pain); sudden or slow onset of any intensity from mild to severe with an anticipated or predictable end and a duration of less than 6 months.

Outcome: COMFORT LEVEL

MAJOR INTERVENTIONS	SUGGESTED INTERVENTIONS	OPTIONAL INTERVENTIONS
Medication Management Pain Management	Acupressure Analgesic Administration Biofeedback Conscious Sedation Coping Enhancement Emotional Support Environmental Management: Comfort Humor Medication Administration Medication Administration: Intramuscular Medication Administration: Intravenous Medication Administration: Oral Medication Prescribing Meditation Facilitation Patient-Controlled Analgesia (PCA) Assistance Positioning Presence Simple Guided Imagery Simple Massage Simple Relaxation Therapy Transcutaneous Electrical Nerve Stimulation (TENS)	Analgesic Administration: Intraspinal Animal-Assisted Therapy Anxiety Reduction Autogenic Training Bathing Bowel Management Calming Technique Cutaneous Stimulation Distraction Dying Care Exercise Promotion Heat/Cold Application Hope Instillation Hypnosis Lactation Suppression Music Therapy Oxygen Therapy Progressive Muscle Relaxation Security Enhancement Sleep Enhancement Splinting Therapeutic Touch

Outcome: PAIN CONTROL

MAJOR INTERVENTIONS	SUGGESTED INTERVENTIONS	OPTIONAL INTERVENTIONS
Medication Management Pain Management Patient-Controlled Analgesia (PCA) Assistance	Health Screening Medication Prescribing Mutual Goal Setting Patient Contracting Self-Modification Assistance Self-Responsibility Facilitation Teaching: Disease Process Teaching: Individual Teaching: Prescribed Medication Teaching: Procedure/ Treatment Telephone Consultation	Coping Enhancement Environmental Management: Comfort Family Support Rectal Prolapse Management Support System Enhancement Surveillance

Outcome: PAIN: DISRUPTIVE EFFECTS

MAJOR INTERVENTIONS	SUGGESTED INTERVENTIONS	OPTIONAL INTERVENTIONS
Analgesic Administration Patient-Controlled Analgesia (PCA) Assistance	Coping Enhancement Hope Instillation Medication Administration Medication Administration: Intramuscular Medication Administration: Intravenous Medication Administration: Oral Medication Management Medication Prescribing Mood Management Pain Management Simple Relaxation Therapy Sleep Enhancement	Acupressure Anxiety Reduction Autogenic Training Biofeedback Calming Technique Cutaneous Stimulation Distraction Emotional Support Energy Management Environmental Management Heat/Cold Application Hypnosis Meditation Facilitation Music Therapy Progressive Muscle Relaxation Simple Guided Imagery Simple Massage Therapeutic Touch Transcutaneous Electrical Nerve Stimulation (TENS)

Continued

Outcome: **PAIN LEVEL**

MAJOR INTERVENTIONS	SUGGESTED INTERVENTIONS	OPTIONAL INTERVENTIONS
Analgesic Administration Conscious Sedation Pain Management	Acupressure Anesthesia Administration Analgesic Administration: Intraspinal Cutaneous Stimulation Environmental Management: Comfort Flatulence Reduction Heat/Cold Application Medication Administration Medication Administration: Intramuscular Medication Administration: Intravenous Medication Administration: Oral Medication Management Medication Prescribing Positioning Simple Guided Imagery Splinting Surveillance Transcutaneous Electrical Nerve Stimulation (TENS)	Biofeedback Distraction Hypnosis Music Therapy Presence Progressive Muscle Relaxation Simple Massage Simple Relaxation Therapy Therapeutic Touch Touch Vital Signs Monitoring

Nursing Diagnosis: PAIN, CHRONIC

DEFINITION: An unpleasant sensory and emotional experience arising from actual or potential tissue damage or described in terms of such damage (International Association for the Study of Pain); sudden or slow onset of any intensity from mild to severe, constant or recurring without an anticipated or predictable end and a duration of greater than 6 months.

Outcome: COMFORT LEVEL

MAJOR INTERVENTIONS	SUGGESTED INTERVENTIONS	OPTIONAL INTERVENTIONS
Pain Management	Analgesic Administration	Acupressure
	Environmental Management: Comfort	Analgesic Administration: Intraspinal
	Medication Administration	Autogenic Training
	Medication Management	Biofeedback
	Medication Prescribing	Cutaneous Stimulation
	Positioning	Distraction
	Simple Massage	Dying Care
	Simple Relaxation Therapy	Heat/Cold Application
	Sleep Enhancement	Hypnosis
	Transcutaneous Electrical Nerve Stimulation (TENS)	Meditation Facilitation
		Progressive Muscle Relaxation
		Therapeutic Touch

Outcome: DEPRESSION CONTROL

MAJOR INTERVENTIONS	SUGGESTED INTERVENTIONS	OPTIONAL INTERVENTIONS
Mood Management	Analgesic Administration	Animal-Assisted Therapy
Pain Management	Behavior Management	Art Therapy
Patient Contracting	Behavior Management: Self-Harm	Hope Instillation
	Coping Enhancement	Humor
	Exercise Promotion	Spiritual Support
	Medication Management	
	Sleep Enhancement	
	Teaching: Prescribed Medication	

Continued

Outcome: DEPRESSION LEVEL

MAJOR INTERVENTIONS	SUGGESTED INTERVENTIONS	OPTIONAL INTERVENTIONS

Mood Management
Pain Management
	Analgesic
	  Administration
	Counseling
	Emotional Support
	Hope Instillation
	Medication
	  Administration
	Medication Management
	Sleep Enhancement
	Transcutaneous
	  Electrical Nerve
	  Stimulation (TENS)
		Animal-Assisted
		  Therapy
		Art Therapy
		Biofeedback
		Environmental
		  Management: Comfort
		Humor
		Music Therapy
		Presence
		Touch

Outcome: PAIN CONTROL

MAJOR INTERVENTIONS	SUGGESTED INTERVENTIONS	OPTIONAL INTERVENTIONS

Medication Management
Patient Contracting
	Behavior Modification
	Documentation
	Learning Facilitation
	Learning Readiness
	  Enhancement
	Mutual Goal Setting
	Pain Management
	Self-Modification
	  Assistance
	Self-Responsibility
	  Facilitation
	Teaching: Individual
	Teaching: Prescribed
	  Medication
	Teaching: Procedure/
	  Treatment
	Telephone Consultation
		Environmental
		  Management: Comfort
		Exercise Promotion:
		  Stretching
		Exercise Therapy:
		  Ambulation
		Exercise Therapy: Joint
		  Mobility
		Exercise Therapy:
		  Muscle Control
		Family Involvement
		  Promotion
		Support System
		  Enhancement
		Surveillance

Outcome: PAIN: DISRUPTIVE EFFECTS

MAJOR INTERVENTIONS	SUGGESTED INTERVENTIONS	OPTIONAL INTERVENTIONS
Behavior Modification Coping Enhancement	Analgesic Administration Hope Instillation Medication Administration Medication Management Medication Prescribing Mood Management Nutrition Management Pain Management Self-Care Assistance Simple Relaxation Therapy Sleep Enhancement	Acupressure Anxiety Reduction Autogenic Training Biofeedback Body Mechanics Promotion Cutaneous Stimulation Distraction Emotional Support Energy Management Environmental Management: Comfort Heat/Cold Application Hypnosis Meditation Facilitation Progressive Muscle Relaxation Role Enhancement Simple Guided Imagery Simple Massage Therapeutic Touch Transcutaneous Electrical Nerve Stimulation (TENS)

Continued

Outcome: PAIN LEVEL

MAJOR INTERVENTIONS	SUGGESTED INTERVENTIONS	OPTIONAL INTERVENTIONS

Pain Management	Acupressure
	Analgesic
	  Administration
	Cutaneous Stimulation
	Distraction
	Environmental
	  Management: Comfort
	Heat/Cold Application
	Medication
	  Administration
	Medication Management
	Medication Prescribing
	Positioning
	Presence
	Simple Guided Imagery
	Simple Massage
	Splinting
	Surveillance
	Touch
	Transcutaneous
	  Electrical Nerve
	  Stimulation (TENS)
	Vital Signs Monitoring
		Biofeedback
		Hypnosis
		Progressive Muscle
		  Relaxation
		Simple Relaxation
		  Therapy
		Therapeutic Touch

Outcome: PAIN: PSYCHOLOGICAL RESPONSE

MAJOR INTERVENTIONS	SUGGESTED INTERVENTIONS	OPTIONAL INTERVENTIONS

Cognitive Restructuring
Mood Management
	Analgesic
	  Administration
	Behavior Management
	Coping Enhancement
	Emotional Support
	Hope Instillation
	Medication
	  Administration
	Sleep Enhancement
	Spiritual Support
	Transcutaneous
	  Electrical Nerve
	  Stimulation (TENS)
		Active Listening
		Animal-Assisted
		  Therapy
		Art Therapy
		Humor
		Music Therapy
		Presence
		Simple Guided Imagery
		Touch

Nursing Diagnosis: PARENTAL ROLE CONFLICT

DEFINITION: The state in which a parent experiences role confusion and conflict in response to crisis.

Outcome: CAREGIVER ADAPTATION TO PATIENT INSTITUTIONALIZATION

MAJOR INTERVENTIONS	SUGGESTED INTERVENTIONS	OPTIONAL INTERVENTIONS

Caregiver Support
Role Enhancement
	Active Listening
	Anticipatory Guidance
	Anxiety Reduction
	Coping Enhancement
	Decision-Making
	  Support
	Emotional Support
	Family Integrity
	  Promotion
	Family Integrity
	  Promotion:
	    Childbearing Family
	Family Process
	  Maintenance
	Family Support
	Guilt Work Facilitation
	Health System Guidance
	Support System
	  Enhancement
		Counseling
		Culture Brokerage
		Family Therapy
		Support Group
		Values Clarification
		Visitation Facilitation

Outcome: CAREGIVER HOME CARE READINESS

MAJOR INTERVENTIONS	SUGGESTED INTERVENTIONS	OPTIONAL INTERVENTIONS

Caregiver Support
Family Involvement
  Promotion
Role Enhancement
	Anticipatory Guidance
	Anxiety Reduction
	Childbirth Preparation
	Coping Enhancement
	Decision-Making
	  Support
	Discharge Planning
	Family Mobilization
	Family Process
	  Maintenance
	Family Support
	Mutual Goal Setting
	Normalization
	  Promotion
		Health System Guidance
		Home Maintenance
		  Assistance
		Respite Care
		Risk Identification
		Security Enhancement
		Support System
		  Enhancement
		Teaching: Individual

Continued

Outcome: COPING

MAJOR INTERVENTIONS	SUGGESTED INTERVENTIONS	OPTIONAL INTERVENTIONS

Coping Enhancement
Counseling
Crisis Intervention
	Anxiety Reduction
	Caregiver Support
	Decision-Making
	  Support
	Emotional Support
	Family Support
	Family Therapy
	Grief Work Facilitation:
	  Perinatal Death
	Respite Care
	Self-Esteem
	  Enhancement
	Socialization
	  Enhancement
	Spiritual Support
	Support Group
	Values Clarification
		Limit Setting
		Normalization
		  Promotion
		Parent Education:
		  Adolescent
		Parent Education:
		  Childrearing Family
		Parent Education: Infant
		Parenting Promotion
		Sibling Support
		Support System
		  Enhancement
		Therapy Group

Outcome: FAMILY ENVIRONMENT: INTERNAL

MAJOR INTERVENTIONS	SUGGESTED INTERVENTIONS	OPTIONAL INTERVENTIONS

Family Process
  Maintenance
Parenting Promotion
	Counseling
	Family Integrity
	  Promotion
	Family Integrity
	  Promotion:
	  Childbearing Family
	Socialization
	  Enhancement
		Abuse Protection
		  Support: Child
		Caregiver Support
		Family Therapy
		Support System
		  Enhancement

Outcome: FAMILY FUNCTIONING

MAJOR INTERVENTIONS	SUGGESTED INTERVENTIONS	OPTIONAL INTERVENTIONS
Crisis Intervention Family Process Maintenance	Counseling Decision-Making Support Family Integrity Promotion Family Integrity Promotion: Childbearing Family Family Support Family Therapy Parenting Promotion	Abuse Protection Support: Child Consultation Socialization Enhancement

Outcome: PARENTING

MAJOR INTERVENTIONS	SUGGESTED INTERVENTIONS	OPTIONAL INTERVENTIONS
Crisis Intervention Family Process Maintenance Parenting Promotion	Abuse Protection Support: Child Coping Enhancement Counseling Environmental Management: Attachment Process Family Integrity Promotion: Childbearing Family Family Support Normalization Promotion Role Enhancement Sibling Support Support System Enhancement	Breastfeeding Assistance Emotional Support Family Integrity Promotion Family Therapy Health System Guidance High-Risk Pregnancy Care Home Maintenance Assistance Self-Esteem Enhancement Socialization Enhancement Support Group

Continued

Outcome: ROLE PERFORMANCE

MAJOR INTERVENTIONS	SUGGESTED INTERVENTIONS	OPTIONAL INTERVENTIONS

Role Enhancement	Behavior Modification
	Caregiver Support
	Counseling
	Emotional Support
	Self-Awareness
	  Enhancement
	Values Clarification
		Attachment Promotion
		Childbirth Preparation
		Decision-Making
		  Support
		Family Integrity
		  Promotion
		Family Therapy
		Self-Esteem
		  Enhancement
		Support Group
		Support System
		  Enhancement

Nursing Diagnosis: PARENTING, ALTERED

DEFINITION: Inability of the primary caretaker to create an environment that promotes the optimum growth and development of the child.

Outcome: CHILD DEVELOPMENT: 2 MONTHS

MAJOR INTERVENTIONS	SUGGESTED INTERVENTIONS	OPTIONAL INTERVENTIONS
Family Integrity Promotion: Childbearing Family Parent Education: Infant Parenting Promotion	Anticipatory Guidance Attachment Promotion Bottle Feeding Breastfeeding Assistance Family Involvement Promotion Family Process Maintenance Family Support Infant Care Lactation Counseling Parent Education: Infant Role Enhancement Teaching: Infant Nutrition Teaching: Infant Safety	Abuse Protection Support: Child Behavior Modification Caregiver Support Environmental Management: Attachment Process Health System Guidance Newborn Care Respite Care Sibling Support Support System Enhancement Surveillance

Outcome: CHILD DEVELOPMENT: 4 MONTHS

MAJOR INTERVENTIONS	SUGGESTED INTERVENTIONS	OPTIONAL INTERVENTIONS
Family Integrity Promotion: Childbearing Family Parent Education: Infant Parenting Promotion	Anticipatory Guidance Bottle Feeding Family Involvement Promotion Family Process Maintenance Family Support Infant Care Lactation Counseling Parent Education: Infant Role Enhancement Security Enhancement Teaching: Infant Nutrition Teaching: Infant Safety	Abuse Protection Support: Child Attachment Promotion Behavior Modification Caregiver Support Environmental Management: Safety Family Mobilization Health System Guidance Respite Care Sibling Support Support System Enhancement Surveillance Sustenance Support

Continued

Outcome: CHILD DEVELOPMENT: 6 MONTHS

MAJOR INTERVENTIONS	SUGGESTED INTERVENTIONS	OPTIONAL INTERVENTIONS
Parent Education: Infant Parenting Promotion	Anticipatory Guidance Bottle Feeding Family Integrity Promotion: Childbearing Family Family Involvement Promotion Family Process Maintenance Family Support Infant Care Lactation Counseling Role Enhancement Security Enhancement Teaching: Infant Nutrition Teaching: Infant Safety	Abuse Protection Support: Child Attachment Promotion Caregiver Support Environmental Management: Safety Health System Guidance Respite Care Sibling Support Support System Enhancement Surveillance Sustenance Support

Outcome: CHILD DEVELOPMENT: 12 MONTHS

MAJOR INTERVENTIONS	SUGGESTED INTERVENTIONS	OPTIONAL INTERVENTIONS
Parenting Promotion	Anticipatory Guidance Bottle Feeding Developmental Enhancement: Child Family Integrity Promotion: Childbearing Family Family Involvement Promotion Family Process Maintenance Family Support Infant Care Lactation Counseling Parent Education: Childrearing Family Parent Education: Infant Role Enhancement Security Enhancement Socialization Enhancement Teaching: Toddler Nutrition Teaching: Toddler Safety	Abuse Protection Support: Child Attachment Promotion Caregiver Support Environmental Management: Safety Health System Guidance Nutrition Management Respite Care Sibling Support Support System Enhancement Surveillance Sustenance Support Therapeutic Play

Outcome: CHILD DEVELOPMENT: 2 YEARS

MAJOR INTERVENTIONS	SUGGESTED INTERVENTIONS	OPTIONAL INTERVENTIONS
Developmental Enhancement: Child Environmental Management: Safety Parenting Promotion	Anticipatory Guidance Family Integrity Promotion Family Involvement Promotion Parent Education: Childrearing Family Role Enhancement Security Enhancement Socialization Enhancement Teaching: Toddler Nutrition Teaching: Toddler Safety	Abuse Protection Support: Child Bowel Training Counseling Family Process Maintenance Family Support Family Therapy Health System Guidance Sibling Support Support System Enhancement Surveillance Sustenance Support Urinary Habit Training

Continued

Outcome: CHILD DEVELOPMENT: 3 YEARS

MAJOR INTERVENTIONS	SUGGESTED INTERVENTIONS	OPTIONAL INTERVENTIONS
Developmental Enhancement: Child Environmental Management: Safety Parenting Promotion	Anticipatory Guidance Bowel Management Bowel Training Family Integrity Promotion Family Involvement Promotion Parent Education: Childrearing Family Role Enhancement Security Enhancement Socialization Enhancement Support System Enhancement Urinary Habit Training	Abuse Protection Support: Child Behavior Management: Overactivity/ Inattention Counseling Family Process Maintenance Family Support Family Therapy Health System Guidance Sibling Support Sleep Enhancement Surveillance Sustenance Support Urinary Incontinence Care: Enuresis

Outcome: CHILD DEVELOPMENT: 4 YEARS

MAJOR INTERVENTIONS	SUGGESTED INTERVENTIONS	OPTIONAL INTERVENTIONS
Developmental Enhancement: Child Parenting Promotion	Anticipatory Guidance Environmental Management: Safety Family Integrity Promotion Family Involvement Promotion Parent Education: Childrearing Family Security Enhancement Socialization Enhancement Support System Enhancement	Abuse Protection Support: Child Behavior Management: Overactivity/ Inattention Counseling Family Process Maintenance Family Support Family Therapy Health System Guidance Sibling Support Sustenance Support Urinary Habit Training Urinary Incontinence Care: Enuresis

Outcome: CHILD DEVELOPMENT: 5 YEARS

MAJOR INTERVENTIONS	SUGGESTED INTERVENTIONS	OPTIONAL INTERVENTIONS
Developmental Enhancement: Child Parent Education: Childrearing Family Parenting Promotion	Anticipatory Guidance Environmental Management: Safety Family Integrity Promotion Family Involvement Promotion Security Enhancement Socialization Enhancement Support System Enhancement	Abuse Protection Support: Child Behavior Management: Overactivity/ Inattention Counseling Family Process Maintenance Family Support Family Therapy Health System Guidance Sibling Support Sustenance Support Urinary Incontinence Care: Enuresis

Outcome: CHILD DEVELOPMENT: MIDDLE CHILDHOOD (6-11 YEARS)

MAJOR INTERVENTIONS	SUGGESTED INTERVENTIONS	OPTIONAL INTERVENTIONS
Developmental Enhancement: Child Parent Education: Childrearing Family Parenting Promotion	Anticipatory Guidance Family Integrity Promotion Family Involvement Promotion Mutual Goal Setting Spiritual Support Substance Use Prevention Teaching: Individual Values Clarification	Abuse Protection Support: Child Counseling Family Process Maintenance Family Support Family Therapy Health System Guidance Sibling Support Sports-Injury Prevention: Youth Sustenance Support

Continued

Outcome: CHILD DEVELOPMENT: ADOLESCENCE (12-17 YEARS)

MAJOR INTERVENTIONS	SUGGESTED INTERVENTIONS	OPTIONAL INTERVENTIONS
Developmental Enhancement: Adolescent Parenting Promotion	Anticipatory Guidance Family Integrity Promotion Family Involvement Promotion Health System Guidance Mutual Goal Setting Parent Education: Adolescent Role Enhancement Spiritual Support Substance Use Prevention Teaching: Individual Values Clarification	Abuse Protection Support Counseling Family Process Maintenance Family Support Family Therapy Sibling Support Sports-Injury Prevention: Youth Support System Enhancement Sustenance Support

Outcome: FAMILY COPING

MAJOR INTERVENTIONS	SUGGESTED INTERVENTIONS	OPTIONAL INTERVENTIONS
Coping Enhancement Family Process Maintenance Family Support	Caregiver Support Counseling Family Integrity Promotion Family Therapy Grief Work Facilitation Normalization Promotion Parenting Promotion	Abuse Protection Support: Child Family Involvement Promotion Financial Resource Assistance Guilt Work Facilitation Home Maintenance Assistance Respite Care

Outcome: FAMILY ENVIRONMENT: INTERNAL

MAJOR INTERVENTIONS	SUGGESTED INTERVENTIONS	OPTIONAL INTERVENTIONS
Family Integrity Promotion Family Integrity Promotion: Childbearing Family	Abuse Protection Support: Child Attachment Promotion Family Process Maintenance Family Support Parenting Promotion	Coping Enhancement Family Therapy Resiliency Promotion

Outcome: FAMILY FUNCTIONING

MAJOR INTERVENTIONS	SUGGESTED INTERVENTIONS	OPTIONAL INTERVENTIONS
Developmental Enhancement: Adolescent Developmental Enhancement: Child Family Process Maintenance	Family Integrity Promotion Family Support Family Therapy Parent Education: Childrearing Family Parenting Promotion	Childbirth Preparation Sibling Support

Outcome: PARENT-INFANT ATTACHMENT

MAJOR INTERVENTIONS	SUGGESTED INTERVENTIONS	OPTIONAL INTERVENTIONS
Attachment Promotion Environmental Management: Attachment Process Kangaroo Care	Breastfeeding Assistance Family Integrity Promotion Infant Care Intrapartal Care Lactation Counseling Parent Education: Infant Risk Identification: Childbearing Family	Anticipatory Guidance Coping Enhancement Emotional Support Role Enhancement

Continued

Outcome: PARENTING

MAJOR INTERVENTIONS	SUGGESTED INTERVENTIONS	OPTIONAL INTERVENTIONS
Abuse Protection Support: Child Developmental Enhancement: Child Parenting Promotion	Anticipatory Guidance Anxiety Reduction Caregiver Support Coping Enhancement Counseling Developmental Enhancement: Adolescent Family Integrity Promotion Family Involvement Promotion Family Support Normalization Promotion Parent Education: Adolescent Parent Education: Childrearing Family Respite Care Role Enhancement Support System Enhancement Surveillance Values Clarification	Breastfeeding Assistance Emotional Support Family Integrity Promotion Family Process Maintenance Family Therapy Health System Guidance Home Maintenance Assistance Parent Education: Infant Prenatal Care Security Enhancement Self-Esteem Enhancement Socialization Enhancement Support Group Telephone Consultation

Outcome: PARENTING: SOCIAL SAFETY

MAJOR INTERVENTIONS	SUGGESTED INTERVENTIONS	OPTIONAL INTERVENTIONS
Abuse Protection Support: Child Parent Education: Adolescent Parent Education: Childrearing Family Risk Identification: Childbearing Family	Anticipatory Guidance Developmental Enhancement: Child Family Integrity Promotion Family Integrity Promotion: Childbearing Family Health Screening Risk Identification Socialization Enhancement Surveillance: Safety	Counseling Emotional Support Family Support Family Therapy Mutual Goal Setting Parent Education: Infant Self-Esteem Enhancement Self-Modification Assistance Self-Responsibility Facilitation Substance Use Prevention Support Group Teaching: Individual

Outcome: ROLE PERFORMANCE

MAJOR INTERVENTIONS	SUGGESTED INTERVENTIONS	OPTIONAL INTERVENTIONS
Role Enhancement	Anticipatory Guidance Behavior Modification Caregiver Support Counseling Decision-Making Support Emotional Support Self-Awareness Enhancement Values Clarification	Attachment Promotion Childbirth Preparation Family Integrity Promotion Family Therapy Health Education Parent Education: Adolescent Parent Education: Childrearing Family Parent Education: Infant Self-Esteem Enhancement Support Group Support System Enhancement

Continued

Outcome: SAFETY BEHAVIOR: HOME PHYSICAL ENVIRONMENT

MAJOR INTERVENTIONS	SUGGESTED INTERVENTIONS	OPTIONAL INTERVENTIONS
Environmental Management: Safety Surveillance: Safety	Environmental Management: Violence Prevention Home Maintenance Assistance Risk Identification Teaching: Infant Safety Teaching: Toddler Safety	Patient Contracting Parent Education: Childrearing Family Parent Education: Infant Vehicle Safety Promotion

Outcome: SOCIAL SUPPORT

MAJOR INTERVENTIONS	SUGGESTED INTERVENTIONS	OPTIONAL INTERVENTIONS
Family Involvement Promotion Support Group Support System Enhancement	Caregiver Support Emotional Support Family Support Referral Telephone Consultation	Coping Enhancement Financial Resource Assistance Spiritual Support Sustenance Support Therapy Group

Nursing Diagnosis: PERSONAL IDENTITY DISTURBANCE

DEFINITION: Inability to distinguish between self and nonself.

Outcome: DISTORTED THOUGHT CONTROL

MAJOR INTERVENTIONS	SUGGESTED INTERVENTIONS	OPTIONAL INTERVENTIONS

Delusion Management
Hallucination
  Management
	Anxiety Reduction
	Cognitive Restructuring
	Delirium Management
	Dementia Management
	Medication Management
	Reality Orientation
	Therapy Group
		Active Listening
		Art Therapy
		Body Image
		  Enhancement
		Environmental
		  Management

Outcome: IDENTITY

MAJOR INTERVENTIONS	SUGGESTED INTERVENTIONS	OPTIONAL INTERVENTIONS

Reality Orientation
Self-Esteem
  Enhancement
	Body Image
	  Enhancement
	Counseling
	Developmental
	  Enhancement:
	  Adolescent
	Developmental
	  Enhancement: Child
	Medication Management
	Self-Awareness
	  Enhancement
	Sexual Counseling
	Socialization
	  Enhancement
	Substance Use
	  Prevention
		Assertiveness Training
		Cognitive Restructuring
		Complex Relationship
		  Building
		Delirium Management
		Delusion Management
		Dementia Management
		Eating Disorders
		  Management
		Hallucination
		  Management
		Hypnosis
		Spiritual Support
		Substance Use Treatment
		Therapy Group
		Values Clarification

Continued

Outcome: **SELF-MUTILATION RESTRAINT**

MAJOR INTERVENTIONS	SUGGESTED INTERVENTIONS	OPTIONAL INTERVENTIONS
Behavior Management: Self-Harm Environmental Management: Violence Prevention	Anger Control Assistance Anxiety Reduction Behavior Management Behavior Modification Cognitive Restructuring Coping Enhancement Counseling Decision-Making Support Emotional Support Environmental Management: Safety Impulse Control Training Limit Setting Mood Management Mutual Goal Setting Patient Contracting Physical Restraint Seclusion Security Enhancement Self-Responsibility Facilitation Suicide Prevention Surveillance: Safety	Active Listening Calming Technique Delirium Management Delusion Management Hallucination Management Substance Use Treatment

Nursing Diagnosis: PHYSICAL MOBILITY, IMPAIRED

DEFINITION: A limitation in independent, purposeful physical movement of the body or of one or more extremities.

Outcome: AMBULATION: WALKING

MAJOR INTERVENTIONS	SUGGESTED INTERVENTIONS	OPTIONAL INTERVENTIONS
Exercise Therapy: Ambulation	Body Mechanics Promotion Energy Management Exercise Promotion Exercise Promotion: Strength Training Exercise Promotion: Stretching Exercise Therapy: Balance Exercise Therapy: Joint Mobility Exercise Therapy: Muscle Control Teaching: Prescribed Activity/Exercise	Activity Therapy Environmental Management: Safety Fall Prevention Pain Management Surveillance: Safety Weight Reduction Assistance

Outcome: AMBULATION: WHEELCHAIR

MAJOR INTERVENTIONS	SUGGESTED INTERVENTIONS	OPTIONAL INTERVENTIONS
Exercise Promotion: Strength Training Positioning: Wheelchair	Body Mechanics Promotion Energy Management Environmental Management: Safety Exercise Therapy: Balance Exercise Therapy: Joint Mobility Exercise Therapy: Muscle Control Fall Prevention Self-Care Assistance Teaching: Prescribed Activity/Exercise	Environmental Management Exercise Promotion Pain Management Surveillance: Safety Weight Reduction Assistance

Continued

Outcome: JOINT MOVEMENT: ACTIVE

MAJOR INTERVENTIONS	SUGGESTED INTERVENTIONS	OPTIONAL INTERVENTIONS
Exercise Therapy: Joint Mobility	Energy Management Exercise Promotion: Strength Training Exercise Promotion: Stretching Exercise Therapy: Muscle Control	Analgesic Administration Body Mechanics Promotion Exercise Promotion Exercise Therapy: Ambulation Exercise Therapy: Balance Pain Management Progressive Muscle Relaxation Teaching: Prescribed Activity/Exercise

Outcome: MOBILITY LEVEL

MAJOR INTERVENTIONS	SUGGESTED INTERVENTIONS	OPTIONAL INTERVENTIONS
Exercise Therapy: Ambulation Exercise Therapy: Balance Exercise Therapy: Joint Mobility Exercise Therapy: Muscle Control	Body Mechanics Promotion Energy Management Exercise Promotion Exercise Promotion: Strength Training Exercise Promotion: Stretching Fall Prevention Pain Management Positioning Traction/Immobilization Care	Activity Therapy Analgesic Administration Cast Care: Maintenance Circulatory Precautions Neurologic Monitoring Peripheral Sensation Management Positioning: Intraoperative Positioning: Neurologic Positioning: Wheelchair Pressure Management Skin Surveillance Teaching: Prescribed Activity/Exercise

Outcome: TRANSFER PERFORMANCE

MAJOR INTERVENTIONS	SUGGESTED INTERVENTIONS	OPTIONAL INTERVENTIONS
Exercise Promotion: Strength Training Exercise Therapy: Balance Exercise Therapy: Muscle Control	Body Mechanics Promotion Energy Management Exercise Therapy: Joint Mobility Fall Prevention Positioning Positioning: Wheelchair Teaching: Psychomotor Skill	Anxiety Reduction Environmental Management: Safety Exercise Promotion Exercise Promotion: Stretching Pain Management Physical Restraint Self-Care Assistance Surveillance: Safety Teaching: Prescribed Activity/Exercise

Nursing Diagnosis: POST-TRAUMA SYNDROME

DEFINITION: A sustained maladaptive response to a traumatic overwhelming event.

Outcome: ABUSE RECOVERY: EMOTIONAL

MAJOR INTERVENTIONS	SUGGESTED INTERVENTIONS	OPTIONAL INTERVENTIONS
Counseling Support System Enhancement	Anger Control Assistance Anxiety Reduction Coping Enhancement Emotional Support Forgiveness Facilitation Mood Management Self-Esteem Enhancement Simple Relaxation Therapy Socialization Enhancement Suicide Prevention Support Group	Assertiveness Training Behavior Management: Self-Harm Family Support Security Enhancement Spiritual Support

Outcome: ABUSE RECOVERY: FINANCIAL

MAJOR INTERVENTIONS	SUGGESTED INTERVENTIONS	OPTIONAL INTERVENTIONS
Coping Enhancement Counseling Financial Resource Assistance	Assertiveness Training Decision-Making Support Patient Rights Protection Security Enhancement Support System Enhancement	Self-Esteem Enhancement Support Group

Outcome: ABUSE RECOVERY: SEXUAL

MAJOR INTERVENTIONS	SUGGESTED INTERVENTIONS	OPTIONAL INTERVENTIONS

Counseling
Rape-Trauma Treatment
Support System
  Enhancement
	Active Listening
	Anger Control
	  Assistance
	Anxiety Reduction
	Coping Enhancement
	Emotional Support
	Forgiveness Facilitation
	Guilt Work Facilitation
	Self-Esteem
	  Enhancement
	Sexual Counseling
	Simple Relaxation
	  Therapy
	Substance Use
	  Prevention
		Assertiveness Training
		Behavior Management:
		  Self-Harm
		Behavior Management:
		  Sexual
		Grief Work Facilitation
		Hope Instillation
		Mood Management
		Presence
		Progressive Muscle
		  Relaxation
		Self-Awareness
		  Enhancement
		Socialization
		  Enhancement
		Spiritual Support
		Suicide Prevention
		Support Group

Outcome: COPING

MAJOR INTERVENTIONS	SUGGESTED INTERVENTIONS	OPTIONAL INTERVENTIONS

Coping Enhancement
Counseling
	Anxiety Reduction
	Emotional Support
	Grief Work Facilitation
	Hope Instillation
	Progressive Muscle
	  Relaxation
	Simple Relaxation
	  Therapy
	Spiritual Support
	Support Group
	Support System
	  Enhancement
		Behavior Management:
		  Self-Harm
		Mood Management
		Reminiscence Therapy
		Sibling Support
		Socialization
		  Enhancement

Continued

Outcome: **FEAR CONTROL**

MAJOR INTERVENTIONS	SUGGESTED INTERVENTIONS	OPTIONAL INTERVENTIONS

Coping Enhancement
Counseling
Security Enhancement
	Anticipatory Guidance
	Anxiety Reduction
	Calming Technique
	Emotional Support
	Environmental
	  Management
	Support System
	  Enhancement
		Abuse Protection
		  Support
		Active Listening
		Animal-Assisted
		  Therapy
		Assertiveness Training
		Simple Relaxation
		  Therapy

Outcome: **IMPULSE CONTROL**

MAJOR INTERVENTIONS	SUGGESTED INTERVENTIONS	OPTIONAL INTERVENTIONS

Impulse Control Training	Anger Control
	  Assistance
	Anxiety Reduction
	Behavior Management:
	  Self-Harm
	Environmental
	  Management: Safety
	Patient Contracting
		Coping Enhancement
		Emotional Support
		Mood Management
		Security Enhancement
		Substance Use
		  Prevention
		Suicide Prevention
		Support Group
		Support System
		  Enhancement

Outcome: SELF-MUTILATION RESTRAINT

MAJOR INTERVENTIONS	SUGGESTED INTERVENTIONS	OPTIONAL INTERVENTIONS
Behavior Management: Self-Harm Counseling	Anger Control Assistance Anxiety Reduction Behavior Management Behavior Modification Cognitive Restructuring Coping Enhancement Environmental Management: Safety Impulse Control Training Limit Setting Mood Management Mutual Goal Setting Patient Contracting Security Enhancement Suicide Prevention Surveillance: Safety	Area Restriction Emotional Support Environmental Management Milieu Therapy Reality Orientation

Nursing Diagnosis: POWERLESSNESS

DEFINITION: Perception that one's own actions will not significantly affect an outcome; a perceived lack of control over a current situation or immediate happening.

Outcome: DEPRESSION CONTROL

MAJOR INTERVENTIONS	SUGGESTED INTERVENTIONS	OPTIONAL INTERVENTIONS

Cognitive Restructuring
Mood Management
Self-Esteem
  Enhancement
	Activity Therapy
	Animal-Assisted
	  Therapy
	Art Therapy
	Complex Relationship
	  Building
	Emotional Support
	Hope Instillation
	Presence
	Self-Awareness
	  Enhancement
	Support Group
		Coping Enhancement
		Crisis Intervention
		Grief Work Facilitation
		Guilt Work Facilitation
		Humor
		Meditation Facilitation
		Reminiscence Therapy
		Therapy Group

Outcome: FAMILY PARTICIPATION IN PROFESSIONAL CARE

MAJOR INTERVENTIONS	SUGGESTED INTERVENTIONS	OPTIONAL INTERVENTIONS

Decision-Making
  Support
Family Involvement
  Promotion
	Family Planning:
	  Unplanned Pregnancy
	Family Support
	Health Care Information
	  Exchange
	Health System Guidance
		Anticipatory Guidance
		Culture Brokerage
		Health Education
		Insurance Authorization
		Normalization
		  Promotion
		Patient Rights Protection
		Risk Identification

Outcome: HEALTH BELIEFS

MAJOR INTERVENTIONS	SUGGESTED INTERVENTIONS	OPTIONAL INTERVENTIONS

Health Education
Values Clarification
	Bibliotherapy
	Cognitive Restructuring
	Hope Instillation
	Risk Identification
	Self-Awareness
	  Enhancement
	Self-Esteem
	  Enhancement
	Self-Modification
	  Assistance
		Culture Brokerage
		Health System Guidance
		Learning Facilitation
		Mutual Goal Setting
		Patient Contracting
		Spiritual Support
		Teaching: Individual

Outcome: HEALTH BELIEFS: PERCEIVED ABILITY TO PERFORM

MAJOR INTERVENTIONS	SUGGESTED INTERVENTIONS	OPTIONAL INTERVENTIONS
Mutual Goal Setting Self-Esteem Enhancement	Health System Guidance Patient Contracting Risk Identification Self-Awareness Enhancement Self-Modification Assistance Teaching: Individual Values Clarification	Coping Enhancement Culture Brokerage Learning Facilitation Self-Care Assistance Support System Enhancement

Outcome: HEALTH BELIEFS: PERCEIVED CONTROL

MAJOR INTERVENTIONS	SUGGESTED INTERVENTIONS	OPTIONAL INTERVENTIONS
Decision-Making Support Self-Responsibility Facilitation	Emotional Support Health System Guidance Patient Rights Protection Self-Esteem Enhancement Self-Modification Assistance Support System Enhancement Teaching: Individual Values Clarification	Assertiveness Training Counseling Culture Brokerage Hope Instillation Insurance Authorization

Outcome: HEALTH BELIEFS: PERCEIVED RESOURCES

MAJOR INTERVENTIONS	SUGGESTED INTERVENTIONS	OPTIONAL INTERVENTIONS
Financial Resource Assistance Health System Guidance	Culture Brokerage Health Care Information Exchange Insurance Authorization Patient Rights Protection Referral Support System Enhancement Sustenance Support	Environmental Management Teaching: Individual

Continued

Outcome: PARTICIPATION: HEALTH CARE DECISIONS

MAJOR INTERVENTIONS	SUGGESTED INTERVENTIONS	OPTIONAL INTERVENTIONS
Decision-Making Support Health System Guidance Self-Responsibility Facilitation	Active Listening Admission Care Assertiveness Training Complex Relationship Building Culture Brokerage Discharge Planning Patient Rights Protection Values Clarification	Anticipatory Guidance Anxiety Reduction Coping Enhancement Family Involvement Promotion Health Care Information Exchange Insurance Authorization Patient Rights Protection Referral

Nursing Diagnosis: PROTECTION, ALTERED

DEFINITION: The state in which an individual experiences a decrease in the ability to guard the self from internal or external threats such as illness or injury.

Outcome: ABUSE PROTECTION

MAJOR INTERVENTIONS	SUGGESTED INTERVENTIONS	OPTIONAL INTERVENTIONS
Abuse Protection Support Abuse Protection Support: Child Abuse Protection Support: Domestic Partner Abuse Protection Support: Elder	Environmental Management: Safety Environmental Management: Violence Prevention Risk Identification Security Enhancement Surveillance: Safety	Anticipatory Guidance Caregiver Support Coping Enhancement Decision-Making Support Emotional Support Self-Responsibility Facilitation

Outcome: COAGULATION STATUS

MAJOR INTERVENTIONS	SUGGESTED INTERVENTIONS	OPTIONAL INTERVENTIONS
Bleeding Precautions	Bleeding Reduction Blood Products Administration Emergency Care Hemorrhage Control	Autotransfusion Surgical Precautions

Outcome: ENDURANCE

MAJOR INTERVENTIONS	SUGGESTED INTERVENTIONS	OPTIONAL INTERVENTIONS
Energy Management	Exercise Promotion Nutrition Management Self-Care Assistance Sleep Enhancement	Nutrition Management Nutrition Therapy Nutritional Counseling Support System Enhancement Teaching: Prescribed Activity/Exercise Teaching: Prescribed Diet

Continued

Outcome: FETAL STATUS: ANTEPARTUM

MAJOR INTERVENTIONS	SUGGESTED INTERVENTIONS	OPTIONAL INTERVENTIONS
Electronic Fetal Monitoring: Antepartum Ultrasonography: Limited Obstetric	High-Risk Pregnancy Care Surveillance: Late Pregnancy	Labor Suppression Prenatal Care Resuscitation: Fetus

Outcome: FETAL STATUS: INTRAPARTUM

MAJOR INTERVENTIONS	SUGGESTED INTERVENTIONS	OPTIONAL INTERVENTIONS
Electronic Fetal Monitoring: Intrapartum	Amnioinfusion Intrapartal Care: High-Risk Delivery	Intrapartal Care Labor Induction

Outcome: IMMUNE STATUS

MAJOR INTERVENTIONS	SUGGESTED INTERVENTIONS	OPTIONAL INTERVENTIONS
Allergy Management Immunization/ Vaccination Management Infection Protection	Health Education Infection Control Latex Precautions Medication Administration Risk Identification Surveillance Teaching: Individual Teaching: Prescribed Medication	Pruritus Management

Outcome: IMMUNIZATION BEHAVIOR

MAJOR INTERVENTIONS	SUGGESTED INTERVENTIONS	OPTIONAL INTERVENTIONS
Immunization/ Vaccination Management Risk Identification	Anticipatory Guidance Decision-Making Support Health Education Health System Guidance Infection Protection	Parent Education: Infant

Outcome: NEUROLOGICAL STATUS: CONSCIOUSNESS

MAJOR INTERVENTIONS	SUGGESTED INTERVENTIONS	OPTIONAL INTERVENTIONS
Cerebral Profusion Promotion	Airway Management	Dementia Management
Emergency Care	Aspiration Precautions	Positioning
Environmental Management: Safety	Environmental Management	Pressure Management
Neurologic Monitoring	Patient Rights Protection	Pressure Ulcer Prevention
	Postanesthesia Care	Shock Management
	Respiratory Monitoring	Skin Surveillance
	Seizure Precautions	Substance Use Treatment
	Surveillance	
	Vital Signs Monitoring	

Nursing Diagnosis: RAPE-TRAUMA SYNDROME

DEFINITION: Sustained maladaptive response to a forced, violent sexual penetration against the victim's will and consent.

Outcome: ABUSE PROTECTION

MAJOR INTERVENTIONS	SUGGESTED INTERVENTIONS	OPTIONAL INTERVENTIONS
Abuse Protection Support Abuse Protection Support: Child Abuse Protection Support: Domestic Partner Abuse Protection Support: Elder	Counseling Environmental Management: Safety Environmental Management: Violence Prevention Risk Identification Security Enhancement Self-Esteem Enhancement Surveillance: Safety	Anticipatory Guidance Caregiver Support Decision-Making Support Documentation Emotional Support Self-Awareness Enhancement

Outcome: ABUSE RECOVERY: EMOTIONAL

MAJOR INTERVENTIONS	SUGGESTED INTERVENTIONS	OPTIONAL INTERVENTIONS
Coping Enhancement Counseling Rape-Trauma Treatment	Crisis Intervention Emotional Support Mood Management Self-Esteem Enhancement Support Group	Abuse Protection Support Anger Control Assistance Anxiety Reduction Family Support Security Enhancement Self-Awareness Enhancement Spiritual Support Support System Enhancement

Outcome: ABUSE RECOVERY: SEXUAL

MAJOR INTERVENTIONS	SUGGESTED INTERVENTIONS	OPTIONAL INTERVENTIONS

Counseling
Rape-Trauma Treatment
	Anger Control
	  Assistance
	Anxiety Reduction
	Calming Technique
	Crisis Intervention
	Decision-Making
	  Support
	Emotional Support
	Hope Instillation
	Presence
	Referral
	Self-Esteem
	  Enhancement
	Sexual Counseling
	Specimen Management
	Support Group
	Support System
	  Enhancement
	Therapy Group
	Vital Signs Monitoring
	Wound Care
		Abuse Protection
		  Support
		Anticipatory Guidance
		Art Therapy
		Behavior Management:
		  Self-Harm
		Behavior Management:
		  Sexual
		Coping Enhancement
		Family Therapy
		Grief Work Facilitation
		Guilt Work Facilitation
		Health System Guidance
		Pain Management
		Role Enhancement
		Security Enhancement
		Spiritual Support
		Substance Use
		  Prevention

Outcome: COPING

MAJOR INTERVENTIONS	SUGGESTED INTERVENTIONS	OPTIONAL INTERVENTIONS

Coping Enhancement
Crisis Intervention
Rape-Trauma Treatment
	Anxiety Reduction
	Calming Technique
	Counseling
	Decision-Making
	  Support
	Emotional Support
	Family Support
	Grief Work Facilitation
	Guilt Work Facilitation
	Hope Instillation
	Pain Management
	Presence
	Simple Relaxation
	  Therapy
	Spiritual Support
	Support Group
		Art Therapy
		Behavior Management:
		  Self-Harm
		Family Therapy
		Support System
		  Enhancement
		Therapeutic Play
		Therapy Group

Nursing Diagnosis: RAPE-TRAUMA SYNDROME: COMPOUND REACTION

Definition: Forced violent sexual penetration against the victim's will and consent. The trauma syndrome that develops from this attack or attempted attack includes an acute phase of disorganization of the victim's lifestyle and a long-term process or reorganization of lifestyle.

Outcome: ABUSE PROTECTION

MAJOR INTERVENTIONS	SUGGESTED INTERVENTIONS	OPTIONAL INTERVENTIONS
Abuse Protection Support Abuse Protection Support: Child Abuse Protection Support: Domestic Partner Abuse Protection Support: Elder	Assertiveness Training Counseling Environmental Management: Safety Environmental Management: Violence Prevention Risk Identification Security Enhancement Self-Esteem Enhancement Surveillance: Safety	Anticipatory Guidance Caregiver Support Decision-Making Support Documentation Emotional Support Self-Awareness Enhancement Self-Responsibility Facilitation Values Clarification

Outcome: ABUSE RECOVERY: EMOTIONAL

MAJOR INTERVENTIONS	SUGGESTED INTERVENTIONS	OPTIONAL INTERVENTIONS
Coping Enhancement Counseling Rape-Trauma Treatment	Assertiveness Training Crisis Intervention Emotional Support Mood Management Self-Esteem Enhancement Socialization Enhancement Suicide Prevention Support Group	Abuse Protection Support Anger Control Assistance Anxiety Reduction Behavior Management: Self-Harm Behavior Modification: Social Skills Complex Relationship Building Family Support Role Enhancement Security Enhancement Self-Awareness Enhancement Spiritual Support Support System Enhancement

Outcome: ABUSE RECOVERY: SEXUAL

MAJOR INTERVENTIONS	SUGGESTED INTERVENTIONS	OPTIONAL INTERVENTIONS
Crisis Intervention Rape-Trauma Treatment	Anger Control Assistance Anticipatory Guidance Anxiety Reduction Calming Technique Coping Enhancement Counseling Decision-Making Support Emotional Support Forgiveness Facilitation Hope Instillation Mood Management Presence Referral Self-Esteem Enhancement Sexual Counseling Substance Use Prevention Support Group Support System Enhancement Therapy Group	Abuse Protection Support Activity Therapy Animal-Assisted Therapy Art Therapy Assertiveness Training Behavior Management: Self-Harm Behavior Management: Sexual Body Image Enhancement Complex Relationship Building Eating Disorders Management Family Therapy Grief Work Facilitation Guilt Work Facilitation Health System Guidance Hypnosis Music Therapy Simple Relaxation Therapy Socialization Enhancement Spiritual Support Suicide Prevention Therapeutic Play

Continued

Outcome: COPING

MAJOR INTERVENTIONS	SUGGESTED INTERVENTIONS	OPTIONAL INTERVENTIONS
Coping Enhancement Crisis Intervention Rape-Trauma Treatment	Anxiety Reduction Calming Technique Counseling Decision-Making Support Emotional Support Family Support Grief Work Facilitation Guilt Work Facilitation Hope Instillation Pain Management Presence Simple Relaxation Therapy Spiritual Support Support Group	Animal-Assisted Therapy Art Therapy Behavior Management: Self-Harm Bibliotherapy Body Image Enhancement Family Therapy Hypnosis Mood Management Music Therapy Recreation Therapy Sibling Support Support System Enhancement Therapeutic Play Therapy Group

Outcome: IMPULSE CONTROL

MAJOR INTERVENTIONS	SUGGESTED INTERVENTIONS	OPTIONAL INTERVENTIONS
Anger Control Assistance Impulse Control Training	Anxiety Reduction Behavior Management Behavior Management: Self-Harm Behavior Modification Behavior Modification: Social Skills Environmental Management: Safety Environmental Management: Violence Prevention Limit Setting Milieu Therapy Patient Contracting Self-Modification Assistance Self-Responsibility Facilitation	Coping Enhancement Emotional Support Mood Management Security Enhancement Substance Use Prevention Support Group Support System Enhancement Surveillance: Safety Teaching: Safe Sex Therapy Group

Outcome: SELF-MUTILATION RESTRAINT

MAJOR INTERVENTIONS	SUGGESTED INTERVENTIONS	OPTIONAL INTERVENTIONS
Behavior Management: Self-Harm Environmental Management: Violence Prevention Suicide Prevention	Anger Control Assistance Anxiety Reduction Behavior Management Behavior Modification Coping Enhancement Counseling Crisis Intervention Emotional Support Environmental Management: Safety Impulse Control Training Limit Setting Mood Management Patient Contracting Security Enhancement Surveillance: Safety	Active Listening Family Involvement Promotion Mutual Goal Setting Presence Teaching: Individual

Nursing Diagnosis: RAPE-TRAUMA SYNDROME: SILENT REACTION

Definition: Forced violent sexual penetration against the victim's will and consent. The trauma syndrome that develops from this attack or attempted attack includes an acute phase of disorganization of the victim's lifestyle and a long-term process of reorganization of lifestyle.

Outcome: ABUSE PROTECTION

MAJOR INTERVENTIONS	SUGGESTED INTERVENTIONS	OPTIONAL INTERVENTIONS
Abuse Protection Support Abuse Protection Support: Child Abuse Protection Support: Domestic Partner Abuse Protection Support: Elder	Assertiveness Training Counseling Environmental Management: Safety Environmental Management: Violence Prevention Risk Identification Security Enhancement Self-Esteem Enhancement Surveillance: Safety	Anticipatory Guidance Caregiver Support Decision-Making Support Documentation Emotional Support Self-Awareness Enhancement Self-Responsibility Facilitation Values Clarification

Outcome: ABUSE RECOVERY: EMOTIONAL

MAJOR INTERVENTIONS	SUGGESTED INTERVENTIONS	OPTIONAL INTERVENTIONS
Abuse Protection Support Coping Enhancement Counseling Rape-Trauma Treatment	Assertiveness Training Crisis Intervention Emotional Support Mood Management Self-Esteem Enhancement Socialization Enhancement Suicide Prevention Support Group	Anger Control Assistance Anxiety Reduction Behavior Management: Self-Harm Behavior Modification: Social Skills Complex Relationship Building Family Support Role Enhancement Security Enhancement Self-Awareness Enhancement Spiritual Support Support System Enhancement

Outcome: ABUSE RECOVERY: SEXUAL

MAJOR INTERVENTIONS	SUGGESTED INTERVENTIONS	OPTIONAL INTERVENTIONS
Counseling Rape-Trauma Treatment	Anger Control Assistance Anticipatory Guidance Art Therapy Anxiety Reduction Calming Technique Coping Enhancement Crisis Intervention Decision-Making Support Emotional Support Hope Instillation Presence Referral Security Enhancement Sexual Counseling Support Group Support System Enhancement Therapy Group	Abuse Protection Support Animal-Assisted Therapy Behavior Management: Self-Harm Behavior Management: Sexual Body Image Enhancement Complex Relationship Building Family Therapy Grief Work Facilitation Guilt Work Facilitation Health System Guidance Self-Esteem Enhancement Simple Relaxation Therapy Socialization Enhancement Spiritual Support Substance Use Prevention Suicide Prevention Therapeutic Play

Continued

Outcome: COPING

MAJOR INTERVENTIONS	SUGGESTED INTERVENTIONS	OPTIONAL INTERVENTIONS

Coping Enhancement
Rape-Trauma Treatment
	Anxiety Reduction
	Calming Technique
	Counseling
	Crisis Intervention
	Decision-Making
	  Support
	Emotional Support
	Family Support
	Grief Work Facilitation
	Guilt Work Facilitation
	Hope Instillation
	Pain Management
	Presence
	Simple Relaxation
	  Therapy
	Spiritual Support
	Support Group
		Animal-Assisted
		  Therapy
		Art Therapy
		Behavior Management:
		  Self-Harm
		Bibliotherapy
		Body Image
		  Enhancement
		Family Therapy
		Hypnosis
		Mood Management
		Music Therapy
		Recreation Therapy
		Sibling Support
		Support System
		  Enhancement
		Therapeutic Play
		Therapy Group

Outcome: IMPULSE CONTROL

MAJOR INTERVENTIONS	SUGGESTED INTERVENTIONS	OPTIONAL INTERVENTIONS

Anger Control
  Assistance
Impulse Control Training
	Anxiety Reduction
	Behavior Management
	Behavior Management:
	  Self-Harm
	Behavior Modification
	Behavior Modification:
	  Social Skills
	Environmental
	  Management: Safety
	Environmental
	  Management: Violence
	  Prevention
	Limit Setting
	Milieu Therapy
	Patient Contracting
	Self-Modification
	  Assistance
	Self-Responsibility
	  Facilitation
		Coping Enhancement
		Emotional Support
		Mood Management
		Security Enhancement
		Substance Use
		  Prevention
		Support Group
		Support System
		  Enhancement
		Surveillance: Safety
		Teaching: Group
		Teaching: Individual
		Teaching: Safe Sex
		Therapy Group

Outcome: SELF-MUTILATION RESTRAINT

MAJOR INTERVENTIONS	SUGGESTED INTERVENTIONS	OPTIONAL INTERVENTIONS
Behavior Management: Self-Harm Environmental Management: Violence Prevention Suicide Prevention	Anger Control Assistance Anxiety Reduction Behavior Management Behavior Modification Coping Enhancement Counseling Crisis Intervention Emotional Support Environmental Management: Safety Impulse Control Training Limit Setting Mood Management Patient Contracting Security Enhancement Suicide Prevention Surveillance: Safety	Active Listening Family Involvement Promotion Mutual Goal Setting Presence Teaching: Individual

Nursing Diagnosis: RELOCATION STRESS SYNDROME

DEFINITION: Physiological and/or psychosocial disturbances as a result of transfer from one environment to another.

Outcome: ANXIETY CONTROL

MAJOR INTERVENTIONS	SUGGESTED INTERVENTIONS	OPTIONAL INTERVENTIONS

Anxiety Reduction	Active Listening
	Animal-Assisted
	  Therapy
	Anticipatory Guidance
	Calming Technique
	Coping Enhancement
	Counseling
	Discharge Planning
	Presence
	Progressive Muscle
	  Relaxation
	Security Enhancement
	Simple Guided Imagery
	Simple Massage
	Simple Relaxation
	  Therapy
	Spiritual Support
	Support System
	  Enhancement
	Touch
		Decision-Making
		  Support
		Environmental
		  Management
		Family Mobilization
		Sleep Enhancement
		Support Group
		Truth Telling

Outcome: CHILD ADAPTATION TO HOSPITALIZATION

MAJOR INTERVENTIONS	SUGGESTED INTERVENTIONS	OPTIONAL INTERVENTIONS
Coping Enhancement Security Enhancement	Active Listening Admission Care Culture Brokerage Emotional Support Environmental Management Family Integrity Promotion Family Involvement Promotion Family Mobilization Family Process Maintenance Family Support Patient Rights Protection Self-Care Assistance Sibling Support Sleep Enhancement Support System Enhancement Therapeutic Play Touch Truth Telling Visitation Facilitation	Animal-Assisted Therapy Anticipatory Guidance Anxiety Reduction Art Therapy Calming Technique Developmental Enhancement: Child Humor Limit Setting Music Therapy Preparatory Sensory Information Presence Recreation Therapy Spiritual Support Support Group Teaching: Individual Teaching: Procedure/Treatment

Continued

Outcome: COPING

MAJOR INTERVENTIONS	SUGGESTED INTERVENTIONS	OPTIONAL INTERVENTIONS
Coping Enhancement Counseling	Active Listening Anticipatory Guidance Anxiety Reduction Calming Technique Caregiver Support Discharge Planning Emotional Support Family Mobilization Family Support Hope Instillation Humor Presence Recreation Therapy Resiliency Promotion Self-Responsibility Facilitation Spiritual Support Support Group Touch	Animal-Assisted Therapy Art Therapy Family Support Mood Management Music Therapy Reminiscence Therapy Sibling Support Simple Guided Imagery Simple Massage Simple Relaxation Therapy Support System Enhancement Therapeutic Play Therapy Group Visitation Facilitation

Outcome: DEPRESSION CONTROL

MAJOR INTERVENTIONS	SUGGESTED INTERVENTIONS	OPTIONAL INTERVENTIONS
Mood Management	Activity Therapy Exercise Promotion Medication Management Nutrition Management Resiliency Promotion Self-Modification Assistance Sleep Enhancement	Discharge Planning Mutual Goal Setting Patient Contracting

Outcome: DEPRESSION LEVEL

MAJOR INTERVENTIONS	SUGGESTED INTERVENTIONS	OPTIONAL INTERVENTIONS

Hope Instillation
Mood Management
	Behavior Management:
	  Self-Harm
	Counseling
	Emotional Support
	Exercise Promotion
	Medication Management
	Self-Modification
	  Assistance
	Sleep Enhancement
		Activity Therapy
		Animal-Assisted
		  Therapy
		Nutrition Management
		Nutritional Monitoring
		Recreation Therapy
		Spiritual Support
		Support System
		  Enhancement

Outcome: LONELINESS

MAJOR INTERVENTIONS	SUGGESTED INTERVENTIONS	OPTIONAL INTERVENTIONS

Family Involvement
  Promotion
Socialization
  Enhancement
Spiritual Support
	Active Listening
	Activity Therapy
	Animal-Assisted
	  Therapy
	Counseling
	Emotional Support
	Environmental
	  Management
	Presence
	Recreation Therapy
	Socialization
	  Enhancement
	Support System
	  Enhancement
	Therapeutic Play
	Touch
	Visitation Facilitation
		Art Therapy
		Bibliotherapy
		Music Therapy

Continued

Outcome: PSYCHOSOCIAL ADJUSTMENT: LIFE CHANGE

MAJOR INTERVENTIONS	SUGGESTED INTERVENTIONS	OPTIONAL INTERVENTIONS

Anticipatory Guidance
Coping Enhancement
	Active Listening
	Anger Control
	  Assistance
	Counseling
	Discharge Planning
	Emotional Support
	Health Education
	Resiliency Promotion
	Role Enhancement
		Decision-Making
		  Support
		Dementia Management
		Family Integrity
		  Promotion
		Family Mobilization
		Family Process
		  Maintenance
		Humor
		Spiritual Support

Outcome: QUALITY OF LIFE

MAJOR INTERVENTIONS	SUGGESTED INTERVENTIONS	OPTIONAL INTERVENTIONS

Values Clarification	Active Listening
	Coping Enhancement
	Counseling
	Decision-Making
	  Support
	Emotional Support
	Family Integrity
	  Promotion
	Family Involvement
	  Promotion
	Family Support
	Hope Instillation
	Humor
	Role Enhancement
	Security Enhancement
	Socialization
	  Enhancement
	Spiritual Support
	Support System
	  Enhancement
		Culture Brokerage
		Mood Management
		Reminiscence Therapy
		Support Group
		Truth Telling

Nursing Diagnosis: ROLE PERFORMANCE, ALTERED

DEFINITION: The patterns of behavior and self-expression do not match the environmental context, norms, and expectations.

Outcome: CAREGIVER LIFESTYLE DISRUPTION

MAJOR INTERVENTIONS	SUGGESTED INTERVENTIONS	OPTIONAL INTERVENTIONS

Coping Enhancement
Role Enhancement
	Anticipatory Guidance
	Caregiver Support
	Decision-Making
	  Support
	Emotional Support
	Family Support
	Health System Guidance
	Mutual Goal Setting
	Support Group
	Support System
	  Enhancement
		Family Involvement
		  Promotion
		Insurance Authorization

Outcome: COPING

MAJOR INTERVENTIONS	SUGGESTED INTERVENTIONS	OPTIONAL INTERVENTIONS

Coping Enhancement	Anticipatory Guidance
	Caregiver Support
	Counseling
	Decision-Making
	  Support
	Emotional Support
	Family Support
	Role Enhancement
	Spiritual Support
	Support Group
	Values Clarification
		Body Image
		  Enhancement
		Cognitive Restructuring
		Family Therapy
		Mood Management
		Normalization
		  Promotion
		Socialization
		  Enhancement
		Spiritual Support
		Substance Use
		  Prevention
		Support Group
		Support System
		  Enhancement

Continued

Outcome: DEPRESSION LEVEL

MAJOR INTERVENTIONS	SUGGESTED INTERVENTIONS	OPTIONAL INTERVENTIONS

Hope Instillation
Mood Management
	Activity Therapy
	Cognitive Restructuring
	Counseling
	Emotional Support
	Exercise Promotion
	Medication Management
	Patient Contracting
	Self-Awareness
	  Enhancement
	Self-Esteem
	  Enhancement
	Self-Modification
	  Assistance
	Sleep Enhancement
	Support Group
	Therapy Group
		Mutual Goal Setting
		Spiritual Support
		Support System
		  Enhancement

Outcome: PSYCHOMOTOR ENERGY

MAJOR INTERVENTIONS	SUGGESTED INTERVENTIONS	OPTIONAL INTERVENTIONS

Mood Management	Coping Enhancement
	Counseling
	Emotional Support
	Energy Management
	Self-Awareness
	  Enhancement
	Self-Esteem
	  Enhancement
	Self-Modification
	  Assistance
		Activity Therapy
		Body Image
		  Enhancement
		Nutrition Management
		Role Enhancement
		Spiritual Support

Outcome: PSYCHOSOCIAL ADJUSTMENT: LIFE CHANGE

MAJOR INTERVENTIONS	SUGGESTED INTERVENTIONS	OPTIONAL INTERVENTIONS

Anticipatory Guidance
Coping Enhancement
	Counseling
	Emotional Support
	Parent Education:
	  Adolescent
	Parent Education:
	  Childrearing Family
	Parent Education: Infant
	Role Enhancement
		Decision-Making
		  Support
		Family Mobilization
		Family Process
		  Maintenance
		Family Therapy
		Humor
		Spiritual Support

Outcome: ROLE PERFORMANCE

MAJOR INTERVENTIONS	SUGGESTED INTERVENTIONS	OPTIONAL INTERVENTIONS
Role Enhancement	Anticipatory Guidance	Active Listening
	Caregiver Support	Attachment Promotion
	Cognitive Restructuring	Body Image
	Complex Relationship	Enhancement
	Building	Childbirth Preparation
	Emotional Support	Counseling
	Parent Education:	Decision-Making
	Adolescent	Support
	Parent Education:	Family Therapy
	Childrearing Family	Normalization
	Parent Education: Infant	Promotion
	Parenting Promotion	Support Group
	Self-Awareness	Support System
	Enhancement	Enhancement
	Self-Esteem	Teaching: Sexuality
	Enhancement	
	Values Clarification	

Nursing Diagnosis: SELF-CARE DEFICIT: BATHING/HYGIENE

DEFINITION: Impaired ability to perform or complete bathing/hygiene activities for oneself.

Outcome: SELF-CARE: ACTIVITIES OF DAILY LIVING (ADL)

MAJOR INTERVENTIONS	SUGGESTED INTERVENTIONS	OPTIONAL INTERVENTIONS
Self-Care Assistance: Bathing/Hygiene	Energy Management Self-Care Assistance Self-Responsibility Facilitation	Behavior Modification Exercise Promotion Exercise Promotion: Stretching Exercise Therapy: Ambulation Exercise Therapy: Balance Exercise Therapy: Joint Mobility Exercise Therapy: Muscle Control Fall Prevention

Outcome: SELF-CARE: BATHING

MAJOR INTERVENTIONS	SUGGESTED INTERVENTIONS	OPTIONAL INTERVENTIONS
Self-Care Assistance: Bathing/Hygiene	Bathing Ear Care Foot Care Hair Care Nail Care Perineal Care Teaching: Individual	Energy Management Environmental Management: Comfort Environmental Management: Safety Exercise Promotion Fall Prevention

Outcome: SELF-CARE: HYGIENE

MAJOR INTERVENTIONS	SUGGESTED INTERVENTIONS	OPTIONAL INTERVENTIONS
Self-Care Assistance: Bathing/Hygiene	Bathing Ear Care Oral Health Maintenance Perineal Care Teaching: Individual	Contact Lens Care Energy Management Foot Care Hair Care Nail Care Oral Health Promotion Oral Health Restoration

Nursing Diagnosis: SELF-CARE DEFICIT: DRESSING/GROOMING

DEFINITION: An impaired ability to perform or complete dressing and grooming activities for oneself.

Outcome: SELF-CARE: ACTIVITIES OF DAILY LIVING (ADL)

MAJOR INTERVENTIONS	SUGGESTED INTERVENTIONS	OPTIONAL INTERVENTIONS
Self-Care Assistance: Dressing/Grooming	Energy Management Environmental Management Self-Care Assistance	Exercise Promotion Exercise Promotion: Stretching Exercise Therapy: Ambulation Exercise Therapy: Balance Exercise Therapy: Joint Mobility Exercise Therapy: Muscle Control Fall Prevention Pain Management

Outcome: SELF-CARE: DRESSING

MAJOR INTERVENTIONS	SUGGESTED INTERVENTIONS	OPTIONAL INTERVENTIONS
Dressing Self-Care Assistance: Dressing/Grooming	Environmental Management Self-Care Assistance Teaching: Individual	Communication Enhancement: Visual Deficit Energy Management Environmental Management: Comfort Environmental Management: Safety Exercise Promotion Fall Prevention

Outcome: SELF-CARE: GROOMING

MAJOR INTERVENTIONS	SUGGESTED INTERVENTIONS	OPTIONAL INTERVENTIONS
Hair Care Self-Care Assistance: Dressing/Grooming	Bathing Body Image Enhancement Dressing Nail Care Self-Care Assistance: Bathing/Hygiene Teaching: Individual	Energy Management Environmental Management: Comfort Exercise Promotion Foot Care Oral Health Promotion

Nursing Diagnosis: SELF-CARE DEFICIT: FEEDING

Definition: An impaired ability to perform or complete feeding activities.

Outcome: NUTRITIONAL STATUS

MAJOR INTERVENTIONS	SUGGESTED INTERVENTIONS	OPTIONAL INTERVENTIONS

Feeding
Nutrition Management
Nutritional Counseling
Nutritional Monitoring
	Nutrition Therapy
	Self-Care Assistance:
	  Feeding
		Enteral Tube Feeding
		Gastrointestinal
		  Intubation
		Sustenance Support
		Teaching: Individual
		Total Parenteral
		  Nutrition (TPN)
		  Administration
		Weight Management

Outcome: NUTRITIONAL STATUS: FOOD & FLUID INTAKE

MAJOR INTERVENTIONS	SUGGESTED INTERVENTIONS	OPTIONAL INTERVENTIONS

Feeding
Nutritional Monitoring
	Bottle Feeding
	Fluid Management
	Fluid Monitoring
	Nutrition Management
	Self-Care Assistance:
	  Feeding
		Enteral Tube Feeding
		Intravenous (IV)
		  Therapy
		Oral Health Maintenance
		Swallowing Therapy
		Total Parenteral
		  Nutrition (TPN)
		  Administration
		Weight Management

Outcome: SELF-CARE: ACTIVITIES OF DAILY LIVING (ADL)

MAJOR INTERVENTIONS	SUGGESTED INTERVENTIONS	OPTIONAL INTERVENTIONS

Self-Care Assistance:
  Feeding
	Feeding
	Self-Care Assistance
		Energy Management
		Environmental
		  Management
		Exercise Promotion
		Exercise Therapy: Joint
		  Mobility
		Exercise Therapy:
		  Muscle Control
		Family Involvement
		  Promotion

Outcome: SELF-CARE: EATING

MAJOR INTERVENTIONS	SUGGESTED INTERVENTIONS	OPTIONAL INTERVENTIONS
Self-Care Assistance: Feeding	Environmental Management Feeding Nutrition Management Nutritional Monitoring Positioning Teaching: Prescribed Diet	Aspiration Precautions Family Involvement Promotion Oral Health Maintenance Pain Management Swallowing Therapy

Outcome: SWALLOWING STATUS

MAJOR INTERVENTIONS	SUGGESTED INTERVENTIONS	OPTIONAL INTERVENTIONS
Swallowing Therapy	Aspiration Precautions Feeding Nutritional Monitoring Positioning Self-Care Assistance: Feeding Teaching: Individual	Anxiety Reduction Enteral Tube Feeding Family Involvement Promotion Nutrition Management Oral Health Maintenance Total Parenteral Nutrition (TPN) Administration

Nursing Diagnosis: SELF-CARE DEFICIT: TOILETING

DEFINITION: An impaired ability to perform or complete own toileting activities.

Outcome: SELF-CARE: ACTIVITIES OF DAILY LIVING (ADL)

MAJOR INTERVENTIONS	SUGGESTED INTERVENTIONS	OPTIONAL INTERVENTIONS
Self-Care Assistance: Toileting	Energy Management Environmental Management Self-Care Assistance	Exercise Promotion Exercise Promotion: Stretching Exercise Therapy: Ambulation Exercise Therapy: Balance Exercise Therapy: Joint Mobility Exercise Therapy: Muscle Control Fall Prevention

Outcome: SELF-CARE: HYGIENE

MAJOR INTERVENTIONS	SUGGESTED INTERVENTIONS	OPTIONAL INTERVENTIONS
Self-Care Assistance: Bathing/Hygiene	Bathing Patient Contracting Perineal Care Self-Care Assistance: Toileting Teaching: Individual	Bowel Irrigation Ostomy Care Skin Surveillance

Outcome: SELF-CARE: TOILETING

MAJOR INTERVENTIONS	SUGGESTED INTERVENTIONS	OPTIONAL INTERVENTIONS
Bowel Training Self-Care Assistance: Toileting	Bowel Incontinence Care: Encopresis Bowel Management Urinary Elimination Management	Bowel Irrigation Constipation/Impaction Management Ostomy Care Perineal Care Skin Surveillance Urinary Incontinence Care

Nursing Diagnosis: SELF-ESTEEM, CHRONIC LOW

Definition: Long standing negative self-evaluation/feelings about self or self-capabilities.

Outcome: DEPRESSION LEVEL

MAJOR INTERVENTIONS	SUGGESTED INTERVENTIONS	OPTIONAL INTERVENTIONS

Hope Instillation
Mood Management
	Behavior Management:
	  Self-Harm
	Counseling
	Emotional Support
	Grief Work Facilitation
	Guilt Work Facilitation
	Milieu Therapy
	Self-Awareness
	  Enhancement
	Self-Esteem
	  Enhancement
	Self-Modification
	  Assistance
	Support Group
	Therapy Group
		Crisis Intervention
		Spiritual Support
		Substance Use
		  Prevention
		Support System
		  Enhancement
		Therapeutic Play

Outcome: QUALITY OF LIFE

MAJOR INTERVENTIONS	SUGGESTED INTERVENTIONS	OPTIONAL INTERVENTIONS

Self-Esteem
  Enhancement
Values Clarification
	Active Listening
	Body Image
	  Enhancement
	Coping Enhancement
	Counseling
	Decision-Making
	  Support
	Emotional Support
	Hope Instillation
	Role Enhancement
	Security Enhancement
	Self-Awareness
	  Enhancement
	Socialization
	  Enhancement
	Spiritual Support
	Support System
	  Enhancement
		Anxiety Reduction
		Culture Brokerage
		Genetic Counseling
		Grief Work Facilitation
		Guilt Work Facilitation
		Mood Management
		Support Group

Continued

Outcome: **SELF-ESTEEM**

MAJOR INTERVENTIONS	SUGGESTED INTERVENTIONS	OPTIONAL INTERVENTIONS
Self-Esteem Enhancement	Body Image Enhancement Cognitive Restructuring Counseling Developmental Enhancement: Child Emotional Support Resiliency Promotion Self-Awareness Enhancement Socialization Enhancement Support System Enhancement	Active Listening Assertiveness Training Complex Relationship Building Coping Enhancement Eating Disorders Management Family Mobilization Role Enhancement Security Enhancement Self-Modification Assistance Spiritual Support Substance Use Prevention Suicide Prevention Support Group Weight Management

Nursing Diagnosis: **Self-Esteem Disturbance**

Definition: Negative self-evaluation/feelings about self or self-capabilities, which may be directly or indirectly expressed.

Outcome: **Child Development: 4 Years**

MAJOR INTERVENTIONS	SUGGESTED INTERVENTIONS	OPTIONAL INTERVENTIONS
Developmental Enhancement: Child Parent Education: Childrearing Family Risk Identification	Abuse Protection Support: Child Bowel Incontinence Care: Encopresis Family Integrity Promotion Security Enhancement Socialization Enhancement Support System Enhancement Teaching: Psychomotor Skill Urinary Habit Training Urinary Incontinence Care: Enuresis	Behavior Management Behavior Management: Overactivity/ Inattention Family Process Maintenance Family Support Family Therapy Health System Guidance Parenting Promotion Sibling Support Sleep Enhancement Sustenance Support Therapeutic Play

Outcome: **Child Development: 5 Years**

MAJOR INTERVENTIONS	SUGGESTED INTERVENTIONS	OPTIONAL INTERVENTIONS
Developmental Enhancement: Child Parent Education: Childrearing Family Risk Identification	Abuse Protection Support: Child Family Integrity Promotion Family Involvement Promotion Security Enhancement Socialization Enhancement Support System Enhancement Teaching: Psychomotor Skill	Behavior Management Behavior Management: Overactivity/ Inattention Family Process Maintenance Family Support Family Therapy Health System Guidance Parenting Promotion Sibling Support Sleep Enhancement Sustenance Support Therapeutic Play Urinary Habit Training Urinary Incontinence Care: Enuresis

Continued

Outcome: CHILD DEVELOPMENT: MIDDLE CHILDHOOD (6-11 YEARS)

MAJOR INTERVENTIONS	SUGGESTED INTERVENTIONS	OPTIONAL INTERVENTIONS
Developmental Enhancement: Child Risk Identification	Abuse Protection Support: Child Body Image Enhancement Exercise Promotion Family Integrity Promotion Family Involvement Promotion Learning Facilitation Mutual Goal Setting Nutritional Monitoring Patient Contracting Self-Awareness Enhancement Self-Esteem Enhancement Self-Modification Assistance Self-Responsibility Facilitation Socialization Enhancement Spiritual Support Substance Use Prevention Teaching: Individual Teaching: Sexuality Values Clarification	Behavior Management Behavior Modification Family Process Maintenance Family Support Family Therapy Health System Guidance Parenting Promotion Sibling Support Therapeutic Play Weight Management

Outcome: CHILD DEVELOPMENT: ADOLESCENCE (12-17 YEARS)

MAJOR INTERVENTIONS	SUGGESTED INTERVENTIONS	OPTIONAL INTERVENTIONS
Developmental Enhancement: Adolescent	Abuse Protection Support	Behavior Management
Parent Education: Adolescent	Anticipatory Guidance	Behavior Modification
Self-Esteem Enhancement	Body Image Enhancement	Bibliotherapy
Self-Responsibility Facilitation	Exercise Promotion	Counseling
	Family Integrity Promotion	Eating Disorders Management
	Family Involvement Promotion	Family Process Maintenance
	Health System Guidance	Family Support
	Mutual Goal Setting	Family Therapy
	Risk Identification	Parenting Promotion
	Role Enhancement	Sexual Counseling
	Self-Awareness Enhancement	Sibling Support
	Self-Modification Assistance	Support System Enhancement
	Socialization Enhancement	Sustenance Support
	Spiritual Support	Weight Management
	Substance Use Prevention	
	Teaching: Individual	
	Teaching: Safe Sex	
	Teaching: Sexuality	
	Values Clarification	

Continued

Outcome: DEPRESSION LEVEL

MAJOR INTERVENTIONS	SUGGESTED INTERVENTIONS	OPTIONAL INTERVENTIONS

Hope Instillation
Mood Management
	Behavior Management:
	  Self-Harm
	Counseling
	Emotional Support
	Grief Work Facilitation
	Guilt Work Facilitation
	Milieu Therapy
	Self-Awareness
	  Enhancement
	Self-Esteem
	  Enhancement
	Self-Modification
	  Assistance
	Support Group
	Therapy Group
		Crisis Intervention
		Spiritual Support
		Substance Use
		  Prevention
		Support System
		  Enhancement
		Therapeutic Play

Outcome: QUALITY OF LIFE

MAJOR INTERVENTIONS	SUGGESTED INTERVENTIONS	OPTIONAL INTERVENTIONS

Self-Esteem
  Enhancement
Values Clarification
	Active Listening
	Body Image
	  Enhancement
	Coping Enhancement
	Counseling
	Decision-Making
	  Support
	Emotional Support
	Hope Instillation
	Role Enhancement
	Security Enhancement
	Self-Awareness
	  Enhancement
	Socialization
	  Enhancement
	Spiritual Support
	Support System
	  Enhancement
		Anxiety Reduction
		Culture Brokerage
		Genetic Counseling
		Grief Work Facilitation
		Guilt Work Facilitation
		Mood Management
		Support Group

Outcome: SELF-ESTEEM

MAJOR INTERVENTIONS	SUGGESTED INTERVENTIONS	OPTIONAL INTERVENTIONS
Self-Esteem Enhancement	Body Image Enhancement Cognitive Restructuring Counseling Developmental Enhancement: Adolescent Developmental Enhancement: Child Emotional Support Mood Management Resiliency Promotion Self-Awareness Enhancement Socialization Enhancement Substance Use Prevention Substance Use Treatment Support Group Therapy Group Weight Management	Active Listening Animal-Assisted Therapy Assertiveness Training Complex Relationship Building Coping Enhancement Eating Disorders Management Family Mobilization Parent Education: Adolescent Parent Education: Childrearing Family Parenting Promotion Security Enhancement Self-Care Assistance Spiritual Support

Nursing Diagnosis: SELF-ESTEEM, SITUATIONAL LOW

DEFINITION: Negative self-evaluation/feelings about self that develop in response to a loss or change in an individual who previously had a positive self-evaluation.

Outcome: DECISION MAKING

MAJOR INTERVENTIONS	SUGGESTED INTERVENTIONS	OPTIONAL INTERVENTIONS
Decision-Making Support	Counseling Emotional Support Family Involvement Promotion Support System Enhancement	Culture Brokerage Family Support

Outcome: GRIEF RESOLUTION

MAJOR INTERVENTIONS	SUGGESTED INTERVENTIONS	OPTIONAL INTERVENTIONS
Grief Work Facilitation Grief Work Facilitation: Perinatal Death	Active Listening Coping Enhancement Counseling Emotional Support Hope Instillation Support Group	Animal-Assisted Therapy Bibliotherapy Decision-Making Support Guilt Work Facilitation Sibling Support Spiritual Support

Outcome: PSYCHOSOCIAL ADJUSTMENT: LIFE CHANGE

MAJOR INTERVENTIONS	SUGGESTED INTERVENTIONS	OPTIONAL INTERVENTIONS
Anticipatory Guidance Coping Enhancement	Body Image Enhancement Cognitive Restructuring Counseling Emotional Support Role Enhancement Self-Esteem Enhancement	Complex Relationship Building Decision-Making Support Developmental Enhancement: Adolescent Developmental Enhancement: Child

Outcome: SELF-ESTEEM

MAJOR INTERVENTIONS	SUGGESTED INTERVENTIONS	OPTIONAL INTERVENTIONS
Self-Esteem Enhancement	Active Listening Body Image Enhancement Cognitive Restructuring Coping Enhancement Counseling Developmental Enhancement: Adolescent Developmental Enhancement: Child Emotional Support Mood Management Self-Awareness Enhancement Socialization Enhancement Support Group	Assertiveness Training Behavior Modification Behavior Modification: Social Skills Bibliotherapy Complex Relationship Building Eating Disorders Management Grief Work Facilitation Guilt Work Facilitation Role Enhancement Security Enhancement Self-Care Assistance Self-Modification Assistance Spiritual Support Weight Management

Nursing Diagnosis: SENSORY/PERCEPTUAL ALTERATIONS: AUDITORY

Dᴇꜰɪɴɪᴛɪᴏɴ: A state in which an individual experiences a change in the amount or patterning of incoming stimuli accompanied by a diminished, exaggerated, distorted or impaired response to such stimuli.

Outcome: COGNITIVE ORIENTATION

MAJOR INTERVENTIONS	SUGGESTED INTERVENTIONS	OPTIONAL INTERVENTIONS
Cognitive Stimulation Reality Orientation	Cerebral Perfusion Promotion Cognitive Restructuring Communication Enhancement: Hearing Deficit Communication Enhancement: Speech Deficit Delirium Management Delusion Management Dementia Management Hallucination Management Medication Management	Activity Therapy Environmental Management Neurologic Monitoring Sleep Enhancement Surveillance: Safety

Outcome: COMMUNICATION: RECEPTIVE ABILITY

MAJOR INTERVENTIONS	SUGGESTED INTERVENTIONS	OPTIONAL INTERVENTIONS
Communication Enhancement: Hearing Deficit	Active Listening Communication Enhancement: Speech Deficit Learning Readiness Enhancement	Cognitive Stimulation Ear Care Environmental Management Reality Orientation

Outcome: DISTORTED THOUGHT CONTROL

MAJOR INTERVENTIONS	SUGGESTED INTERVENTIONS	OPTIONAL INTERVENTIONS

Delusion Management
Hallucination
  Management
	Anxiety Reduction
	Cognitive Restructuring
	Delirium Management
	Dementia Management
	Medication Management
	Milieu Therapy
	Reality Orientation
	Therapy Group
		Active Listening
		Activity Therapy
		Animal-Assisted
		  Therapy
		Cognitive Stimulation
		Communication
		  Enhancement: Hearing
		  Deficit
		Communication
		  Enhancement: Speech
		  Deficit
		Environmental
		  Management

Outcome: HEARING COMPENSATION BEHAVIOR

MAJOR INTERVENTIONS	SUGGESTED INTERVENTIONS	OPTIONAL INTERVENTIONS

Communication
  Enhancement:
  Hearing Deficit
	Cognitive Stimulation
	Communication
	  Enhancement: Speech
	  Deficit
	Ear Care
	Emotional Support
	Environmental
	  Management
	Exercise Therapy:
	  Balance
	Medication
	  Administration: Ear
	Positioning
		Activity Therapy
		Fall Prevention
		Fluid Management
		Self-Esteem
		  Enhancement
		Sleep Enhancement

Nursing Diagnosis: SENSORY/PERCEPTUAL ALTERATIONS: GUSTATORY

DEFINITION: A state in which an individual experiences a change in the amount or patterning of incoming stimuli accompanied by a diminished, exaggerated, distorted or impaired response to such stimuli.

Outcome: COGNITIVE ORIENTATION

MAJOR INTERVENTIONS	SUGGESTED INTERVENTIONS	OPTIONAL INTERVENTIONS
Reality Orientation	Cognitive Stimulation Delirium Management Delusion Management Dementia Management Hallucination Management Medication Management	Environmental Management Neurologic Monitoring Substance Use Treatment

Outcome: DISTORTED THOUGHT CONTROL

MAJOR INTERVENTIONS	SUGGESTED INTERVENTIONS	OPTIONAL INTERVENTIONS
Delusion Management Hallucination Management	Anxiety Reduction Dementia Management Medication Management Reality Orientation	Cognitive Stimulation Environmental Management

Outcome: NUTRITIONAL STATUS: FOOD & FLUID INTAKE

MAJOR INTERVENTIONS	SUGGESTED INTERVENTIONS	OPTIONAL INTERVENTIONS
Fluid Monitoring Nausea Management Nutritional Monitoring	Feeding Fluid Management Nutrition Management Self-Care Assistance: Feeding Vomiting Management	Bottle Feeding Medication Management Oral Health Restoration Swallowing Therapy Weight Gain Assistance Weight Management

Outcome: SENSORY FUNCTION: TASTE & SMELL

MAJOR INTERVENTIONS	SUGGESTED INTERVENTIONS	OPTIONAL INTERVENTIONS

Cognitive Stimulation
Nausea Management
Nutrition Management
	Cerebral Perfusion
	  Promotion
	Electrolyte Management
	Environmental
	  Management
	Feeding
	Fluid Management
	Fluid Monitoring
	Nutrition Management
	Vomiting Management
	Weight Management
		Medication Management
		Neurologic Monitoring
		Nutritional Monitoring
		Swallowing Therapy

Nursing Diagnosis: **SENSORY/PERCEPTUAL ALTERATIONS: KINESTHETIC**

DEFINITION: A state in which an individual experiences a change in the amount or patterning of incoming stimuli accompanied by a diminished, exaggerated, distorted or impaired response to such stimuli.

Outcome: **BALANCE**

MAJOR INTERVENTIONS	SUGGESTED INTERVENTIONS	OPTIONAL INTERVENTIONS
Exercise Therapy: Balance	Body Mechanics Promotion Energy Management Exercise Therapy: Ambulation Exercise Therapy: Joint Mobility Exercise Therapy: Muscle Control Fall Prevention Surveillance: Safety	Environmental Management: Safety Exercise Promotion Positioning Teaching: Prescribed Activity/Exercise

Outcome: **BODY POSITIONING: SELF-INITIATED**

MAJOR INTERVENTIONS	SUGGESTED INTERVENTIONS	OPTIONAL INTERVENTIONS
Body Mechanics Promotion Exercise Promotion: Strength Training	Exercise Promotion Exercise Promotion: Stretching Exercise Therapy: Ambulation Exercise Therapy: Balance Exercise Therapy: Joint Mobility Exercise Therapy: Muscle Control Self-Care Assistance Teaching: Prescribed Activity/Exercise	Energy Management Fall Prevention Pain Management Peripheral Sensation Management Positioning Self-Modification Assistance Unilateral Neglect Management

Outcome: COGNITIVE ORIENTATION

MAJOR INTERVENTIONS	SUGGESTED INTERVENTIONS	OPTIONAL INTERVENTIONS

Cognitive Stimulation
Reality Orientation
	Cognitive Restructuring
	Delirium Management
	Delusion Management
	Dementia Management
	Hallucination
	  Management
	Medication Management
		Animal-Assisted
		  Therapy
		Calming Technique
		Environmental
		  Management
		Neurologic Monitoring
		Substance Use Treatment
		Surveillance: Safety

Outcome: DISTORTED THOUGHT CONTROL

MAJOR INTERVENTIONS	SUGGESTED INTERVENTIONS	OPTIONAL INTERVENTIONS

Delusion Management
Hallucination
  Management
	Anxiety Reduction
	Cognitive Restructuring
	Delirium Management
	Dementia Management
	Medication Management
	Reality Orientation
	Therapy Group
		Active Listening
		Activity Therapy
		Animal-Assisted
		  Therapy
		Body Image
		  Enhancement
		Cognitive Stimulation
		Environmental
		  Management

Outcome: MUSCLE FUNCTION

MAJOR INTERVENTIONS	SUGGESTED INTERVENTIONS	OPTIONAL INTERVENTIONS

Body Mechanics
  Promotion
Exercise Promotion:
  Strength Training
	Cutaneous Stimulation
	Energy Management
	Exercise Promotion:
	  Stretching
	Exercise Therapy:
	  Balance
	Exercise Therapy:
	  Muscle Control
	Progressive Muscle
	  Relaxation
	Simple Massage
	Simple Relaxation
	  Therapy
		Exercise Promotion
		Exercise Therapy: Joint
		  Mobility
		Nutrition Management
		Pain Management
		Sleep Enhancement
		Teaching: Prescribed
		  Activity/Exercise

Continued

Outcome: NEUROLOGICAL STATUS: CENTRAL MOTOR CONTROL

MAJOR INTERVENTIONS	SUGGESTED INTERVENTIONS	OPTIONAL INTERVENTIONS
Neurologic Monitoring	Cerebral Profusion Promotion Electrolyte Management Electrolyte Monitoring Energy Management Environmental Management Exercise Promotion: Strength Training Exercise Promotion: Stretching Exercise Therapy: Balance Exercise Therapy: Muscle Control Medication Administration Medication Management Surveillance	Dysreflexia Management Exercise Therapy: Joint Mobility Surveillance: Safety

Outcome: SENSORY FUNCTION: PROPRIOCEPTION

MAJOR INTERVENTIONS	SUGGESTED INTERVENTIONS	OPTIONAL INTERVENTIONS
Body Mechanics Promotion	Activity Therapy Exercise Promotion Exercise Promotion: Strength Training Exercise Therapy: Ambulation Exercise Therapy: Balance Exercise Therapy: Muscle Control Positioning Neurologic Monitoring	Cerebral Perfusion Promotion Developmental Enhancement: Child Exercise Promotion: Stretching Fluid Management Fluid Monitoring

Nursing Diagnosis: SENSORY/PERCEPTUAL ALTERATIONS: OLFACTORY

DEFINITION: A state in which an individual experiences a change in the amount or patterning of incoming stimuli accompanied by a diminished, exaggerated, distorted or impaired response to such stimuli.

Outcome: COGNITIVE ORIENTATION

MAJOR INTERVENTIONS	SUGGESTED INTERVENTIONS	OPTIONAL INTERVENTIONS
Cognitive Stimulation Reality Orientation	Delirium Management Delusion Management Dementia Management Hallucination Management Medication Management	Environmental Management Neurologic Monitoring Substance Use Treatment

Outcome: DISTORTED THOUGHT CONTROL

MAJOR INTERVENTIONS	SUGGESTED INTERVENTIONS	OPTIONAL INTERVENTIONS
Delusion Management Hallucination Management	Anxiety Reduction Delirium Management Dementia Management Medication Management Reality Orientation	Cognitive Stimulation Environmental Management

Outcome: NUTRITIONAL STATUS: FOOD & FLUID INTAKE

MAJOR INTERVENTIONS	SUGGESTED INTERVENTIONS	OPTIONAL INTERVENTIONS
Nutrition Management	Environmental Management Feeding Fluid Management Fluid Monitoring Nausea Management Nutritional Monitoring Vomiting Management	Bottle Feeding Medication Management Oral Health Restoration Weight Management

Continued

Outcome: SENSORY FUNCTION: TASTE & SMELL

MAJOR INTERVENTIONS	SUGGESTED INTERVENTIONS	OPTIONAL INTERVENTIONS
Cognitive Stimulation Nutrition Management	Cerebral Perfusion Promotion Environmental Management Feeding Nausea Management Nutritional Monitoring Weight Management	Fluid Management Fluid Monitoring Medication Management Neurologic Monitoring

Nursing Diagnosis: SENSORY/PERCEPTUAL ALTERATIONS: TACTILE

DEFINITION: A state in which an individual experiences a change in the amount or patterning of incoming stimuli accompanied by a diminished, exaggerated, distorted or impaired response to such stimuli.

Outcome: COGNITIVE ORIENTATION

MAJOR INTERVENTIONS	SUGGESTED INTERVENTIONS	OPTIONAL INTERVENTIONS
Cognitive Stimulation Reality Orientation	Delirium Management Delusion Management Dementia Management Hallucination Management Medication Management	Environmental Management Neurologic Monitoring Substance Use Treatment

Outcome: DISTORTED THOUGHT CONTROL

MAJOR INTERVENTIONS	SUGGESTED INTERVENTIONS	OPTIONAL INTERVENTIONS
Delusion Management Hallucination Management	Anxiety Reduction Delirium Management Dementia Management Medication Management Reality Orientation Sleep Enhancement Therapy Group	Active Listening Activity Therapy Body Image Enhancement Cognitive Stimulation Environmental Management

Outcome: NEUROLOGICAL STATUS: SPINAL SENSORY/MOTOR FUNCTION

MAJOR INTERVENTIONS	SUGGESTED INTERVENTIONS	OPTIONAL INTERVENTIONS
Environmental Management: Safety Peripheral Sensation Management	Dysreflexia Management Electrolyte Monitoring Laboratory Data Interpretation Medication Administration Medication Management Neurologic Monitoring Pressure Ulcer Prevention Traction/Immobilization Care Skin Surveillance Surveillance	Exercise Promotion: Stretching Exercise Therapy; Ambulation Exercise Therapy: Balance Risk Identification Skin Care: Topical Treatments Splinting

Continued

Outcome: Sᴇɴsᴏʀʏ Fᴜɴᴄᴛɪᴏɴ: Cᴜᴛᴀɴᴇᴏᴜs

MAJOR INTERVENTIONS	SUGGESTED INTERVENTIONS	OPTIONAL INTERVENTIONS
Peripheral Sensation Management Surveillance: Safety	Cutaneous Stimulation Electrolyte Management Environmental Management Neurologic Monitoring Pain Management Positioning Pressure Management Skin Surveillance Touch	Cerebral Perfusion Promotion Emotional Support Exercise Therapy: Ambulation Exercise Therapy: Balance Medication Management Prosthesis Care Transcutaneous Electrical Nerve Stimulation (TENS)

Nursing Diagnosis: SENSORY/PERCEPTUAL ALTERATIONS: VISUAL

DEFINITION: A state in which an individual experiences a change in the amount or patterning of incoming stimuli accompanied by a diminished, exaggerated, distorted or impaired response to such stimuli.

Outcome: BODY IMAGE

MAJOR INTERVENTIONS	SUGGESTED INTERVENTIONS	OPTIONAL INTERVENTIONS
Body Image Enhancement Self-Esteem Enhancement	Active Listening Anticipatory Guidance Development Enhancement: Adolescent Development Enhancement: Child Self-Awareness Enhancement Self-Care Assistance	Cognitive Restructuring Coping Enhancement Counseling Family Mobilization Grief Work Facilitation Normalization Promotion Self-Modification Assistance

Outcome: COGNITIVE ORIENTATION

MAJOR INTERVENTIONS	SUGGESTED INTERVENTIONS	OPTIONAL INTERVENTIONS
Cognitive Stimulation Reality Orientation	Cognitive Restructuring Communication Enhancement: Visual Deficit Delirium Management Delusion Management Dementia Management Hallucination Management Medication Management	Activity Therapy Environmental Management Neurologic Monitoring Reminiscence Therapy Substance Use Treatment Surveillance: Safety

Continued

Outcome: DISTORTED THOUGHT CONTROL

MAJOR INTERVENTIONS	SUGGESTED INTERVENTIONS	OPTIONAL INTERVENTIONS

Delusion Management
Hallucination
  Management
	Anxiety Reduction
	Cognitive Restructuring
	Delirium Management
	Dementia Management
	Medication Management
	Reality Orientation
		Activity Therapy
		Body Image
		  Enhancement
		Cognitive Stimulation
		Communication
		  Enhancement: Visual
		  Deficit
		Environmental
		  Management
		Music Therapy
		Recreation Therapy

Outcome: SENSORY FUNCTION: VISION

MAJOR INTERVENTIONS	SUGGESTED INTERVENTIONS	OPTIONAL INTERVENTIONS

Communication
  Enhancement: Visual
  Deficit
	Cerebral Perfusion
	  Promotion
	Cognitive Stimulation
	Environmental
	  Management
	Eye Care
	Medication
	  Administration: Eye
	Surveillance: Safety
		Cerebral Edema
		  Management
		Developmental
		  Enhancement: Child
		Emotional Support
		Neurologic Monitoring
		Medication Management
		Self-Esteem
		  Enhancement

Outcome: VISION COMPENSATION BEHAVIOR

MAJOR INTERVENTIONS	SUGGESTED INTERVENTIONS	OPTIONAL INTERVENTIONS

Communication
  Enhancement: Visual
  Deficit
Environmental
  Management
	Cognitive Restructuring
	Cognitive Stimulation
	Emotional Support
	Exercise Therapy:
	  Balance
	Fall Prevention
	Feeding
	Medication
	  Administration: Eye
	Positioning
	Surveillance: Safety
		Activity Therapy
		Exercise Therapy:
		  Ambulation
		Medication Management

Nursing Diagnosis: SEXUAL DYSFUNCTION

DEFINITION: The state in which an individual experiences a change in sexual function that is viewed as unsatisfying, unrewarding, inadequate.

Outcome: ABUSE RECOVERY: SEXUAL

MAJOR INTERVENTIONS	SUGGESTED INTERVENTIONS	OPTIONAL INTERVENTIONS
Abuse Protection Support Coping Enhancement Counseling Sexual Counseling	Abuse Protection Support: Child Abuse Protection Support: Domestic Partner Abuse Protection Support: Elder Active Listening Emotional Support Health System Guidance Self-Awareness Enhancement Self-Esteem Enhancement Teaching: Sexuality	Anxiety Reduction Behavior Management: Sexual Body Image Enhancement Decision-Making Support Family Therapy Guilt Work Facilitation Resiliency Promotion Role Enhancement Simple Relaxation Therapy Spiritual Support Substance Use Prevention Support Group Support System Enhancement Therapy Group

Outcome: PHYSICAL AGING STATUS

MAJOR INTERVENTIONS	SUGGESTED INTERVENTIONS	OPTIONAL INTERVENTIONS
Sexual Counseling	Emotional Support Exercise Promotion Mutual Goal Setting Self-Modification Assistance Substance Use Prevention Teaching: Sexuality	Behavior Modification Body Image Enhancement Energy Management Medication Management Substance Use Treatment

Continued

Outcome: RISK CONTROL: SEXUALLY TRANSMITTED DISEASES (STD)

MAJOR INTERVENTIONS	SUGGESTED INTERVENTIONS	OPTIONAL INTERVENTIONS
Behavior Modification	Active Listening	Assertiveness Training
Infection Protection	Anticipatory Guidance	Emotional Support
Risk Identification	Behavior Management:	Family Involvement
Teaching: Safe Sex	Sexual	Promotion
	Health Screening	Fertility Preservation
	Health System Guidance	Impulse Control Training
	Patient Contracting	Self-Esteem
	Self-Awareness	Enhancement
	Enhancement	Substance Use
	Self-Modification	Prevention
	Assistance	Substance Use Treatment
	Self-Responsibility	Support Group
	Facilitation	Support System
	Sexual Counseling	Enhancement
	Teaching: Sexuality	
	Values Clarification	

Outcome: SEXUAL FUNCTIONING

MAJOR INTERVENTIONS	SUGGESTED INTERVENTIONS	OPTIONAL INTERVENTIONS
Sexual Counseling	Behavior Management:	Circulatory Care:
	Sexual	Arterial Insufficiency
	Self-Awareness	Energy Management
	Enhancement	Family Planning:
	Self-Esteem	Contraception
	Enhancement	Family Planning:
	Self-Responsibility	Infertility
	Facilitation	Medication Management
	Teaching: Safe Sex	Reproductive
	Teaching: Sexuality	Technology
	Values Clarification	Management
		Substance Use Treatment

Nursing Diagnosis: SEXUALITY PATTERNS, ALTERED

DEFINITION: The state in which an individual expresses concern regarding his/her sexuality.

Outcome: ABUSE RECOVERY: SEXUAL

MAJOR INTERVENTIONS	SUGGESTED INTERVENTIONS	OPTIONAL INTERVENTIONS
Coping Enhancement Counseling	Active Listening Anger Control Assistance Anxiety Reduction Emotional Support Presence Self-Esteem Enhancement Sexual Counseling Teaching: Sexuality Therapy Group	Behavior Management: Sexual Body Image Enhancement Complex Relationship Building Decision-Making Support Guilt Work Facilitation Role Enhancement Self-Awareness Enhancement Socialization Enhancement Spiritual Support Suicide Prevention Support Group Support System Enhancement

Outcome: BODY IMAGE

MAJOR INTERVENTIONS	SUGGESTED INTERVENTIONS	OPTIONAL INTERVENTIONS
Body Image Enhancement	Active Listening Anticipatory Guidance Emotional Support Self-Awareness Enhancement Self-Esteem Enhancement Values Clarification	Cognitive Restructuring Coping Enhancement Counseling Postpartal Care Prenatal Care

Continued

Outcome: CHILD DEVELOPMENT: MIDDLE CHILDHOOD (6-11 YEARS)

MAJOR INTERVENTIONS	SUGGESTED INTERVENTIONS	OPTIONAL INTERVENTIONS
Developmental Enhancement: Child Parent Education: Childrearing Family	Anticipatory Guidance Body Image Enhancement Self-Awareness Enhancement Self-Esteem Enhancement Self-Responsibility Facilitation Socialization Enhancement Spiritual Support Substance Use Prevention Teaching: Safe Sex Teaching: Sexuality Values Clarification	Abuse Protection Support: Child Behavior Management Behavior Modification Counseling Health Education

Outcome: CHILD DEVELOPMENT: ADOLESCENCE (12-17 YEARS)

MAJOR INTERVENTIONS	SUGGESTED INTERVENTIONS	OPTIONAL INTERVENTIONS
Parent Education: Adolescent Self-Esteem Enhancement Self-Responsibility Facilitation	Anticipatory Guidance Behavior Management: Sexual Body Image Enhancement Role Enhancement Self-Awareness Enhancement Sexual Counseling Spiritual Support Teaching: Safe Sex Teaching: Sexuality Values Clarification	Counseling Health Education Socialization Enhancement Substance Use Prevention Support System Enhancement

Outcome: ROLE PERFORMANCE

MAJOR INTERVENTIONS	SUGGESTED INTERVENTIONS	OPTIONAL INTERVENTIONS
Family Planning: Contraception Role Enhancement Teaching: Safe Sex	Anticipatory Guidance Behavior Modification Childbirth Preparation Counseling Self-Awareness Enhancement Sexual Counseling Values Clarification	Active Listening Body Image Enhancement Health Education Pessary Management Self-Esteem Enhancement Support Group Support System Enhancement Teaching: Sexuality

Outcome: SELF-ESTEEM

MAJOR INTERVENTIONS	SUGGESTED INTERVENTIONS	OPTIONAL INTERVENTIONS
Self-Esteem Enhancement	Active Listening Body Image Enhancement Counseling Developmental Enhancement: Adolescent Developmental Enhancement: Child Self-Awareness Enhancement Socialization Enhancement Support Group	Assertiveness Training Complex Relationship Building Coping Enhancement Fertility Preservation

Continued

Outcome: Sexual Identity: Acceptance

MAJOR INTERVENTIONS	SUGGESTED INTERVENTIONS	OPTIONAL INTERVENTIONS
Sexual Counseling	Anxiety Reduction Body Image Enhancement Developmental Enhancement: Adolescent Role Enhancement Self-Awareness Enhancement Self-Esteem Enhancement Values Clarification	Anticipatory Guidance Behavior Management: Sexual Coping Enhancement Counseling Support System Enhancement Teaching: Sexuality

Nursing Diagnosis: SKIN INTEGRITY, IMPAIRED

DEFINITION: A state in which the individual has altered epidermis and/or dermis.

Outcome: TISSUE INTEGRITY: SKIN & MUCOUS MEMBRANES

MAJOR INTERVENTIONS	SUGGESTED INTERVENTIONS	OPTIONAL INTERVENTIONS
Pressure Management	Bathing	Amputation Care
Pressure Ulcer Care	Bed Rest Care	Cast Care: Maintenance
Skin Surveillance	Circulatory Care:	Diarrhea Management
	Arterial Insufficiency	Fluid/Electrolyte
	Circulatory Precautions	Management
	Cutaneous Stimulation	Incision Site Care
	Foot Care	Ostomy Care
	Infection Protection	Perineal Care
	Medication	Positioning:
	Administration: Skin	Intraoperative
	Medication Management	Positioning: Wheelchair
	Nutrition Management	Prosthesis Care
	Positioning	Self-Care Assistance:
	Pressure Ulcer	Bathing/Hygiene
	Prevention	Self-Care Assistance:
	Radiation Therapy	Toileting
	Management	Simple Massage
	Skin Care: Topical	Traction/Immobilization
	Treatments	Care
	Urinary Incontinence	Wound Irrigation
	Care	
	Wound Care	

Continued

Outcome: WOUND HEALING: PRIMARY INTENTION

MAJOR INTERVENTIONS	SUGGESTED INTERVENTIONS	OPTIONAL INTERVENTIONS
Incision Site Care Wound Care	Bleeding Reduction: Wound Circulatory Precautions Fluid/Electrolyte Management Infection Control: Intraoperative Infection Protection Medication Administration Medication Administration: Skin Nutrition Management Nutrition Therapy Skin Care: Topical Treatments Skin Surveillance Splinting Suturing Teaching: Procedure/Treatment Wound Care: Closed Drainage	Bathing Bed Rest Care Cesarean Section Care Perineal Care Teaching: Preoperative Teaching: Psychomotor Skill

Outcome: WOUND HEALING: SECONDARY INTENTION

MAJOR INTERVENTIONS	SUGGESTED INTERVENTIONS	OPTIONAL INTERVENTIONS

Pressure Ulcer Care
Wound Care
	Circulatory Care:
	  Arterial Insufficiency
	Circulatory Care: Venous
	  Insufficiency
	Circulatory Precautions
	Fluid Management
	Infection Control
	Infection Protection
	Medication
	  Administration
	Medication
	  Administration: Skin
	Nutrition Therapy
	Skin Care: Topical
	  Treatments
	Skin Surveillance
	Splinting
	Transcutaneous
	  Electrical Nerve
	  Stimulation (TENS)
	Wound Care: Closed
	  Drainage
	Wound Irrigation
		Bathing
		Cutaneous Stimulation
		Hyperglycemia
		  Management
		Leech Therapy
		Nutrition Management
		Positioning
		Teaching: Procedure/
		  Treatment
		Teaching: Psychomotor
		  Skill
		Total Parenteral
		  Nutrition (TPN)
		  Administration

Nursing Diagnosis: SLEEP DEPRIVATION

DEFINITION: Prolonged periods of time without sustained natural, periodic suspension of relative unconsciousness.

Outcome: REST

MAJOR INTERVENTIONS	SUGGESTED INTERVENTIONS	OPTIONAL INTERVENTIONS

Energy Management
Sleep Enhancement
	Autogenic Training
	Biofeedback
	Exercise Promotion
	Pain Management
	Simple Guided Imagery
	Simple Relaxation
	   Therapy
		Environmental
		   Management: Comfort
		Music Therapy
		Progressive Muscle
		   Relaxation
		Surveillance: Safety

Outcome: SLEEP

MAJOR INTERVENTIONS	SUGGESTED INTERVENTIONS	OPTIONAL INTERVENTIONS

Sleep Enhancement	Anxiety Reduction
	Coping Enhancement
	Energy Management
	Environmental
	   Management
	Environmental
	   Management: Comfort
	Medication Management
	Meditation Facilitation
	Pain Management
	Progressive Muscle
	   Relaxation
	Simple Guided Imagery
	Simple Massage
		Dementia Management
		Exercise Promotion
		Music Therapy
		Nausea Management
		Simple Relaxation
		   Therapy
		Urinary Incontinence
		   Care: Enuresis
		Vomiting Management

Outcome: SYMPTOM SEVERITY

MAJOR INTERVENTIONS	SUGGESTED INTERVENTIONS	OPTIONAL INTERVENTIONS

Sleep Enhancement	Anxiety Reduction
	Coping Enhancement
	Energy Management
	Medication
	   Administration
	Medication Management
	Pain Management
	Positioning
		Progressive Muscle
		   Relaxation
		Simple Guided Imagery
		Simple Massage
		Simple Relaxation
		   Therapy

Nursing Diagnosis: SLEEP PATTERN DISTURBANCE

DEFINITION: Time limited disruption of sleep (natural, periodic suspension of consciousness) amount and quality.

Outcome: REST

MAJOR INTERVENTIONS	SUGGESTED INTERVENTIONS	OPTIONAL INTERVENTIONS

Energy Management
Sleep Enhancement
	Autogenic Training
	Biofeedback
	Dementia Management
	Exercise Promotion
	Pain Management
	Respite Care
	Simple Guided Imagery
	Simple Relaxation
	   Therapy
		Anxiety Reduction
		Coping Enhancement
		Environmental
		   Management: Comfort
		Meditation Facilitation
		Music Therapy
		Progressive Muscle
		   Relaxation
		Self-Care Assistance

Outcome: SLEEP

MAJOR INTERVENTIONS	SUGGESTED INTERVENTIONS	OPTIONAL INTERVENTIONS

Sleep Enhancement	Calming Technique
	Energy Management
	Environmental
	   Management
	Environmental
	   Management: Comfort
	Exercise Promotion
	Medication
	   Administration
	Medication Management
	Medication Prescribing
	Music Therapy
	Pain Management
	Progressive Muscle
	   Relaxation
	Security Enhancement
	Simple Guided Therapy
	Simple Massage
	Simple Relaxation
	   Therapy
		Anxiety Reduction
		Autogenic Training
		Bathing
		Kangaroo Care
		Laboratory Data
		   Interpretation
		Meditation Facilitation
		Positioning
		Touch

Continued

Outcome: **WELL-BEING**

MAJOR INTERVENTIONS	SUGGESTED INTERVENTIONS	OPTIONAL INTERVENTIONS
Coping Enhancement Sleep Enhancement	Active Listening Developmental Enhancement: Adolescent Developmental Enhancement: Child Emotional Support Hope Instillation Meditation Facilitation Pain Management Security Enhancement Simple Guided Imagery Simple Relaxation Therapy	Abuse Protection Support Dying Care Energy Management Exercise Promotion Substance Use Prevention

Nursing Diagnosis: SOCIAL INTERACTION, IMPAIRED

DEFINITION: The state in which an individual participates in an insufficient or excessive quantity or ineffective quality of social exchange.

Outcome: CHILD DEVELOPMENT: MIDDLE CHILDHOOD (6-11 YEARS)

MAJOR INTERVENTIONS	SUGGESTED INTERVENTIONS	OPTIONAL INTERVENTIONS
Development Enhancement: Child	Anticipatory Guidance Behavior Management: Overactivity/ Inattention Behavior Modification: Social Skills Family Integrity Promotion Family Involvement Promotion Learning Facilitation Mutual Goal Setting Self-Awareness Enhancement Self-Esteem Enhancement Self-Modification Assistance Self-Responsibility Facilitation Socialization Enhancement Spiritual Support Substance Use Prevention Values Clarification	Abuse Protection Support: Child Behavior Management Behavior Modification Counseling Family Process Maintenance Family Support Family Therapy Therapeutic Play

Continued

Outcome: CHILD DEVELOPMENT: ADOLESCENCE (12-17 YEARS)

MAJOR INTERVENTIONS	SUGGESTED INTERVENTIONS	OPTIONAL INTERVENTIONS
Developmental Enhancement: Adolescent Self-Esteem Enhancement Socialization Enhancement	Anticipatory Guidance Behavior Management: Sexual Behavior Modification: Social Skills Family Integrity Promotion Family Involvement Promotion Mutual Goal Setting Role Enhancement Self-Awareness Enhancement Self-Responsibility Facilitation Spiritual Support Substance Use Prevention Values Clarification	Abuse Protection Support Behavior Management Behavior Modification Counseling Eating Disorders Management Family Process Maintenance Family Support Family Therapy Sexual Counseling Support System Enhancement

Outcome: FAMILY ENVIRONMENT: INTERNAL

MAJOR INTERVENTIONS	SUGGESTED INTERVENTIONS	OPTIONAL INTERVENTIONS
Family Integrity Promotion Family Process Maintenance	Abuse Protection Support: Child Abuse Protection Support: Domestic Partner Abuse Protection Support: Elder Counseling Family Support Resiliency Promotion	Attachment Promotion Behavior Management: Overactivity/ Inattention Caregiver Support Family Therapy Support System Enhancement

Outcome: PLAY PARTICIPATION

MAJOR INTERVENTIONS	SUGGESTED INTERVENTIONS	OPTIONAL INTERVENTIONS
Socialization Enhancement Therapeutic Play	Behavior Modification: Social Skills Normalization Promotion Recreation Therapy	Activity Therapy Anger Control Assistance Animal-Assisted Therapy Family Support Family Therapy

Outcome: SOCIAL INTERACTION SKILLS

MAJOR INTERVENTIONS	SUGGESTED INTERVENTIONS	OPTIONAL INTERVENTIONS
Behavior Modification: Social Skills Complex Relationship Building	Active Listening Assertiveness Training Behavior Management: Sexual Counseling Dementia Management Developmental Enhancement: Adolescent Developmental Enhancement: Child Family Integrity Promotion Family Process Maintenance Recreation Therapy Resiliency Promotion Role Enhancement Self-Awareness Enhancement Self-Esteem Enhancement Self-Responsibility Facilitation Support Group Support System Enhancement Therapy Group	Anger Control Assistance Anxiety Reduction Attachment Promotion Communication Enhancement: Hearing Deficit Communication Enhancement: Speech Deficit Coping Enhancement Family Therapy Humor Impulse Control Training Reality Orientation Reminiscence Therapy Visitation Facilitation

Continued

Outcome: **SOCIAL INVOLVEMENT**

MAJOR INTERVENTIONS	SUGGESTED INTERVENTIONS	OPTIONAL INTERVENTIONS
Socialization Enhancement	Activity Therapy Animal-Assisted Therapy Developmental Enhancement: Adolescent Developmental Enhancement: Child Recreation Therapy Reminiscence Therapy Self-Awareness Enhancement Self-Esteem Enhancement Self-Responsibility Facilitation Substance Use Treatment Therapeutic Play Values Clarification Visitation Facilitation	Active Listening Assertiveness Training Behavior Management Communication Enhancement: Hearing Deficit Communication Enhancement: Speech Deficit Complex Relationship Building Counseling Emotional Support Family Therapy Humor Milieu Therapy Mutual Goal Setting Normalization Promotion Pass Facilitation Presence Support Group Support System Enhancement

Nursing Diagnosis: SOCIAL ISOLATION

DEFINITION: Aloneness experienced by the individual and perceived as imposed by others and as a negative or threatened state.

Outcome: FAMILY ENVIRONMENT: INTERNAL

MAJOR INTERVENTIONS	SUGGESTED INTERVENTIONS	OPTIONAL INTERVENTIONS
Family Integrity Promotion	Abuse Protection Support: Child Abuse Protection Support: Domestic Partner Abuse Protection Support: Elder Behavior Modification: Social Skills Caregiver Support Counseling Family Process Maintenance Family Therapy Resiliency Promotion	Attachment Promotion Family Support Grief Work Facilitation: Perinatal Death Support System Enhancement

Outcome: LEISURE PARTICIPATION

MAJOR INTERVENTIONS	SUGGESTED INTERVENTIONS	OPTIONAL INTERVENTIONS
Recreation Therapy	Activity Therapy Animal-Assisted Therapy Socialization Enhancement Therapeutic Play	Art Therapy Bibliotherapy Music Therapy Reminiscence Therapy

Continued

Outcome: LONELINESS

MAJOR INTERVENTIONS	SUGGESTED INTERVENTIONS	OPTIONAL INTERVENTIONS
Socialization Enhancement Support System Enhancement	Active Listening Activity Therapy Animal-Assisted Therapy Complex Relationship Building Counseling Developmental Enhancement: Adolescent Developmental Enhancement: Child Emotional Support Family Support Hope Instillation Milieu Therapy Presence Self-Esteem Enhancement Spiritual Growth Facilitation Therapy Group Touch Visitation Facilitation	Abuse Protection Support: Child Abuse Protection Support: Domestic Partner Abuse Protection Support: Elder Bibliotherapy Communication Enhancement: Hearing Deficit Communication Enhancement: Speech Deficit Environmental Management Family Therapy Grief Work Facilitation Support Group

Outcome: MOOD EQUILIBRIUM

MAJOR INTERVENTIONS	SUGGESTED INTERVENTIONS	OPTIONAL INTERVENTIONS
Mood Management	Active Listening Coping Enhancement Counseling Emotional Support Grief Work Facilitation Guilt Work Facilitation Hope Instillation Medication Management Presence Self-Esteem Enhancement Spiritual Support Support System Enhancement Touch	Animal-Assisted Therapy Anxiety Reduction Art Therapy Bibliotherapy Environmental Management Exercise Promotion Family Support Humor Music Therapy Socialization Enhancement Support Group Therapeutic Play Therapy Group Visitation Facilitation

Outcome: PLAY PARTICIPATION

MAJOR INTERVENTIONS	SUGGESTED INTERVENTIONS	OPTIONAL INTERVENTIONS
Socialization Enhancement Therapeutic Play	Exercise Promotion Recreation Therapy	Activity Therapy Animal-Assisted Therapy Art Therapy Environmental Management Music Therapy

Outcome: SOCIAL INTERACTION SKILLS

MAJOR INTERVENTIONS	SUGGESTED INTERVENTIONS	OPTIONAL INTERVENTIONS
Behavior Modification: Social Skills Complex Relationship Building	Active Listening Counseling Developmental Enhancement: Adolescent Developmental Enhancement: Child Family Integrity Promotion Normalization Promotion Recreation Therapy Self-Awareness Enhancement Self-Esteem Enhancement Touch	Anger Control Assistance Anxiety Reduction Attachment Promotion Communication Enhancement: Hearing Deficit Communication Enhancement: Speech Deficit Coping Enhancement Family Therapy Humor Reminiscence Therapy Therapy Group Visitation Facilitation

Continued

Outcome: SOCIAL INVOLVEMENT

MAJOR INTERVENTIONS	SUGGESTED INTERVENTIONS	OPTIONAL INTERVENTIONS
Socialization Enhancement	Activity Therapy Animal-Assisted Therapy Complex Relationship Building Forgiveness Facilitation Pass Facilitation Recreation Therapy Reminiscence Therapy Self-Awareness Enhancement Self-Esteem Enhancement Therapeutic Play Visitation Facilitation	Active Listening Art Therapy Communication Enhancement: Hearing Deficit Communication Enhancement: Speech Deficit Counseling Culture Brokerage Developmental Enhancement: Adolescent Developmental Enhancement: Child Emotional Support Family Therapy Humor Milieu Therapy Mood Management Normalization Promotion Presence Support Group Support System Enhancement Urinary Elimination Management

Outcome: SOCIAL SUPPORT

MAJOR INTERVENTIONS	SUGGESTED INTERVENTIONS	OPTIONAL INTERVENTIONS
Family Involvement Promotion Support System Enhancement	Referral Socialization Enhancement Support Group Telephone Consultation	Caregiver Support Coping Enhancement Emotional Support Family Support Spiritual Support Therapy Group

Outcome: WELL-BEING

MAJOR INTERVENTIONS	SUGGESTED INTERVENTIONS	OPTIONAL INTERVENTIONS

Coping Enhancement
Self-Awareness
  Enhancement
	Active Listening
	Counseling
	Emotional Support
	Family Integrity
	  Promotion
	Family Support
	Hope Instillation
	Humor
	Security Enhancement
	Self-Esteem
	  Enhancement
	Socialization
	  Enhancement
	Spiritual Support
	Support System
	  Enhancement
	Values Clarification
	Visitation Facilitation
		Abuse Protection
		  Support
		Communication
		  Enhancement: Hearing
		  Deficit
		Communication
		  Enhancement: Speech
		  Deficit
		Communication
		  Enhancement: Visual
		  Deficit
		Dying Care
		Exercise Promotion
		Normalization
		  Promotion
		Pain Management
		Substance Use
		  Prevention
		Weight Management

Nursing Diagnosis: **SORROW, CHRONIC**

DEFINITION: A cyclical, recurring and potentially progressive pattern of pervasive sadness that is experienced (by a client [parent or caregiver, or individual with chronic illness or disability]) in response to continual loss, throughout the trajectory of an illness or disability.

Outcome: **ACCEPTANCE: HEALTH STATUS**

MAJOR INTERVENTIONS	SUGGESTED INTERVENTIONS	OPTIONAL INTERVENTIONS
Coping Enhancement Hope Instillation	Counseling Decision-Making Support Emotional Support Grief Work Facilitation Presence Resiliency Promotion Spiritual Support Support Group Values Clarification	Active Listening Genetic Counseling Grief Work Facilitation: Perinatal Death Normalization Promotion Risk Identification: Genetic Truth Telling

Outcome: **DEPRESSION CONTROL**

MAJOR INTERVENTIONS	SUGGESTED INTERVENTIONS	OPTIONAL INTERVENTIONS
Mood Management	Activity Therapy Behavior Management Exercise Promotion Medication Management Resiliency Promotion Self-Modification Assistance Sleep Enhancement	Grief Work Facilitation Guilt Work Facilitation Substance Use Prevention

Outcome: **DEPRESSION LEVEL**

MAJOR INTERVENTIONS	SUGGESTED INTERVENTIONS	OPTIONAL INTERVENTIONS
Hope Instillation Mood Management	Bibliotherapy Cognitive Restructuring Counseling Emotional Support Exercise Promotion Forgiveness Facilitation Grief Work Facilitation Guilt Work Facilitation Resiliency Promotion Self-Modification Assistance Sleep Enhancement Support Group	Activity Therapy Animal-Assisted Therapy Spiritual Support Substance Use Prevention Support System Enhancement

Outcome: GRIEF RESOLUTION

MAJOR INTERVENTIONS	SUGGESTED INTERVENTIONS	OPTIONAL INTERVENTIONS

Grief Work Facilitation	Active Listening
	Coping Enhancement
	Dying Care
	Emotional Support
	Hope Instillation
	Spiritual Support
	Support Group
		Animal-Assisted
		  Therapy
		Bibliotherapy
		Decision-Making
		  Support
		Forgiveness Facilitation
		Grief Work Facilitation:
		  Perinatal Death
		Guilt Work Facilitation
		Music Therapy
		Presence
		Visitation Facilitation

Outcome: HOPE

MAJOR INTERVENTIONS	SUGGESTED INTERVENTIONS	OPTIONAL INTERVENTIONS

Hope Instillation
Spiritual Support
	Coping Enhancement
	Emotional Support
	Resiliency Promotion
	Self-Awareness
	  Enhancement
	Support Group
	Support System
	  Enhancement
		Counseling
		Family Mobilization
		Forgiveness Facilitation
		Milieu Therapy
		Presence
		Touch

Outcome: MOOD EQUILIBRIUM

MAJOR INTERVENTIONS	SUGGESTED INTERVENTIONS	OPTIONAL INTERVENTIONS

Mood Management	Active Listening
	Coping Enhancement
	Counseling
	Emotional Support
	Grief Work Facilitation
	Hope Instillation
	Medication Management
	Presence
	Resiliency Promotion
	Socialization
	  Enhancement
	Spiritual Support
	Support Group
		Activity Therapy
		Anger Control
		  Assistance
		Animal-Assisted
		  Therapy
		Bibliotherapy
		Exercise Promotion
		Family Support
		Forgiveness Facilitation
		Humor
		Meditation Facilitation
		Music Therapy
		Sleep Enhancement
		Support System
		  Enhancement

Nursing Diagnosis: SPIRITUAL DISTRESS (DISTRESS OF THE HUMAN SPIRIT)

Definition: Disruption in the life principle that pervades a person's entire being and that integrates and transcends one's biological and psychosocial nature.

Outcome: DIGNIFIED DYING

MAJOR INTERVENTIONS	SUGGESTED INTERVENTIONS	OPTIONAL INTERVENTIONS

Dying Care
Spiritual Growth
  Facilitation
Spiritual Support
	Active Listening
	Anticipatory Guidance
	Anxiety Reduction
	Bibliotherapy
	Coping Enhancement
	Counseling
	Decision-Making
	  Support
	Emotional Support
	Family Involvement
	  Promotion
	Forgiveness Facilitation
	Grief Work Facilitation
	Guilt Work Facilitation
	Hope Instillation
	Presence
	Reminiscence Therapy
	Resiliency Promotion
	Security Enhancement
	Support System
	  Enhancement
	Touch
	Truth Telling
	Values Clarification
		Anger Control
		  Assistance
		Animal-Assisted
		  Therapy
		Caregiver Support
		Culture Brokerage
		Meditation Facilitation
		Music Therapy
		Referral
		Self-Awareness
		  Enhancement

Outcome: HOPE

MAJOR INTERVENTIONS	SUGGESTED INTERVENTIONS	OPTIONAL INTERVENTIONS

Hope Instillation
Spiritual Growth
  Facilitation
Spiritual Support
	Coping Enhancement
	Emotional Support
	Self-Awareness
	  Enhancement
	Support Group
	Support System
	  Enhancement
	Values Clarification
		Counseling
		Family Support
		Milieu Therapy
		Presence
		Touch

Outcome: SPIRITUAL WELL-BEING

MAJOR INTERVENTIONS	SUGGESTED INTERVENTIONS	OPTIONAL INTERVENTIONS
Spiritual Growth Facilitation Spiritual Support	Emotional Support Forgiveness Facilitation Grief Work Facilitation Guilt Work Facilitation Hope Instillation Meditation Facilitation Self-Awareness Enhancement Support Group Values Clarification	Abuse Protection Support: Religious Art Therapy Bibliotherapy Counseling Dying Care Family Support Music Therapy Referral Religious Addiction Prevention Self-Esteem Enhancement Socialization Enhancement Support System Enhancement Touch

Nursing Diagnosis: SPIRITUAL WELL-BEING, POTENTIAL FOR ENHANCED

DEFINITION: Spiritual well-being is the process of an individual's developing/unfolding of mystery through harmonious interconnectedness that springs from inner strengths.

Outcome: HOPE

MAJOR INTERVENTIONS	SUGGESTED INTERVENTIONS	OPTIONAL INTERVENTIONS

Hope Installation
Spiritual Growth
   Facilitation
Spiritual Support
	Coping Enhancement
	Emotional Support
	Self-Awareness
	   Enhancement
	Self-Esteem
	   Enhancement
	Support Group
	Values Clarification
		Counseling
		Family Support
		Presence
		Touch

Outcome: QUALITY OF LIFE

MAJOR INTERVENTIONS	SUGGESTED INTERVENTIONS	OPTIONAL INTERVENTIONS

Values Clarification	Active Listening
	Coping Enhancement
	Emotional Support
	Family Support
	Hope Installation
	Humor
	Role Enhancement
	Self-Awareness
	   Enhancement
	Self-Esteem
	   Enhancement
	Self-Responsibility
	   Facilitation
	Spiritual Support
		Body Image
		   Enhancement
		Culture Brokerage
		Reminiscence Therapy
		Support Group

Outcome: SPIRITUAL WELL-BEING

MAJOR INTERVENTIONS	SUGGESTED INTERVENTIONS	OPTIONAL INTERVENTIONS
Spiritual Growth Facilitation Spiritual Support	Bibliotherapy Hope Instillation Meditation Facilitation Religious Ritual Enhancement Resiliency Promotion Self-Awareness Enhancement Self-Esteem Enhancement Self-Modification Assistance Support Group Values Clarification	Autogenic Training Counseling Family Support Music Therapy Religious Addiction Prevention Touch

Outcome: WELL-BEING

MAJOR INTERVENTIONS	SUGGESTED INTERVENTIONS	OPTIONAL INTERVENTIONS
Self-Awareness Enhancement Self-Esteem Enhancement Spiritual Growth Facilitation Spiritual Support	Active Listening Coping Enhancement Counseling Hope Instillation Meditation Facilitation Religious Ritual Enhancement Resiliency Promotion Role Enhancement Self-Modification Assistance Self-Responsibility Facilitation Values Clarification	Autogenic Training Bibliotherapy Family Support Simple Guided Imagery

Nursing Diagnosis: SURGICAL RECOVERY, DELAYED

DEFINITION: An extension of the number of postoperative days required for individuals to initiate and perform on their own behalf activities that maintain life, health, and well-being.

Outcome: ENDURANCE

MAJOR INTERVENTIONS	SUGGESTED INTERVENTIONS	OPTIONAL INTERVENTIONS
Energy Management	Exercise Promotion Exercise Promotion: Strength Training Nutrition Management Sleep Enhancement	Environmental Management Environmental Management: Comfort Exercise Therapy: Ambulation Exercise Therapy: Joint Mobility Exercise Therapy: Muscle Control Self-Care Assistance

Outcome: IMMOBILITY CONSEQUENCES: PHYSIOLOGICAL

MAJOR INTERVENTIONS	SUGGESTED INTERVENTIONS	OPTIONAL INTERVENTIONS
Bed Rest Care	Bowel Management Case Management Circulatory Precautions Constipation/Impaction Management Cough Enhancement Embolus Precautions Exercise Promotion: Stretching Exercise Therapy: Ambulation Exercise Therapy: Joint Mobility Flatulence Reduction Positioning Simple Massage Skin Surveillance Teaching: Prescribed Activity/Exercise Urinary Elimination Management Urinary Retention Care	Airway Management Aspiration Precautions Discharge Planning Environmental Management: Home Preparation Feeding Insurance Authorization Oral Health Maintenance Respiratory Monitoring

Outcome: NUTRITIONAL STATUS

MAJOR INTERVENTIONS	SUGGESTED INTERVENTIONS	OPTIONAL INTERVENTIONS

Nutrition Management
Nutrition Therapy
Nutritional Monitoring
	Diet Staging
	Energy Management
	Enteral Tube Feeding
	Feeding
	Fluid/Electrolyte
	  Management
	Nausea Management
		Bottle Feeding
		Fluid Management
		Gastrointestinal
		  Intubation
		Intravenous (IV)
		  Therapy
		Self-Care Assistance:
		  Feeding
		Total Parenteral
		  Nutrition (TPN)
		  Administration
		Vomiting Management

Outcome: PAIN LEVEL

MAJOR INTERVENTIONS	SUGGESTED INTERVENTIONS	OPTIONAL INTERVENTIONS

Pain Management	Analgesic
	  Administration
	Analgesic
	  Administration:
	  Intraspinal
	Environmental
	  Management: Comfort
	Medication
	  Administration
	Medication Management
	Positioning
	Sleep Enhancement
	Splinting
	Surveillance
	Transcutaneous
	  Electrical Nerve
	  Stimulation (TENS)
	Vital Signs Monitoring
		Energy Management
		Music Therapy
		Simple Massage

Continued

Outcome: SELF-CARE: ACTIVITIES OF DAILY LIVING (ADL)

MAJOR INTERVENTIONS	SUGGESTED INTERVENTIONS	OPTIONAL INTERVENTIONS

Self-Care Assistance	Energy Management
	Exercise Therapy:
	  Ambulation
	Self-Care Assistance:
	  Bathing/Hygiene
	Self-Care Assistance:
	  Dressing/Grooming
	Self-Care Assistance:
	  Feeding
	Self-Care Assistance:
	  Toileting
		Caregiver Support
		Discharge Planning
		Environmental
		  Management: Home
		  Preparation
		Environmental
		  Management: Safety
		Exercise Promotion
		Exercise Therapy: Joint
		  Mobility
		Fall Prevention
		Health Care Information
		  Exchange
		Health System Guidance
		Home Maintenance
		  Assistance
		Multidisciplinary Care
		  Conference
		Telephone Consultation

Outcome: WOUND HEALING: PRIMARY INTENTION

MAJOR INTERVENTIONS	SUGGESTED INTERVENTIONS	OPTIONAL INTERVENTIONS

Incision Site Care
Nutrition Management
Wound Care
	Circulatory Precautions
	Fever Treatment
	Fluid Management
	Infection Control
	Infection Control:
	  Intraoperative
	Infection Protection
	Medication
	  Administration
	Nutrition Therapy
	Skin Surveillance
	Splinting
	Temperature Regulation
	Wound Care: Closed
	  Drainage
		Bathing
		Bed Rest Care
		Cesarean Section Care
		Hyperglycemia
		  Management
		Perineal Care
		Wound Irrigation

Nursing Diagnosis: SWALLOWING, IMPAIRED

DEFINITION: Abnormal functioning of the swallowing mechanism associated with deficits in oral, pharyngeal, or esophageal structure or function.

Outcome: ASPIRATION CONTROL

MAJOR INTERVENTIONS	SUGGESTED INTERVENTIONS	OPTIONAL INTERVENTIONS
Aspiration Precautions	Airway Management Airway Suctioning Positioning Risk Identification Surveillance Swallowing Therapy	Anxiety Reduction Cough Enhancement Enteral Tube Feeding

Outcome: SWALLOWING STATUS

MAJOR INTERVENTIONS	SUGGESTED INTERVENTIONS	OPTIONAL INTERVENTIONS
Aspiration Precautions Swallowing Therapy	Airway Suctioning Progressive Muscle Relaxation Surveillance	Anxiety Reduction Emotional Support Enteral Tube Feeding Feeding Medication Management Nutrition Management Positioning Referral

Outcome: SWALLOWING STATUS: ESOPHAGEAL PHASE

MAJOR INTERVENTIONS	SUGGESTED INTERVENTIONS	OPTIONAL INTERVENTIONS
Positioning	Anxiety Reduction Aspiration Precautions Progressive Muscle Relaxation Surveillance Swallowing Therapy	Airway Suctioning Enteral Tube Feeding

Continued

Outcome: SWALLOWING STATUS: ORAL PHASE

MAJOR INTERVENTIONS	SUGGESTED INTERVENTIONS	OPTIONAL INTERVENTIONS
Swallowing Therapy	Aspiration Precautions Feeding Positioning Self-Care Assistance: Feeding Surveillance	Oral Health Maintenance Oral Health Restoration Nutrition Management Nutrition Therapy

Outcome: SWALLOWING STATUS: PHARYNGEAL

MAJOR INTERVENTIONS	SUGGESTED INTERVENTIONS	OPTIONAL INTERVENTIONS
Aspiration Precautions Swallowing Therapy	Airway Suctioning Positioning Progressive Muscle Relaxation Surveillance	Anxiety Reduction Emotional Support Referral

Nursing Diagnosis: THERMOREGULATION, INEFFECTIVE

DEFINITION: The state in which the individual's temperature fluctuates between hypothermia and hyperthermia.

Outcome: THERMOREGULATION

MAJOR INTERVENTIONS	SUGGESTED INTERVENTIONS	OPTIONAL INTERVENTIONS
Temperature Regulation Temperature Regulation: Intraoperative	Environmental Management Fever Treatment Fluid Management Fluid Monitoring Heat Exposure Treatment Hypothermia Treatment Malignant Hyperthermia Precautions Medication Administration Vital Signs Monitoring	Bathing Emergency Care Hemodynamic Regulation Shock Management

Outcome: THERMOREGULATION: NEONATE

MAJOR INTERVENTIONS	SUGGESTED INTERVENTIONS	OPTIONAL INTERVENTIONS
Newborn Care Temperature Regulation	Environmental Management Fluid Management Fluid Monitoring Medication Administration Newborn Monitoring Vital Signs Monitoring	Acid-Base Management Bathing Dressing Fever Treatment Heat Exposure Treatment Hypoglycemia Management Hypothermia Treatment Phototherapy: Neonate

Nursing Diagnosis: THOUGHT PROCESSES, ALTERED

DEFINITION: A state in which an individual experiences a disruption in cognitive operations and activities.

Outcome: COGNITIVE ABILITY

MAJOR INTERVENTIONS	SUGGESTED INTERVENTIONS	OPTIONAL INTERVENTIONS
Cognitive Stimulation Dementia Management	Cognitive Restructuring Elopement Precautions Environmental Management Environmental Management: Safety Medication Management Memory Training Milieu Therapy Reminiscence Therapy	Active Listening Mood Management Patient Rights Protection Presence Reality Orientation

Outcome: COGNITIVE ORIENTATION

MAJOR INTERVENTIONS	SUGGESTED INTERVENTIONS	OPTIONAL INTERVENTIONS
Reality Orientation	Cognitive Restructuring Cognitive Stimulation Delirium Management Delusion Management Hallucination Management Medication Management Memory Training Surveillance	Animal-Assisted Therapy Calming Technique Environmental Management Milieu Therapy Neurologic Monitoring Reminiscence Therapy Substance Use Treatment

Outcome: CONCENTRATION

MAJOR INTERVENTIONS	SUGGESTED INTERVENTIONS	OPTIONAL INTERVENTIONS
Analgesic Administration Anxiety Reduction Cognitive Stimulation	Cerebral Perfusion Promotion Delirium Management Hallucination Management Hypoglycemia Management Medication Management Milieu Therapy Substance Use Treatment Touch	Active Listening Calming Technique Cognitive Restructuring Delusion Management Dementia Management Environmental Management Reality Orientation

Outcome: DECISION MAKING

MAJOR INTERVENTIONS	SUGGESTED INTERVENTIONS	OPTIONAL INTERVENTIONS
Decision-Making Support	Counseling Emotional Support Patient Rights Protection Support System Enhancement	Family Support Security Enhancement Self-Esteem Enhancement

Outcome: DISTORTED THOUGHT CONTROL

MAJOR INTERVENTIONS	SUGGESTED INTERVENTIONS	OPTIONAL INTERVENTIONS
Delusion Management Hallucination Management	Anxiety Reduction Behavior Management Cognitive Restructuring Delirium Management Dementia Management Elopement Precautions Environmental Management: Safety Medication Management Milieu Therapy Reality Orientation Surveillance: Safety Therapy Group	Active Listening Animal-Assisted Therapy Area Restriction Cognitive Stimulation Environmental Management Memory Training Music Therapy Recreation Therapy Sleep Enhancement

Outcome: IDENTITY

MAJOR INTERVENTIONS	SUGGESTED INTERVENTIONS	OPTIONAL INTERVENTIONS
Cognitive Restructuring Reality Orientation	Body Image Enhancement Counseling Developmental Enhancement: Adolescent Developmental Enhancement: Child Medication Management Self-Awareness Enhancement Self-Esteem Enhancement	Delirium Management Delusion Management Dementia Management Environmental Management: Violence Prevention Family Therapy Hallucination Management Milieu Therapy Therapy Group

Continued

Outcome: INFORMATION PROCESSING

MAJOR INTERVENTIONS	SUGGESTED INTERVENTIONS	OPTIONAL INTERVENTIONS

Cognitive Stimulation	Active Listening
	Calming Technique
	Medication Management
	Memory Training
	Reality Orientation
		Anxiety Reduction
		Cerebral Edema
		  Management
		Cerebral Perfusion
		  Promotion
		Cognitive Restructuring
		Delirium Management
		Delusion Management
		Dementia Management
		Environmental
		  Management
		Fluid/Electrolyte
		  Management
		Hallucination
		  Management
		Milieu Therapy
		Music Therapy
		Oxygen Therapy
		Pain Management
		Reminiscence Therapy
		Sleep Enhancement

Outcome: MEMORY

MAJOR INTERVENTIONS	SUGGESTED INTERVENTIONS	OPTIONAL INTERVENTIONS
Dementia Management Memory Training	Active Listening Cognitive Restructuring Cognitive Stimulation Elopement Precautions Environmental Management: Safety Learning Facilitation Milieu Therapy Reminiscence Therapy	Bibliotherapy Coping Enhancement Medication Management Patient Rights Protection Reality Orientation

Outcome: NEUROLOGICAL STATUS: CONSCIOUSNESS

MAJOR INTERVENTIONS	SUGGESTED INTERVENTIONS	OPTIONAL INTERVENTIONS
Cerebral Perfusion Promotion Environmental Management: Safety Neurologic Monitoring	Cerebral Edema Management Cognitive Stimulation Delirium Management Dementia Management Environmental Management Fluid Resuscitation Intracranial Pressure (ICP) Monitoring Medication Administration Medication Management Patient Rights Protection Surveillance Vital Signs Monitoring	Family Support Patient Rights Protection Physical Restraint Substance Use Treatment Substance Use Treatment: Alcohol Withdrawal Substance Use Treatment: Drug Withdrawal Substance Use Treatment: Overdose Temperature Regulation Therapeutic Touch Touch

Nursing Diagnosis: **Tissue Integrity, Impaired**

DEFINITION: A state in which an individual experiences damage to mucous membrane, corneal, integumentary, or subcutaneous tissue. It is a state in which an individual has altered body tissue.

Outcome: **Tissue Integrity: Skin & Mucous Membranes**

MAJOR INTERVENTIONS	SUGGESTED INTERVENTIONS	OPTIONAL INTERVENTIONS
Eye Care	Bleeding Reduction:	Allergy Management
Oral Health Maintenance	Gastrointestinal	Amputation Care
Pressure Ulcer	Bleeding Reduction:	Bathing
Prevention	Nasal	Blood Products
Wound Care	Bleeding Reduction:	Administration
	Postpartum Uterus	Diarrhea Management
	Chemotherapy	Fluid Management
	Management	Fluid Monitoring
	Circulatory Precautions	Medication Management
	Hemorrhage Control	Perineal Care
	Infection Protection	Pressure Ulcer Care
	Medication	Urinary Incontinence
	Administration: Ear	Care
	Medication	Urinary Incontinence
	Administration: Eye	Care: Enuresis
	Medication	Vital Signs Monitoring
	Administration: Rectal	
	Medication	
	Administration:	
	Vaginal	
	Nutrition Management	
	Oral Health Restoration	
	Pressure Management	
	Radiation Therapy	
	Management	
	Rectal Prolapse	
	Management	
	Simple Massage	

Outcome: WOUND HEALING: PRIMARY INTENTION

MAJOR INTERVENTIONS	SUGGESTED INTERVENTIONS	OPTIONAL INTERVENTIONS

Incision Site Care
Wound Care
	Circulatory Precautions
	Fluid Management
	Infection Control:
	  Intraoperative
	Infection Protection
	Medication
	  Administration
	Nutrition Management
	Splinting
	Suturing
	Wound Care: Closed
	  Drainage
		Cesarean Section Care
		Perineal Care

Outcome: WOUND HEALING: SECONDARY INTENTION

MAJOR INTERVENTIONS	SUGGESTED INTERVENTIONS	OPTIONAL INTERVENTIONS

Wound Care	Circulatory Care:
	  Arterial Insufficiency
	Circulatory Precautions
	Fluid Management
	Infection Control
	Infection Protection
	Medication
	  Administration
	Nutrition Management
	Splinting
	Transcutaneous
	  Electrical Nerve
	  Stimulation (TENS)
	Wound Care: Closed
	  Drainage
	Wound Irrigation
		Bathing
		Cutaneous Stimulation
		Leech Therapy
		Nutrition Management
		Pressure Ulcer Care
		Total Parenteral
		  Nutrition (TPN)
		  Administration

Nursing Diagnosis: TISSUE PERFUSION, ALTERED: CARDIOPULMONARY

DEFINITION: A decrease in oxygen resulting in the failure to nourish the tissues at the capillary level.

Outcome: CARDIAC PUMP EFFECTIVENESS

MAJOR INTERVENTIONS	SUGGESTED INTERVENTIONS	OPTIONAL INTERVENTIONS
Cardiac Care: Acute Dysrhythmia Management Hemodynamic Regulation Shock Management: Cardiac	Cardiac Care Cardiac Care: Rehabilitative Cardiac Precautions Circulatory Precautions Fluid Management Invasive Hemodynamic Monitoring Vital Signs Monitoring	Blood Products Administration Embolus Precautions Fluid Monitoring Resuscitation: Fetus Resuscitation: Neonate Shock Management Shock Prevention Temperature Regulation

Outcome: CIRCULATION STATUS

MAJOR INTERVENTIONS	SUGGESTED INTERVENTIONS	OPTIONAL INTERVENTIONS
Circulatory Care: Arterial Insufficiency Circulatory Care: Venous Insufficiency Circulatory Precautions	Bleeding Precautions Bleeding Reduction Blood Products Administration Cardiac Care: Acute Circulatory Care: Mechanical Assist Device Embolus Care: Peripheral Embolus Care: Pulmonary Embolus Precautions Fluid Management Fluid Monitoring Hemodynamic Regulation Hemorrhage Control Hypovolemia Management Medication Administration Shock Management: Cardiac Shock Management: Vasogenic Shock Prevention	Fluid Resuscitation Invasive Hemodynamic Monitoring Laboratory Data Interpretation Resuscitation Resuscitation: Fetus Resuscitation: Neonate

Outcome: TISSUE PERFUSION: CARDIAC

MAJOR INTERVENTIONS	SUGGESTED INTERVENTIONS	OPTIONAL INTERVENTIONS
Cardiac Care: Acute Hemodynamic Regulation Shock Management: Cardiac	Acid-Base Management Acid-Base Monitoring Cardiac Care Cardiac Precautions Circulatory Care: Arterial Insufficiency Circulatory Care: Mechanical Assist Device Circulatory Care: Venous Insufficiency Circulatory Precautions Dysrhythmia Management Electronic Fetal Monitoring: Intrapartum Fluid/Electrolyte Management Invasive Hemodynamic Monitoring Medication Administration Oxygen Therapy Respiratory Monitoring Resuscitation Resuscitation: Neonate Shock Management Shock Management: Vasogenic Technology Management Vital Signs Monitoring	Acid-Base Management: Metabolic Acidosis Acid-Base Management: Metabolic Alkalosis Acid-Base Management: Respiratory Acidosis Acid-Base Management: Respiratory Alkalosis Bedside Laboratory Testing Bleeding Reduction Blood Products Administration Code Management Embolus Precautions Emergency Care Fluid Management Fluid Monitoring Fluid Resuscitation Hemorrhage Control Laboratory Data Interpretation Medication Management Phlebotomy: Arterial Blood Sample Phlebotomy: Venous Blood Sample Resuscitation Smoking Cessation Assistance Substance Use Treatment

Continued

Outcome: Tissue Perfusion: Pulmonary

MAJOR INTERVENTIONS	SUGGESTED INTERVENTIONS	OPTIONAL INTERVENTIONS
Acid-Base Management: Respiratory Acidosis Acid-Base Management: Respiratory Alkalosis Embolus Care: Pulmonary Hemodynamic Regulation	Acid-Base Monitoring Cardiac Care: Acute Circulatory Care: Arterial Insufficiency Fluid Management Intravenous (IV) Therapy Invasive Hemodynamic Monitoring Medication Administration Medication Management Oxygen Therapy Respiratory Monitoring Vital Signs Monitoring	Electrolyte Management Emergency Care Hemorrhage Control Mechanical Ventilation Resuscitation Resuscitation: Fetus Shock Management Shock Prevention

Outcome: Vital Signs Status

MAJOR INTERVENTIONS	SUGGESTED INTERVENTIONS	OPTIONAL INTERVENTIONS
Hemodynamic Regulation Vital Signs Monitoring	Acid-Base Management Cardiac Care Circulatory Care: Arterial Insufficiency Circulatory Care: Venous Insufficiency Dysrhythmia Management Electrolyte Management Fluid Management Hypovolemia Management Intravenous (IV) Therapy Medication Administration Medication Management Respiratory Monitoring Shock Management Shock Prevention Surveillance Temperature Regulation	Blood Products Administration Emergency Care Hemorrhage Control Oxygen Therapy Pain Management Resuscitation

Nursing Diagnosis: TISSUE PERFUSION, ALTERED: CEREBRAL

DEFINITION: A decrease in oxygen resulting in the failure to nourish the tissues at the capillary level.

Outcome: CIRCULATION STATUS

MAJOR INTERVENTIONS	SUGGESTED INTERVENTIONS	OPTIONAL INTERVENTIONS
Cerebral Perfusion Promotion Circulatory Care: Arterial Insufficiency Circulatory Care: Venous Insufficiency	Bleeding Precautions Bleeding Reduction Circulatory Care: Mechanical Assist Device Embolus Care: Peripheral Embolus Precautions Fluid Monitoring Hemodynamic Regulation Hemorrhage Control Hypovolemia Management Laboratory Data Interpretation Shock Management Shock Prevention	Bedside Laboratory Testing Blood Products Administration Circulatory Precautions Fluid Resuscitation Intravenous (IV) Insertion Intravenous (IV) Therapy Invasive Hemodynamic Monitoring Phlebotomy: Arterial Blood Sample Phlebotomy: Venous Blood Sample Shock Management: Vasogenic Shock Management: Volume Subarachnoid Hemorrhage Precautions

Continued

Outcome: NEUROLOGICAL STATUS		
MAJOR INTERVENTIONS	**SUGGESTED INTERVENTIONS**	**OPTIONAL INTERVENTIONS**
Cerebral Perfusion Promotion Intracranial Pressure (ICP) Monitoring Neurologic Monitoring	Acid-Base Management Acid-Base Management: Metabolic Acidosis Acid-Base Management: Metabolic Alkalosis Acid-Base Management: Respiratory Acidosis Acid-Base Management: Respiratory Alkalosis Acid-Base Monitoring Bedside Laboratory Testing Cerebral Edema Management Code Management Electrolyte Management Electrolyte Monitoring Emergency Care Fluid Management Invasive Hemodynamic Monitoring Laboratory Data Interpretation Medication Administration Medication Management Oxygen Therapy Peripheral Sensation Management Positioning: Neurologic Respiratory Monitoring Resuscitation Seizure Management Seizure Precautions Subarachnoid Hemorrhage Precautions Surveillance Vital Signs Monitoring	Electronic Fetal Monitoring: Intrapartum Nutrition Management Pain Management Peripherally Inserted Central (PIC) Catheter Care Resuscitation: Fetus Resuscitation: Neonate

Outcome: TISSUE PERFUSION: CEREBRAL

MAJOR INTERVENTIONS	SUGGESTED INTERVENTIONS	OPTIONAL INTERVENTIONS
Cerebral Perfusion Promotion Intracranial Pressure (ICP) Management Neurologic Monitoring	Acid-Base Management Acid-Base Monitoring Bleeding Reduction Cerebral Edema Management Fluid Management Fluid Monitoring Fluid Resuscitation Hemorrhage Control Hypovolemia Management Medication Administration Medication Administration: Intravenous Medication Administration: Ventricular Reservoir Medication Management Oxygen Therapy Positioning Seizure Management Seizure Precautions Shock Management Subarachnoid Hemorrhage Precautions Surveillance Vital Signs Monitoring	Blood Products Administration Circulatory Care: Arterial Insufficiency Circulatory Care: Mechanical Assist Device Circulatory Care: Venous Insufficiency Circulatory Precautions Code Management Electrolyte Management Electrolyte Monitoring Embolus Precautions Emergency Care Phlebotomy: Arterial Blood Sample Phlebotomy: Venous Blood Sample Shock Management: Cardiac Shock Management: Vasogenic Shock Management: Volume Technology Management

Nursing Diagnosis: TISSUE PERFUSION, ALTERED: GASTROINTESTINAL

DEFINITION: A decrease in oxygen resulting in the failure to nourish the tissues at the capillary level.

Outcome: CIRCULATION STATUS

MAJOR INTERVENTIONS	SUGGESTED INTERVENTIONS	OPTIONAL INTERVENTIONS
Circulatory Care: Arterial Insufficiency Circulatory Care: Venous Insufficiency	Bleeding Precautions Bleeding Reduction: Gastrointestinal Fluid Monitoring Hemodynamic Regulation Hemorrhage Control Hypovolemia Management Laboratory Data Interpretation Shock Management Vital Signs Monitoring	Bedside Laboratory Testing Blood Products Administration Fluid Resuscitation Intravenous (IV) Insertion Intravenous (IV) Therapy Invasive Hemodynamic Monitoring Peripherally Inserted Central (PIC) Catheter Care Phlebotomy: Arterial Blood Sample Phlebotomy: Venous Blood Sample

Outcome: ELECTROLYTE & ACID/BASE BALANCE

MAJOR INTERVENTIONS	SUGGESTED INTERVENTIONS	OPTIONAL INTERVENTIONS
Electrolyte Management Fluid/Electrolyte Management	Acid-Base Management Acid-Base Monitoring Electrolyte Monitoring Fluid Management Fluid Monitoring Hemodynamic Regulation Intravenous (IV) Therapy Laboratory Data Interpretation Vital Signs Monitoring	Total Parenteral Nutrition (TPN) Administration

Outcome: FLUID BALANCE

MAJOR INTERVENTIONS	SUGGESTED INTERVENTIONS	OPTIONAL INTERVENTIONS
Fluid Management Fluid/Electrolyte Management	Bedside Laboratory Testing Diarrhea Management Electrolyte Management Electrolyte Monitoring Fluid Monitoring Fluid Resuscitation Hypovolemia Management Intravenous (IV) Insertion Intravenous (IV) Therapy Laboratory Data Interpretation Medication Administration Medication Management Nutrition Management Nutritional Monitoring Total Parenteral Nutrition (TPN) Administration Vital Signs Monitoring	Bleeding Reduction Blood Products Administration Hemodynamic Regulation Hemorrhage Control Invasive Hemodynamic Monitoring Shock Management Venous Access Devices (VAD) Maintenance

Outcome: HYDRATION

MAJOR INTERVENTIONS	SUGGESTED INTERVENTIONS	OPTIONAL INTERVENTIONS
Fluid/Electrolyte Management Hypovolemia Management	Diarrhea Management Electrolyte Management Electrolyte Monitoring Fluid Management Fluid Monitoring Fluid Resuscitation Intravenous (IV) Insertion Intravenous (IV) Therapy Nutrition Management Nutritional Monitoring Vital Signs Monitoring	Bleeding Precautions Bleeding Reduction Hemorrhage Control Temperature Regulation

Continued

Outcome: TISSUE PERFUSION: ABDOMINAL ORGANS

MAJOR INTERVENTIONS	SUGGESTED INTERVENTIONS	OPTIONAL INTERVENTIONS
Hypovolemia Management Intravenous (IV) Therapy	Acid-Base Management Acid-Base Monitoring Bedside Laboratory Testing Electrolyte Management Electrolyte Monitoring Flatulence Reduction Fluid Management Fluid Monitoring Fluid/Electrolyte Management Gastrointestinal Intubation Laboratory Data Interpretation Medication Administration: Enteral Medication Management Nausea Management Nutrition Management Oxygen Therapy Pain Management Shock Management Tube Care: Gastrointestinal Vital Signs Monitoring	Bleeding Reduction: Gastrointestinal Bowel Management Enteral Tube Feeding Medication Administration: Intravenous Resuscitation Temperature Regulation

Nursing Diagnosis: TISSUE PERFUSION, ALTERED: PERIPHERAL

DEFINITION: A decrease in oxygen resulting in the failure to nourish the tissues at the capillary level.

Outcome: SENSORY FUNCTION: CUTANEOUS

MAJOR INTERVENTIONS	SUGGESTED INTERVENTIONS	OPTIONAL INTERVENTIONS

Neurologic Monitoring
Peripheral Sensation
  Management
	Circulatory Care:
	  Arterial Insufficiency
	Circulatory Care: Venous
	  Insufficiency
	Cutaneous Stimulation
	Positioning
	Pressure Ulcer
	  Prevention
	Skin Surveillance
		Foot Care
		Pain Management
		Temperature Regulation

Outcome: TISSUE INTEGRITY: SKIN & MUCOUS MEMBRANES

MAJOR INTERVENTIONS	SUGGESTED INTERVENTIONS	OPTIONAL INTERVENTIONS

Circulatory Care:
  Arterial Insufficiency
Circulatory Care: Venous
  Insufficiency
Skin Surveillance
	Bed Rest Care
	Circulatory Precautions
	Foot Care
	Medication
	  Administration: Skin
	Nutrition Management
	Positioning
	Pressure Management
	Pressure Ulcer
	  Prevention
		Amputation Care
		Cast Care: Wet
		Cutaneous Stimulation
		Fluid Management
		Fluid Monitoring
		Medication Management
		Total Parenteral
		  Nutrition (TPN)
		  Administration
		Wound Care

Continued

Outcome: **TISSUE PERFUSION: PERIPHERAL**

MAJOR INTERVENTIONS	SUGGESTED INTERVENTIONS	OPTIONAL INTERVENTIONS
Circulatory Care: Arterial Insufficiency Circulatory Care: Venous Insufficiency Embolus Care: Peripheral	Bedside Laboratory Testing Circulatory Care: Mechanical Assist Device Circulatory Precautions Fluid Management Fluid/Electrolyte Management Hemodynamic Regulation Hypovolemia Management Invasive Hemodynamic Monitoring Medication Administration Medication Prescribing Pneumatic Tourniquet Precautions Positioning Pressure Ulcer Prevention Shock Management Shock Management: Cardiac Shock Management: Vasogenic Shock Management: Volume Skin Surveillance	Bleeding Reduction Blood Products Administration Cardiac Care: Acute Emergency Care Laboratory Data Interpretation Phlebotomy: Arterial Blood Sample Phlebotomy: Venous Blood Sample Positioning: Wheelchair Resuscitation Resuscitation: Neonate

Nursing Diagnosis: TISSUE PERFUSION, ALTERED: RENAL

DEFINITION: A decrease in oxygen resulting in the failure to nourish the tissues at the capillary level.

Outcome: CIRCULATION STATUS

MAJOR INTERVENTIONS	SUGGESTED INTERVENTIONS	OPTIONAL INTERVENTIONS
Circulatory Care: Arterial Insufficiency Circulatory Care: Venous Insufficiency	Bleeding Precautions Bleeding Reduction Fluid Monitoring Hemodynamic Regulation Hemorrhage Control Hypovolemia Management Laboratory Data Interpretation Shock Management Shock Prevention	Bedside Laboratory Testing Blood Products Administration Circulatory Precautions Fluid Resuscitation Intravenous (IV) Insertion Intravenous (IV) Therapy Invasive Hemodynamic Monitoring Oxygen Therapy Resuscitation Shock Management: Cardiac Shock Management: Vasogenic Shock Management: Volume

Continued

Outcome: Electrolyte & Acid/Base Balance

MAJOR INTERVENTIONS	SUGGESTED INTERVENTIONS	OPTIONAL INTERVENTIONS
Electrolyte Management Fluid/Electrolyte Management Hemodialysis Therapy Hemofiltration Therapy Peritoneal Dialysis Therapy	Acid-Base Management Acid-Base Management: Metabolic Acidosis Acid-Base Management: Metabolic Alkalosis Acid-Base Monitoring Electrolyte Monitoring Emergency Care Fluid Management Fluid Monitoring Hemodynamic Regulation Laboratory Data Interpretation Vital Signs Monitoring	Electrolyte Management: Hypercalcemia Electrolyte Management: Hyperkalemia Electrolyte Management: Hypermagnesemia Electrolyte Management: Hypernatremia Intravenous (IV) Insertion Intravenous (IV) Therapy Medication Administration Medication Management Phlebotomy: Arterial Blood Sample Phlebotomy: Venous Blood Sample Specimen Management Total Parenteral Nutrition (TPN) Administration

Outcome: FLUID BALANCE

MAJOR INTERVENTIONS	SUGGESTED INTERVENTIONS	OPTIONAL INTERVENTIONS
Fluid Management Fluid/Electrolyte Management Hemodialysis Therapy Hemofiltration Therapy Peritoneal Dialysis Therapy	Bedside Laboratory Testing Electrolyte Management Electrolyte Monitoring Fluid Monitoring Fluid Resuscitation Hypovolemia Management Intravenous (IV) Insertion Intravenous (IV) Therapy Laboratory Data Interpretation Medication Administration Medication Management Urinary Elimination Management Vital Signs Monitoring	Hemodynamic Regulation Hemorrhage Control Invasive Hemodynamic Monitoring Peripherally Inserted Central (PIC) Catheter Care Respiratory Monitoring Shock Management Shock Management: Volume Shock Prevention Surveillance Total Parenteral Nutrition (TPN) Administration Venous Access Devices (VAD) Maintenance

Outcome: TISSUE PERFUSION: ABDOMINAL ORGANS

MAJOR INTERVENTIONS	SUGGESTED INTERVENTIONS	OPTIONAL INTERVENTIONS
Hypovolemia Management Intravenous (IV) Therapy	Acid-Base Management Acid-Base Monitoring Bleeding Reduction Electrolyte Management Electrolyte Monitoring Laboratory Data Interpretation Medication Management Shock Management Shock Management: Volume Shock Prevention Specimen Management Vital Signs Monitoring	Bleeding Reduction: Gastrointestinal Emergency Care Fluid Resuscitation Hemodynamic Regulation Hemorrhage Control Intravenous (IV) Insertion

Continued

Outcome: URINARY ELIMINATION

MAJOR INTERVENTIONS	SUGGESTED INTERVENTIONS	OPTIONAL INTERVENTIONS
Urinary Elimination Management	Fluid/Electrolyte Management Medication Administration Nutrition Management Self-Care Assistance: Toileting Specimen Management Urinary Catheterization	Fluid Management Tube Care: Urinary Urinary Catheterization: Intermittent Urinary Retention Care

Nursing Diagnosis: TRANSFER ABILITY, IMPAIRED

DEFINITION: Limitation of independent movement between two nearby surfaces.

Outcome: BALANCE

MAJOR INTERVENTIONS	SUGGESTED INTERVENTIONS	OPTIONAL INTERVENTIONS
Exercise Therapy: Balance	Body Mechanics Promotion Energy Management Exercise Therapy: Ambulation Exercise Therapy: Joint Mobility Exercise Therapy: Muscle Control Fall Prevention	Environmental Management: Safety Exercise Promotion Positioning Teaching: Prescribed Activity/Exercise Weight Management

Outcome: BODY POSITIONING: SELF-INITIATED

MAJOR INTERVENTIONS	SUGGESTED INTERVENTIONS	OPTIONAL INTERVENTIONS
Exercise Promotion: Strength Training Exercise Therapy: Muscle Control	Body Mechanics Promotion Exercise Promotion Exercise Promotion: Stretching Exercise Therapy: Ambulation Exercise Therapy: Balance Exercise Therapy: Joint Mobility Self-Care Assistance Teaching: Prescribed Activity/Exercise	Energy Management Fall Prevention Pain Management Positioning Self-Care Assistance: Toileting Unilateral Neglect Management

Continued

Outcome: MOBILITY LEVEL

MAJOR INTERVENTIONS	SUGGESTED INTERVENTIONS	OPTIONAL INTERVENTIONS
Exercise Therapy: Ambulation Exercise Therapy: Balance Exercise Therapy: Joint Mobility Exercise Therapy: Muscle Control	Body Mechanics Promotion Energy Management Exercise Promotion: Strength Training Exercise Promotion: Stretching Fall Prevention Positioning: Wheelchair	Analgesic Administration Environmental Management: Safety Exercise Promotion Medication Management Mutual Goal Setting Pain Management Positioning Simple Relaxation Therapy Teaching: Prescribed Activity/Exercise

Outcome: MUSCLE FUNCTION

MAJOR INTERVENTIONS	SUGGESTED INTERVENTIONS	OPTIONAL INTERVENTIONS
Exercise Promotion: Strength Training	Body Mechanics Promotion Energy Management Exercise Promotion Exercise Promotion: Stretching Exercise Therapy: Balance Exercise Therapy: Joint Mobility Exercise Therapy: Muscle Control	Nutrition Management Pain Management Sleep Enhancement Teaching: Prescribed Activity/Exercise

Outcome: TRANSFER PERFORMANCE

MAJOR INTERVENTIONS	SUGGESTED INTERVENTIONS	OPTIONAL INTERVENTIONS
Exercise Promotion: Strength Training Transport	Body Mechanics Promotion Energy Management Exercise Promotion Exercise Promotion: Stretching Exercise Therapy: Balance Exercise Therapy: Joint Mobility Exercise Therapy: Muscle Control Fall Prevention Positioning Positioning: Wheelchair Teaching: Prescribed Activity/Exercise Teaching: Psychomotor Skill	Environmental Management: Safety Pain Management Self-Care Assistance Surveillance: Safety Weight Management

Nursing Diagnosis: UNILATERAL NEGLECT

DEFINITION: A state in which an individual is perceptually unaware of and inattentive to one side of the body.

Outcome: BODY IMAGE

MAJOR INTERVENTIONS	SUGGESTED INTERVENTIONS	OPTIONAL INTERVENTIONS
Unilateral Neglect Management	Amputation Care Anticipatory Guidance Body Image Enhancement Coping Enhancement Emotional Support Positioning Self-Care Assistance Touch	Caregiver Support Support System Enhancement Teaching: Individual

Outcome: BODY POSITIONING: SELF-INITIATED

MAJOR INTERVENTIONS	SUGGESTED INTERVENTIONS	OPTIONAL INTERVENTIONS
Self-Care Assistance Unilateral Neglect Management	Body Mechanics Promotion Exercise Promotion Exercise Promotion: Stretching Exercise Therapy: Ambulation Exercise Therapy: Balance Exercise Therapy: Joint Mobility Exercise Therapy: Muscle Control Teaching: Individual	Fall Prevention Pain Management Peripheral Sensation Management Positioning

Outcome: SELF-CARE: ACTIVITIES OF DAILY LIVING (ADL)

MAJOR INTERVENTIONS	SUGGESTED INTERVENTIONS	OPTIONAL INTERVENTIONS
Self-Care Assistance	Self-Care Assistance: Bathing/Hygiene Self-Care Assistance: Dressing/Grooming Self-Care Assistance: Feeding Self-Care Assistance: Toileting	Environmental Management: Safety Exercise Promotion Exercise Promotion: Stretching Exercise Therapy: Ambulation Exercise Therapy: Balance Exercise Therapy: Joint Mobility Exercise Therapy: Muscle Control Fall Prevention Home Maintenance Assistance

Nursing Diagnosis: URINARY ELIMINATION, ALTERED

DEFINITION: The state in which an individual experiences a disturbance in urine elimination.

Outcome: URINARY CONTINENCE

MAJOR INTERVENTIONS	SUGGESTED INTERVENTIONS	OPTIONAL INTERVENTIONS

Urinary Bladder Training
Urinary Elimination
  Management
Urinary Incontinence
  Care
	Biofeedback
	Fluid Management
	Fluid Monitoring
	Medication
	  Administration
	Medication Management
	Medication Prescribing
	Pelvic Muscle Exercise
	Pessary Management
	Prompted Voiding
	Self-Care Assistance:
	  Toileting
	Teaching: Prescribed
	  Medication
	Teaching: Procedure/
	  Treatment
	Urinary Catheterization
	Urinary Catheterization:
	  Intermittent
	Urinary Habit Training
	Urinary Incontinence
	  Care: Enuresis
		Anxiety Reduction
		Environmental
		  Management
		Infection Control
		Infection Prevention
		Perineal Care
		Postpartal Care
		Skin Surveillance
		Urinary Retention Care

Outcome: URINARY ELIMINATION

MAJOR INTERVENTIONS	SUGGESTED INTERVENTIONS	OPTIONAL INTERVENTIONS

Urinary Elimination
  Management
	Fluid Management
	Medication Management
	Medication Prescribing
	Self-Care Assistance:
	  Toileting
	Specimen Management
	Urinary Catheterization
	Urinary Catheterization:
	  Intermittent
	Urinary Incontinence
	  Care
	Urinary Incontinence
	  Care: Enuresis
		Hemodialysis Therapy
		Pain Management
		Pelvic Muscle Exercise
		Prompted Voiding
		Tube Care: Urinary
		Urinary Bladder Training
		Urinary Habit Training
		Urinary Retention Care

Nursing Diagnosis: URINARY INCONTINENCE, FUNCTIONAL

DEFINITION: Inability of usually continent person to reach toilet in time to avoid unintentional loss of urine.

Outcome: TISSUE INTEGRITY: SKIN & MUCOUS MEMBRANES

MAJOR INTERVENTIONS	SUGGESTED INTERVENTIONS	OPTIONAL INTERVENTIONS
Perineal Care Urinary Incontinence Care	Bathing Self-Care Assistance: Toileting	Urinary Incontinence Care: Enuresis

Outcome: URINARY CONTINENCE

MAJOR INTERVENTIONS	SUGGESTED INTERVENTIONS	OPTIONAL INTERVENTIONS
Prompted Voiding Urinary Habit Training	Environmental Management Self-Care Assistance: Toileting Urinary Elimination Management Urinary Incontinence Care	Communication Enhancement: Visual Deficit Dressing Exercise Promotion Exercise Therapy: Ambulation Self-Awareness Enhancement Surveillance: Safety

Outcome: URINARY ELIMINATION

MAJOR INTERVENTIONS	SUGGESTED INTERVENTIONS	OPTIONAL INTERVENTIONS
Urinary Elimination Management	Prompted Voiding Self-Care Assistance: Toileting Urinary Habit Training Urinary Incontinence Care	Fluid Management

Nursing Diagnosis: URINARY INCONTINENCE, REFLEX

DEFINITION: An involuntary loss of urine at somewhat predictable intervals when a specific bladder volume is reached.

Outcome: TISSUE INTEGRITY: SKIN & MUCOUS MEMBRANES

MAJOR INTERVENTIONS	SUGGESTED INTERVENTIONS	OPTIONAL INTERVENTIONS

Perineal Care
Urinary Incontinence
  Care
	Bathing
	Self-Care Assistance:
	  Toileting
		Skin Surveillance

Outcome: URINARY CONTINENCE

MAJOR INTERVENTIONS	SUGGESTED INTERVENTIONS	OPTIONAL INTERVENTIONS

Urinary Bladder Training
Urinary Catheterization:
  Intermittent
	Pelvic Muscle Exercise
	Tube Care: Urinary
	Urinary Catheterization
	Urinary Elimination
	  Management
	Urinary Habit Training
	Urinary Incontinence
	  Care
	Urinary Retention Care
		Fluid Management
		Fluid Monitoring
		Self-Care Assistance:
		  Toileting
		Teaching:
		  Procedure/Treatment

Outcome: URINARY ELIMINATION

MAJOR INTERVENTIONS	SUGGESTED INTERVENTIONS	OPTIONAL INTERVENTIONS

Urinary Elimination
  Management
	Pelvic Muscle Exercise
	Self-Care Assistance:
	  Toileting
	Urinary Bladder Training
	Urinary Catheterization:
	  Intermittent
		Fluid Management
		Tube Care: Urinary
		Urinary Catheterization
		Urinary Incontinence
		  Care
		Urinary Retention Care

Nursing Diagnosis: **URINARY INCONTINENCE, STRESS**

DEFINITION: The state in which an individual experiences a loss of urine of less than 50 ml occurring with increased abdominal pressure.

Outcome: **TISSUE INTEGRITY: SKIN & MUCOUS MEMBRANES**

MAJOR INTERVENTIONS	SUGGESTED INTERVENTIONS	OPTIONAL INTERVENTIONS
Perineal Care Urinary Incontinence Care	Self-Care Assistance: Toileting	Bathing

Outcome: **URINARY CONTINENCE**

MAJOR INTERVENTIONS	SUGGESTED INTERVENTIONS	OPTIONAL INTERVENTIONS
Pelvic Muscle Exercise Urinary Incontinence Care	Biofeedback Medication Management Pessary Management Urinary Elimination Management Urinary Habit Training Weight Management	Environmental Management Postpartal Care Respiratory Monitoring Self-Care Assistance: Toileting

Outcome: **URINARY ELIMINATION**

MAJOR INTERVENTIONS	SUGGESTED INTERVENTIONS	OPTIONAL INTERVENTIONS
Urinary Elimination Management	Medication Administration Pelvic Muscle Exercise Teaching: Individual Teaching: Prescribed Medication Urinary Habit Training Urinary Incontinence Care	Self-Care Assistance: Toileting

Nursing Diagnosis: URINARY INCONTINENCE, TOTAL

DEFINITION: The state in which an individual experiences a continuous and unpredictable loss of urine.

Outcome: TISSUE INTEGRITY: SKIN & MUCOUS MEMBRANES

MAJOR INTERVENTIONS	SUGGESTED INTERVENTIONS	OPTIONAL INTERVENTIONS

Perineal Care
Urinary Incontinence
  Care
	Bathing
	Self-Care Assistance:
	  Toileting
		Skin Surveillance
		Skin Care: Topical
		  Treatments

Outcome: URINARY CONTINENCE

MAJOR INTERVENTIONS	SUGGESTED INTERVENTIONS	OPTIONAL INTERVENTIONS

Urinary Incontinence
  Care
	Environmental
	  Management
	Self-Care Assistance:
	  Toileting
	Tube Care: Urinary
	Urinary Catheterization
		Fluid Management
		Fluid Monitoring
		Teaching:
		  Procedure/Treatment

Outcome: URINARY ELIMINATION

MAJOR INTERVENTIONS	SUGGESTED INTERVENTIONS	OPTIONAL INTERVENTIONS

Urinary Elimination
  Management
	Self-Care Assistance:
	  Toileting
	Urinary Catheterization
	Urinary Incontinence
	  Care
		Fluid Management
		Tube Care: Urinary

Nursing Diagnosis: URINARY INCONTINENCE, URGE

DEFINITION: The state in which an individual experiences involuntary passage of urine occurring soon after a strong sense of urgency to void.

Outcome: TISSUE INTEGRITY: SKIN & MUCOUS MEMBRANES

MAJOR INTERVENTIONS	SUGGESTED INTERVENTIONS	OPTIONAL INTERVENTIONS
Perineal Care Urinary Incontinence Care	Bathing Self-Care Assistance: Toileting	

Outcome: URINARY CONTINENCE

MAJOR INTERVENTIONS	SUGGESTED INTERVENTIONS	OPTIONAL INTERVENTIONS
Urinary Habit Training Urinary Incontinence Care	Biofeedback Environmental Management Fluid Management Fluid Monitoring Medication Management Urinary Elimination Management	Medication Administration Medication Prescribing Pelvic Muscle Exercise Self-Care Assistance: Toileting Teaching: Prescribed Medication Teaching: Procedure/ Treatment Tube Care: Urinary Urinary Catheterization Urinary Catheterization: Intermittent

Outcome: URINARY ELIMINATION

MAJOR INTERVENTIONS	SUGGESTED INTERVENTIONS	OPTIONAL INTERVENTIONS
Urinary Elimination Management Urinary Habit Training	Medication Administration Self-Care Assistance: Toileting Urinary Incontinence Care	Fluid Management Pelvic Muscle Exercise

Nursing Diagnosis: URINARY RETENTION

DEFINITION: The state in which the individual experiences incomplete emptying of the bladder.

Outcome: URINARY CONTINENCE

MAJOR INTERVENTIONS	SUGGESTED INTERVENTIONS	OPTIONAL INTERVENTIONS
Urinary Bladder Training Urinary Catheterization: Intermittent	Bladder Irrigation Fluid Management Fluid Monitoring Medication Administration Medication Management Tube Care: Urinary Urinary Catheterization Urinary Elimination Management Urinary Habit Training Urinary Incontinence Care Urinary Incontinence Care: Enuresis Urinary Retention Care	Anxiety Reduction Exercise Promotion Perineal Care Postpartal Care Simple Relaxation Therapy

Outcome: URINARY ELIMINATION

MAJOR INTERVENTIONS	SUGGESTED INTERVENTIONS	OPTIONAL INTERVENTIONS
Urinary Elimination Management Urinary Retention Care	Fluid Management Fluid Monitoring Medication Administration Medication Management Self-Care Assistance: Toileting Specimen Management Urinary Catheterization: Intermittent	Pelvic Muscle Exercise Tube Care: Urinary Urinary Bladder Training Urinary Catheterization Urinary Habit Training

Nursing Diagnosis: VENTILATION, INABILITY TO SUSTAIN SPONTANEOUS

DEFINITION: A state in which the response pattern of decreased energy reserves results in an individual's inability to maintain breathing adequate to support life.

Outcome: RESPIRATORY STATUS: GAS EXCHANGE

MAJOR INTERVENTIONS	SUGGESTED INTERVENTIONS	OPTIONAL INTERVENTIONS
Artificial Airway Management Mechanical Ventilation Respiratory Monitoring	Acid-Base Management Acid-Base Management: Respiratory Acidosis Acid-Base Management: Respiratory Alkalosis Acid-Base Monitoring Airway Insertion and Stabilization Airway Management Airway Suctioning Anxiety Reduction Chest Physiotherapy Energy Management Oxygen Therapy Positioning Ventilation Assistance	Aspiration Precautions Cough Enhancement Laboratory Data Interpretation

Outcome: RESPIRATORY STATUS: VENTILATION

MAJOR INTERVENTIONS	SUGGESTED INTERVENTIONS	OPTIONAL INTERVENTIONS
Airway Management Artificial Airway Management Mechanical Ventilation Respiratory Monitoring Ventilation Assistance	Acid-Base Monitoring Airway Insertion and Stabilization Airway Suctioning Anxiety Reduction Aspiration Precautions Calming Technique Chest Physiotherapy Emotional Support Energy Management Fluid Management Mechanical Ventilatory Weaning Oxygen Therapy Positioning Resuscitation: Neonate Vital Signs Monitoring	Coping Enhancement Emergency Care Endotracheal Extubation Phlebotomy: Arterial Blood Sample Simple Relaxation Therapy Surveillance Technology Management Tube Care: Chest

Continued

Outcome: VITAL SIGNS STATUS

MAJOR INTERVENTIONS	SUGGESTED INTERVENTIONS	OPTIONAL INTERVENTIONS
Respiratory Monitoring Vital Signs Monitoring	Acid-Base Management Airway Management Anxiety Reduction Environmental Management Fluid Management Fluid/Electrolyte Management Intravenous (IV) Insertion Intravenous (IV) Therapy Medication Administration Medication Management Ventilation Assistance	Emergency Care Exercise Promotion Infection Control Infection Protection Oxygen Therapy Pain Management Resuscitation

Nursing Diagnosis: VENTILATORY WEANING RESPONSE, DYSFUNCTIONAL

DEFINITION: A state in which an individual cannot adjust to lowered levels of mechanical ventilator support, which interrupts and prolongs the weaning process.

Outcome: ANXIETY CONTROL

MAJOR INTERVENTIONS	SUGGESTED INTERVENTIONS	OPTIONAL INTERVENTIONS
Anxiety Reduction Preparatory Sensory Information	Calming Technique Coping Enhancement Counseling Distraction Medication Administration Meditation Facilitation Music Therapy Presence Security Enhancement Simple Guided Imagery Simple Relaxation Therapy	Biofeedback Environmental Management Risk Identification

Outcome: RESPIRATORY STATUS: GAS EXCHANGE

MAJOR INTERVENTIONS	SUGGESTED INTERVENTIONS	OPTIONAL INTERVENTIONS
Respiratory Monitoring Ventilation Assistance	Acid-Base Management: Respiratory Acidosis Acid-Base Management: Respiratory Alkalosis Acid-Base Monitoring Airway Management Anxiety Reduction Artificial Airway Management Aspiration Precautions Mechanical Ventilation Oxygen Therapy Positioning	Airway Insertion and Stabilization Airway Suctioning Chest Physiotherapy Cough Enhancement Energy Management Laboratory Data Interpretation Phlebotomy: Arterial Blood Sample

Continued

Outcome: RESPIRATORY STATUS: VENTILATION

MAJOR INTERVENTIONS	SUGGESTED INTERVENTIONS	OPTIONAL INTERVENTIONS

Mechanical Ventilation
Mechanical Ventilatory
  Weaning
Respiratory Monitoring
	Airway Insertion and
	  Stabilization
	Airway Management
	Airway Suctioning
	Artificial Airway
	  Management
	Aspiration Precautions
	Energy Management
	Environmental
	  Management: Safety
	Positioning
	Ventilation Assistance
		Acid-Base Monitoring
		Anxiety Reduction
		Calming Technique
		Cough Enhancement
		Emotional Support
		Oxygen Therapy
		Presence
		Simple Relaxation
		  Therapy

Outcome: VITAL SIGNS STATUS

MAJOR INTERVENTIONS	SUGGESTED INTERVENTIONS	OPTIONAL INTERVENTIONS

Respiratory Monitoring
Vital Signs Monitoring
	Acid-Base Management
	Airway Management
	Anxiety Reduction
	Electrolyte Management
	Environmental
	  Management
	Medication
	  Administration
	Medication Management
	Ventilation Assistance
		Environmental
		  Management: Comfort
		Music Therapy
		Oxygen Therapy
		Pain Management
		Resuscitation
		Simple Relaxation
		  Therapy

Nursing Diagnosis: WALKING, IMPAIRED

Definition: Limitation of independent movement within the environment on foot.

Outcome: AMBULATION: WALKING

MAJOR INTERVENTIONS	SUGGESTED INTERVENTIONS	OPTIONAL INTERVENTIONS
Exercise Therapy: Ambulation	Body Mechanics Promotion Energy Management Exercise Promotion Exercise Promotion: Strength Training Exercise Promotion: Stretching Exercise Therapy: Balance Exercise Therapy: Joint Mobility Exercise Therapy: Muscle Control Teaching: Prescribed Activity/Exercise Transport	Environmental Management Environmental Management: Safety Fall Prevention Medication Management Pain Management Positioning Weight Reduction Assistance

Outcome: ENDURANCE

MAJOR INTERVENTIONS	SUGGESTED INTERVENTIONS	OPTIONAL INTERVENTIONS
Energy Management	Exercise Promotion Nutrition Management Sleep Enhancement Teaching: Prescribed Activity/Exercise	Environmental Management Exercise Therapy: Ambulation Exercise Therapy: Balance Exercise Therapy: Joint Mobility Exercise Therapy: Muscle Control Mutual Goal Setting Weight Management

Continued

Outcome: **MOBILITY LEVEL**		
MAJOR INTERVENTIONS	**SUGGESTED INTERVENTIONS**	**OPTIONAL INTERVENTIONS**
Exercise Therapy: Ambulation	Body Mechanics Promotion Energy Management Exercise Promotion: Strength Training Exercise Therapy: Balance Exercise Therapy: Joint Mobility Exercise Therapy: Muscle Control	Analgesic Administration Environmental Management: Safety Exercise Promotion Exercise Promotion: Stretching Pain Management Positioning Teaching: Prescribed Activity/Exercise

Outcome: **SELF-CARE: ACTIVITIES OF DAILY LIVING (ADL)**		
MAJOR INTERVENTIONS	**SUGGESTED INTERVENTIONS**	**OPTIONAL INTERVENTIONS**
Self-Care Assistance	Energy Management Environmental Management: Safety Exercise Promotion Exercise Promotion: Strength Training Exercise Therapy: Ambulation	Body Mechanics Promotion Exercise Promotion: Stretching Exercise Therapy: Balance Exercise Therapy: Joint Mobility Exercise Therapy: Muscle Control Fall Prevention Home Maintenance Assistance

Nursing Diagnosis: WHEELCHAIR MOBILITY, IMPAIRED

Definition: Limitation of independent operation of wheelchair within environment.

Outcome: AMBULATION: WHEELCHAIR

MAJOR INTERVENTIONS	SUGGESTED INTERVENTIONS	OPTIONAL INTERVENTIONS
Exercise Promotion: Strength Training Positioning: Wheelchair	Body Mechanics Promotion Energy Management Environmental Management: Safety Exercise Promotion Exercise Promotion: Stretching Exercise Therapy: Balance Exercise Therapy: Muscle Control Fall Prevention Positioning Teaching: Prescribed Activity/Exercise Transport	Medication Management Pain Management Positioning: Neurologic Weight Management

Outcome: BALANCE

MAJOR INTERVENTIONS	SUGGESTED INTERVENTIONS	OPTIONAL INTERVENTIONS
Exercise Therapy: Balance	Body Mechanics Promotion Energy Management Exercise Therapy: Muscle Control Fall Prevention	Environmental Management: Safety Exercise Promotion Positioning Teaching: Prescribed Activity/Exercise Weight Management

Continued

Outcome: MOBILITY LEVEL

MAJOR INTERVENTIONS	SUGGESTED INTERVENTIONS	OPTIONAL INTERVENTIONS
Exercise Promotion: Strength Training Positioning: Wheelchair	Body Mechanics Promotion Energy Management Exercise Therapy: Balance Exercise Therapy: Muscle Control Fall Prevention Transport	Analgesic Administration Environmental Management: Safety Exercise Promotion Exercise Promotion: Stretching Mutual Goal Setting Pain Management Positioning Teaching: Prescribed Activity/Exercise

Outcome: MUSCLE FUNCTION

MAJOR INTERVENTIONS	SUGGESTED INTERVENTIONS	OPTIONAL INTERVENTIONS
Exercise Therapy: Muscle Control	Body Mechanics Promotion Energy Management Exercise Promotion: Strength Training Exercise Promotion: Stretching Exercise Therapy: Balance	Exercise Promotion Nutrition Management Pain Management Sleep Enhancement Teaching: Prescribed Activity/Exercise

Nursing Diagnosis: ACTIVITY INTOLERANCE, RISK FOR

DEFINITION: A state in which an individual is at risk of experiencing insufficient physiological or psychological energy to endure or complete required or desired daily activities.

Outcome: ACTIVITY TOLERANCE

MAJOR INTERVENTIONS	SUGGESTED INTERVENTIONS	OPTIONAL INTERVENTIONS
Energy Management Exercise Promotion: 　Strength Training	Activity Therapy Exercise Promotion Exercise Therapy: 　Ambulation Exercise Therapy: Joint 　Mobility Exercise Therapy: 　Muscle Control Nutrition Management Pain Management Security Enhancement Sleep Enhancement Smoking Cessation 　Assistance Vital Signs Monitoring	Dementia Management Emotional Support Hope Instillation Medication Management Oxygen Therapy Self-Esteem 　Enhancement Teaching: Prescribed 　Activity/Exercise Weight Reduction 　Assistance

Outcome: ENDURANCE

MAJOR INTERVENTIONS	SUGGESTED INTERVENTIONS	OPTIONAL INTERVENTIONS
Energy Management Exercise Promotion: 　Strength Training	Activity Therapy Emotional Support Exercise Promotion Exercise Promotion: 　Stretching Health Screening Nutrition Management Oxygen Therapy Pain Management Risk Identification Sleep Enhancement Smoking Cessation 　Assistance Teaching: Prescribed 　Activity/Exercise Teaching: 　Prescribed Diet Vital Signs Monitoring	Cardiac Care: 　Rehabilitative Counseling Dementia Management Eating Disorders 　Management Exercise Therapy: 　Ambulation Exercise Therapy: 　Balance Exercise Therapy: Joint 　Mobility Exercise Therapy: 　Muscle Control Mood Management Mutual Goal Setting Support System 　Enhancement Weight Management

Continued

Outcome: Energy Conservation

MAJOR INTERVENTIONS	SUGGESTED INTERVENTIONS	OPTIONAL INTERVENTIONS
Energy Management	Body Mechanics Promotion Environmental Management Environmental Management: Comfort Exercise Promotion Nutrition Management Nutritional Monitoring Pain Management Sleep Enhancement Teaching: Prescribed Activity/Exercise	Exercise Therapy: Ambulation Exercise Therapy: Balance Exercise Therapy: Joint Mobility Exercise Therapy: Muscle Control Mood Management Oxygen Therapy Simple Relaxation Therapy Smoking Cessation Assistance Weight Management

For interventions and outcomes related to specific risk factors refer to the following diagnoses: Breathing Pattern, Ineffective; Cardiac Output, Decreased; Failure to Thrive, Adult; Fatigue; Gas Exchange, Impaired; Health Maintenance, Altered.

Nursing Diagnosis: ASPIRATION, RISK FOR

DEFINITION: The state in which an individual is at risk for entry of gastrointestinal secretions, oropharyngeal secretions, or solids or fluids into tracheobronchial passages.

Outcome: ASPIRATION CONTROL

MAJOR INTERVENTIONS	SUGGESTED INTERVENTIONS	OPTIONAL INTERVENTIONS
Aspiration Precautions Swallowing Therapy Vomiting Management	Airway Suctioning Amnioinfusion Artificial Airway Management Conscious Sedation Gastrointestinal Intubation Positioning Postanesthesia Care Respiratory Monitoring Resuscitation: Neonate Surveillance	Enteral Tube Feeding Feeding Medication Administration: Enteral Neurologic Monitoring Vital Signs Monitoring

Outcome: RESPIRATORY STATUS: VENTILATION

MAJOR INTERVENTIONS	SUGGESTED INTERVENTIONS	OPTIONAL INTERVENTIONS
Airway Management Aspiration Precautions Respiratory Monitoring	Airway Suctioning Mechanical Ventilation Positioning	Anxiety Reduction Chest Physiotherapy Cough Enhancement Mechanical Ventilatory Weaning

Outcome: SWALLOWING STATUS

MAJOR INTERVENTIONS	SUGGESTED INTERVENTIONS	OPTIONAL INTERVENTIONS
Aspiration Precautions Swallowing Therapy	Enteral Tube Feeding Feeding Oral Health Maintenance Positioning Self-Care Assistance: Feeding Surveillance	Airway Management Airway Suctioning Vomiting Management

For interventions and outcomes related to specific risk factors refer to the following diagnoses: Confusion, Acute; Confusion, Chronic; Infant Feeding Pattern, Ineffective; Physical Mobility, Impaired; Self-Care Deficit: Feeding.

Nursing Diagnosis: AUTONOMIC DYSREFLEXIA, RISK FOR

DEFINITION: A lifelong threatening uninhibited response of the sympathetic nervous system for an individual with a spinal cord injury or lesion at T8 or above, and having recovered from spinal shock.

Outcome: NEUROLOGICAL STATUS: AUTONOMIC

MAJOR INTERVENTIONS	SUGGESTED INTERVENTIONS	OPTIONAL INTERVENTIONS

Dysreflexia Management
Neurologic Monitoring
Vital Signs Monitoring
	Airway Management
	Anxiety Reduction
	Emergency Care
	Fluid Monitoring
	Infection Control
	Intravenous (IV)
	  Therapy
	Medication
	  Administration
	Medication Management
	Positioning
	Respiratory Monitoring
	Shock Management
	Surveillance: Safety
	Temperature Regulation
	Urinary Elimination
	  Management
		Bowel Management
		Fever Treatment
		Heat Exposure
		  Treatment
		Infection Protection
		Skin Surveillance
		Urinary Catheterization
		Urinary Catheterization:
		  Intermittent
		Urinary Elimination
		  Management

Outcome: SYMPTOM SEVERITY

MAJOR INTERVENTIONS	SUGGESTED INTERVENTIONS	OPTIONAL INTERVENTIONS

Dysreflexia Management	Anxiety Reduction
	Energy Management
	Medication
	  Administration
	Medication Management
	Pain Management
	Positioning
	Pressure Management
	Temperature Regulation
		Flatulence Reduction
		Peripheral Sensation
		  Management

Outcome: VITAL SIGNS STATUS

MAJOR INTERVENTIONS	SUGGESTED INTERVENTIONS	OPTIONAL INTERVENTIONS
Vital Signs Monitoring	Airway Management Anxiety Reduction Dysrhythmia Management Environmental Management Fever Treatment Fluid Management Heat Exposure Treatment Hemodynamic Regulation Medication Administration Medication Management Medication Prescribing Respiratory Monitoring Shock Management Shock Prevention Temperature Regulation	Cough Enhancement Emergency Care Exercise Promotion Infection Protection Intravenous (IV) Insertion Intravenous (IV) Therapy Nutrition Management Pain Management

For interventions and outcomes related to specific risk factors refer to the following diagnoses: Body Temperature, Risk for Altered; Constipation; Fluid Volume Excess; Gas Exchange, Impaired; Hyperthermia; Infection, Risk for; Pain; Sexual Dysfunction; Skin Integrity, Impaired; Thermoregulation, Ineffective; Urinary Retention.

Nursing Diagnosis: BODY TEMPERATURE, RISK FOR ALTERED

DEFINITION: The state in which the individual is at risk for failure to maintain body temperature within normal range.

Outcome: THERMOREGULATION

MAJOR INTERVENTIONS	SUGGESTED INTERVENTIONS	OPTIONAL INTERVENTIONS
Temperature Regulation	Cerebral Edema	Bathing
Temperature Regulation:	Management	Emergency Care
Intraoperative	Environmental	Energy Management
Vital Signs Monitoring	Management	Environmental
	Fever Treatment	Management: Comfort
	Fluid Management	Fluid Monitoring
	Heat Exposure	Heat/Cold Application
	Treatment	Hemodynamic
	Malignant Hyperthermia	Regulation
	Precautions	
	Medication	
	Administration	
	Postanesthesia Care	

Outcome: THERMOREGULATION: NEONATE

MAJOR INTERVENTIONS	SUGGESTED INTERVENTIONS	OPTIONAL INTERVENTIONS
Newborn Care	Environmental	Dressing
Temperature Regulation	Management	Environmental
Vital Signs Monitoring	Fluid Management	Management: Comfort
	Newborn Monitoring	Fever Treatment
		Heat Exposure
		Treatment
		Kangaroo Care
		Parent Education: Infant
		Phototherapy: Neonate
		Resuscitation: Neonate

For interventions and outcomes related to specific risk factors refer to the following diagnoses: Fluid Volume Deficit; Infant Behavior, Disorganized; Infection, Risk For; Protection, Altered; Skin Integrity, Impaired; Surgical Recovery, Delayed; Urinary Retention.

Nursing Diagnosis: **CAREGIVER ROLE STRAIN, RISK FOR**

DEFINITION: A caregiver is vulnerable for felt difficulty in performing the family caregiver role.

Outcome: **CAREGIVER EMOTIONAL HEALTH**

MAJOR INTERVENTIONS	SUGGESTED INTERVENTIONS	OPTIONAL INTERVENTIONS
Caregiver Support	Active Listening	Family Integrity
Emotional Support	Anger Control	Promotion
Respite Care	Assistance	Family Mobilization
	Anticipatory Guidance	Family Process
	Coping Enhancement	Maintenance
	Decision-Making	Family Support
	Support	Referral
	Family Involvement	Simple Relaxation
	Promotion	Therapy
	Grief Work Facilitation	Support Group
	Guilt Work Facilitation	Support System
	Hope Instillation	Enhancement
	Socialization	
	Enhancement	
	Spiritual Support	

Continued

Outcome: Caregiver Home Care Readiness

MAJOR INTERVENTIONS	SUGGESTED INTERVENTIONS	OPTIONAL INTERVENTIONS

Caregiver Support
Family Involvement
  Promotion
Parenting Promotion
	Anticipatory Guidance
	Anxiety Reduction
	Coping Enhancement
	Decision-Making
	  Support
	Discharge Planning
	Emotional Support
	Environmental
	  Management: Home
	  Preparation
	Family Mobilization
	Family Process
	  Maintenance
	Family Support
	Health System Guidance
	Home Maintenance
	  Assistance
	Normalization
	  Promotion
	Parent Education:
	  Adolescent
	Parent Education:
	  Childrearing Family
	Parent Education: Infant
	Referral
	Respite Care
	Support System
	  Enhancement
		Financial Resource
		  Assistance
		Insurance Authorization
		Teaching: Disease
		  Process
		Teaching: Infant
		  Nutrition
		Teaching: Infant Safety
		Teaching: Prescribed
		  Activity/Exercise
		Teaching:
		  Prescribed Diet
		Teaching: Prescribed
		  Medication
		Teaching: Procedure/
		  Treatment
		Teaching: Psychomotor
		  Skill
		Teaching: Toddler
		  Nutrition
		Teaching: Toddler Safety

Outcome: Caregiver Physical Health

MAJOR INTERVENTIONS	SUGGESTED INTERVENTIONS	OPTIONAL INTERVENTIONS

Energy Management
Health Screening
Respite Care
	Coping Enhancement
	Family Mobilization
	Infection Protection
	Nutrition Management
	Risk Identification
	Sleep Enhancement
	Weight Management
		Body Mechanics
		  Promotion
		Caregiver Support
		Exercise Promotion
		Family Involvement
		  Promotion
		Family Support
		Health System Guidance
		Medication Management
		Referral

Outcome: CAREGIVER STRESSORS

MAJOR INTERVENTIONS	SUGGESTED INTERVENTIONS	OPTIONAL INTERVENTIONS

Caregiver Support
Coping Enhancement
	Decision-Making
	  Support
	Emotional Support
	Family Involvement
	  Promotion
	Family Mobilization
	Family Support
	Home Maintenance
	  Assistance
	Meditation Facilitation
	Normalization
	  Promotion
	Recreation Therapy
	Respite Care
	Simple Relaxation
	  Therapy
	Support Group
	Support System
	  Enhancement
		Active Listening
		Anticipatory Guidance
		Counseling
		Energy Management
		Family Integrity
		  Promotion
		Family Process
		  Maintenance
		Family Therapy
		Financial Resource
		  Assistance
		Guilt Work Facilitation
		Referral
		Spiritual Support

Outcome: CAREGIVING ENDURANCE POTENTIAL

MAJOR INTERVENTIONS	SUGGESTED INTERVENTIONS	OPTIONAL INTERVENTIONS

Caregiver Support
Coping Enhancement
	Decision-Making
	  Support
	Energy Management
	Exercise Promotion
	Family Involvement
	  Promotion
	Parenting Promotion
	Respite Care
	Spiritual Support
	Support Group
	Support System
	  Enhancement
		Assertiveness Training
		Emotional Support
		Family Mobilization
		Family Support
		Recreation Therapy
		Simple Relaxation
		  Therapy

Continued

Outcome: PARENTING

MAJOR INTERVENTIONS	SUGGESTED INTERVENTIONS	OPTIONAL INTERVENTIONS
Parent Education: Childrearing Family Parent Education: Infant Parenting Promotion	Abuse Protection Support: Child Anticipatory Guidance Coping Enhancement Counseling Family Integrity Promotion Family Mobilization Family Process Maintenance Family Support Parent Education: Adolescent Respite Care Risk Identification Role Enhancement Support System Enhancement	Emotional Support Family Therapy Health System Guidance Home Maintenance Assistance Self-Esteem Enhancement Socialization Enhancement Support Group

For interventions and outcomes related to specific risk factors refer to the following diagnoses: Decisional Conflict; Diversional Activity Deficit; Families, Management of Therapeutic Regimen, Ineffective; Family Processes, Altered; Fatigue; Grieving, Dysfunctional; Home Maintenance Management, Impaired; Hopelessness; Knowledge Deficit; Parenteral Role Conflict; Powerlessness; Role Performance, Altered; Sleep Deprivation; Social Interaction, Impaired; Social Isolation.

Nursing Diagnosis: CONSTIPATION, RISK OF

DEFINITION: At risk for a decrease in a person's normal frequency of defecation accompanied by difficult or incomplete passage of stool and/or passage of excessively hard, dry stool.

Outcome: BOWEL ELIMINATION

MAJOR INTERVENTIONS	SUGGESTED INTERVENTIONS	OPTIONAL INTERVENTIONS
Constipation/Impaction Management	Bowel Irrigation Bowel Management Bowel Training Diet Staging Exercise Therapy: Ambulation Fluid Management Fluid Monitoring Medication Management Medication Prescribing Nutrition Management Nutritional Monitoring	Exercise Promotion Flatulence Reduction Medication Administration: Oral Ostomy Care Pain Management Rectal Prolapse Management

Outcome: SELF-CARE: TOILETING

MAJOR INTERVENTIONS	SUGGESTED INTERVENTIONS	OPTIONAL INTERVENTIONS
Self-Care Assistance: Toileting	Constipation/Impaction Management Bowel Management Bowel Training	Anxiety Reduction Exercise Promotion Perineal Care Simple Relaxation Therapy

For interventions and outcomes related to specific risk factors refer to the following diagnoses: Health Maintenance, Altered; Fluid Volume Deficit; Nutrition, Altered: Less Than Body Requirements; Physical Mobility, Impaired; Self-Care Deficit, Feeding; Self-Care Deficit, Toileting; Sorrow, Chronic.

Nursing Diagnosis: DEVELOPMENT, RISK FOR ALTERED

DEFINITION: At risk for delay of 25% or more in one or more of the areas of social or self-regulatory behavior, or cognitive, language, gross or fine motor skills.

Outcome: CHILD DEVELOPMENT: 12 MONTHS

MAJOR INTERVENTIONS	SUGGESTED INTERVENTIONS	OPTIONAL INTERVENTIONS

Infant Care
Parent Education: Infant
Risk Identification:
  Genetic
	Anticipatory Guidance
	Attachment Promotion
	Developmental
	  Enhancement: Child
	Family Integrity
	  Promotion:
	  Childbearing Family
	Family Support
	Health Screening
	Immunization/
	  Vaccination
	  Management
	Lactation Counseling
	Nutritional Counseling
	Security Enhancement
	Sleep Enhancement
	Socialization
	  Enhancement
		Abuse Protection
		  Support: Child
		Caregiver Support
		Environmental
		  Management: Safety
		Health System Guidance
		Nutrition Management
		Nutritional Monitoring
		Respite Care
		Sibling Support
		Support System
		  Enhancement
		Surveillance
		Sustenance Support
		Therapeutic Play

Outcome: CHILD DEVELOPMENT: 2 YEARS

MAJOR INTERVENTIONS	SUGGESTED INTERVENTIONS	OPTIONAL INTERVENTIONS
Developmental Enhancement: Child Environmental Management: Safety Risk Identification	Anticipatory Guidance Caregiver Support Family Integrity Promotion Family Involvement Promotion Health Screening Nutrition Management Parenting Promotion Security Enhancement Sleep Enhancement Socialization Enhancement Teaching: Toddler Nutrition Teaching: Toddler Safety	Abuse Protection Support: Child Behavior Management Bowel Training Counseling Family Process Maintenance Family Support Family Therapy Health System Guidance Nutritional Counseling Nutritional Monitoring Respite Care Sibling Support Support System Enhancement Surveillance: Safety Sustenance Support Therapeutic Play Urinary Habit Training

Outcome: CHILD DEVELOPMENT: 3 YEARS

MAJOR INTERVENTIONS	SUGGESTED INTERVENTIONS	OPTIONAL INTERVENTIONS
Developmental Enhancement: Child Environmental Management: Safety Health Screening Risk Identification	Anticipatory Guidance Bowel Management Bowel Training Family Integrity Promotion Family Involvement Promotion Nutrition Management Parenting Promotion Security Enhancement Socialization Enhancement Urinary Habit Training Urinary Incontinence Care: Enuresis	Abuse Protection Support: Child Behavior Management Behavior Modification Counseling Family Process Maintenance Family Support Family Therapy Health System Guidance Nutritional Monitoring Sibling Support Sleep Enhancement Surveillance: Safety Therapeutic Play

Continued

Outcome: CHILD DEVELOPMENT: 4 YEARS

MAJOR INTERVENTIONS	SUGGESTED INTERVENTIONS	OPTIONAL INTERVENTIONS
Developmental Enhancement: Child Health Screening Risk Identification	Anticipatory Guidance Environmental Management: Safety Family Integrity Promotion Family Involvement Promotion Learning Facilitation Nutrition Management Security Enhancement Socialization Enhancement Support System Enhancement	Abuse Protection Support: Child Behavior Management Behavior Management: Overactivity/ Inattention Behavior Modification Counseling Energy Management Family Process Maintenance Family Support Family Therapy Health System Guidance Sibling Support Sleep Enhancement Sustenance Support Therapeutic Play Urinary Habit Training Urinary Incontinence Care: Enuresis

Outcome: CHILD DEVELOPMENT: 5 YEARS

MAJOR INTERVENTIONS	SUGGESTED INTERVENTIONS	OPTIONAL INTERVENTIONS
Developmental Enhancement: Child Health Screening Risk Identification	Anticipatory Guidance Environmental Management: Safety Family Integrity Promotion Family Involvement Promotion Learning Facilitation Nutrition Management Parenting Promotion Security Enhancement Socialization Enhancement Support System Enhancement	Abuse Protection Support: Child Behavior Management Behavior Management: Overactivity/ Inattention Behavior Modification Counseling Energy Management Family Process Maintenance Family Support Family Therapy Health System Guidance Nutritional Counseling Nutritional Monitoring Sibling Support Sleep Enhancement Sustenance Support Therapeutic Play Urinary Habit Training Urinary Incontinence Care: Enuresis

Continued

Outcome: CHILD DEVELOPMENT: MIDDLE CHILDHOOD (6-11 YEARS)

MAJOR INTERVENTIONS	SUGGESTED INTERVENTIONS	OPTIONAL INTERVENTIONS
Development Enhancement: Child	Anticipatory Guidance	Abuse Protection Support: Child
Health Screening	Behavior Modification: Social Skills	Behavior Management
Risk Identification	Body Image Enhancement	Behavior Modification
	Exercise Promotion	Counseling
	Family Integrity Promotion	Eating Disorders Management
	Family Involvement Promotion	Family Process Maintenance
	Impulse Control Training	Family Support
	Learning Facilitation	Family Therapy
	Nutrition Management	Fire-Setting Precautions
	Nutritional Monitoring	Health System Guidance
	Parenting Promotion	Sibling Support
	Self-Awareness Enhancement	Sustenance Support
	Self-Esteem Enhancement	Therapeutic Play
	Self-Modification Assistance	Weight Management
	Self-Responsibility Facilitation	
	Socialization Enhancement	
	Spiritual Support	
	Substance Use Prevention	
	Teaching: Individual	
	Teaching: Safe Sex	
	Teaching: Sexuality	

Outcome: Child Development: Adolescence (12-17 Years)

MAJOR INTERVENTIONS	SUGGESTED INTERVENTIONS	OPTIONAL INTERVENTIONS
Developmental Enhancement: Adolescent Parent Education: Adolescent Risk Identification	Anticipatory Guidance Body Image Enhancement Exercise Promotion Health Screening Health System Guidance Learning Readiness Enhancement Mutual Goal Setting Nutrition Management Nutritional Counseling Role Enhancement Self-Awareness Enhancement Self-Esteem Enhancement Self-Modification Assistance Self-Responsibility Facilitation Sleep Enhancement Socialization Enhancement Spiritual Support Substance Use Prevention Teaching: Individual Teaching: Safe Sex Teaching: Sexuality Values Clarification	Abuse Protection Support Behavior Management: Sexual Behavior Modification Counseling Decision-Making Support Eating Disorders Management Family Process Management Family Support Family Therapy Sexual Counseling Support System Enhancement Weight Management

Continued

Outcome: GROWTH

MAJOR INTERVENTIONS	SUGGESTED INTERVENTIONS	OPTIONAL INTERVENTIONS
Developmental Enhancement: Adolescent Developmental Enhancement: Child Health Screening	Anticipatory Guidance Bottle Feeding Breastfeeding Assistance Counseling Eating Disorders Management Energy Management Environmental Management Family Involvement Promotion Health Education Infant Care Lactation Counseling Nutrition Management Nutrition Therapy Nutritional Counseling Nutritional Monitoring Prenatal Care Self-Esteem Enhancement Teaching: Infant Nutrition Teaching: Toddler Nutrition Weight Management	Abuse Protection Support: Child Family Therapy High-Risk Pregnancy Care Parent Education: Adolescent Preconception Counseling Referral Substance Use Prevention Substance Use Treatment Support Group Support System Enhancement Sustenance Support

Outcome: SOCIAL INTERACTION SKILLS

MAJOR INTERVENTIONS	SUGGESTED INTERVENTIONS	OPTIONAL INTERVENTIONS
Behavior Modification: Social Skills Developmental Enhancement: Adolescent Developmental Enhancement: Child	Active Listening Assertiveness Training Complex Relationship Building Counseling Family Integrity Promotion Family Process Maintenance Recreation Therapy Role Enhancement Self-Awareness Enhancement Self-Esteem Enhancement Self-Responsibility Facilitation	Anger Control Assistance Anxiety Reduction Attachment Promotion Body Image Enhancement Coping Enhancement Family Therapy Impulse Control Training Sexual Counseling Therapy Group

For interventions and outcomes related to specific risk factors refer to the following diagnoses: Breastfeeding, Ineffective; Caregiver Role Strain; Infant Feeding Pattern, Ineffective; Parenting, Altered; Parental Role Conflict; Social Isolation; Spiritual Distress.

Nursing Diagnosis: DISUSE SYNDROME, RISK FOR

DEFINITION: A state in which an individual is at risk for deterioration of body systems as the result of prescribed or unavoidable musculoskeletal inactivity. Complications from immobility can include pressure ulcer; constipation; stasis of pulmonary secretions; thrombosis; urinary tract infection/retention; decreased strength/endurance; orthostatic hypotension; decreased range of joint motion; disorientation; body image disturbance and powerlessness.

Outcome: ENDURANCE

MAJOR INTERVENTIONS	SUGGESTED INTERVENTIONS	OPTIONAL INTERVENTIONS
Activity Therapy Energy Management	Exercise Promotion Exercise Promotion: Strength Training Nutrition Management Risk Identification Sleep Enhancement Teaching: Prescribed Activity/Exercise	Environmental Management Exercise Therapy: Ambulation Exercise Therapy: Balance Exercise Therapy: Joint Mobility Exercise Therapy: Muscle Control Pain Management

Outcome: IMMOBILITY CONSEQUENCES: PHYSIOLOGICAL

MAJOR INTERVENTIONS	SUGGESTED INTERVENTIONS	OPTIONAL INTERVENTIONS
Energy Management	Bowel Management Embolus Precautions Exercise Promotion: Stretching Exercise Therapy: Joint Mobility Exercise Therapy: Muscle Control Fluid Management Fluid Monitoring Positioning Pressure Ulcer Prevention Simple Massage Skin Surveillance	Environmental Management Exercise Therapy: Ambulation Fall Prevention Physical Restraint Positioning: Wheelchair Surveillance

Outcome: IMMOBILITY CONSEQUENCES: PSYCHO-COGNITIVE

MAJOR INTERVENTIONS	SUGGESTED INTERVENTIONS	OPTIONAL INTERVENTIONS
Cognitive Stimulation Environmental Management	Coping Enhancement Emotional Support Presence Simple Relaxation Therapy Sleep Enhancement	Animal-Assisted Therapy Counseling Environmental Management: Comfort Humor Mood Management Progressive Muscle Relaxation Reality Orientation

Outcome: MOBILITY LEVEL

MAJOR INTERVENTIONS	SUGGESTED INTERVENTIONS	OPTIONAL INTERVENTIONS
Exercise Therapy: Ambulation Exercise Therapy: Balance Exercise Therapy: Joint Mobility Exercise Therapy: Muscle Control	Activity Therapy Body Mechanics Promotion Energy Management Exercise Promotion Exercise Promotion: Strength Training Exercise Promotion: Stretching Fall Prevention	Analgesic Administration Environmental Management Pain Management Positioning Positioning: Wheelchair Teaching: Prescribed Activity/Exercise

For interventions and outcomes related to specific risk factors refer to the following diagnoses: Confusion, Chronic; Fatigue; Pain; Physical Mobility, Impaired; Thought Processes, Altered; Walking, Impaired.

Nursing Diagnosis: **FLUID VOLUME DEFICIT, RISK FOR**

DEFINITION: The state in which an individual is at risk for experiencing vascular, cellular, or intracellular dehydration.

Outcome: **ELECTROLYTE & ACID/BASE BALANCE**

MAJOR INTERVENTIONS	SUGGESTED INTERVENTIONS	OPTIONAL INTERVENTIONS

Electrolyte Management
Fluid Management
Fluid/Electrolyte
  Management
	Acid-Base Management
	Acid-Base Monitoring
	Electrolyte Monitoring
	Fluid Monitoring
	Hemodynamic
	  Regulation
	Intravenous (IV)
	  Therapy
	Laboratory Data
	  Interpretation
	Vital Signs Monitoring
		Electrolyte Management:
		  Hypercalcemia
		Electrolyte Management:
		  Hyperkalemia
		Electrolyte Management:
		  Hypermagnesemia
		Electrolyte Management:
		  Hypernatremia
		Electrolyte Management:
		  Hyperphosphatemia
		Electrolyte Management:
		  Hypocalcemia
		Electrolyte Management:
		  Hypokalemia
		Electrolyte Management:
		  Hypomagnesemia
		Electrolyte Management:
		  Hyponatremia
		Electrolyte Management:
		  Hypophosphatemia

Outcome: FLUID BALANCE

MAJOR INTERVENTIONS	SUGGESTED INTERVENTIONS	OPTIONAL INTERVENTIONS
Fluid Management Fluid Monitoring Hypovolemia Management Intravenous (IV) Therapy	Autotransfusion Bedside Laboratory Testing Diarrhea Management Electrolyte Management Electrolyte Monitoring Fluid Resuscitation Fluid/Electrolyte Management Intravenous (IV) Insertion Laboratory Data Interpretation Nutrition Management Nutritional Monitoring Shock Management: Volume Total Parenteral Nutrition (TPN) Administration Urinary Elimination Management Venous Access Devices (VAD) Maintenance Vital Signs Monitoring	Bleeding Precautions Bleeding Reduction Blood Products Administration Cardiac Care: Acute Hemodynamic Regulation Hemorrhage Control Peripherally Inserted Central (PIC) Catheter Care Shock Prevention Surveillance

Continued

Outcome: HYDRATION

MAJOR INTERVENTIONS	SUGGESTED INTERVENTIONS	OPTIONAL INTERVENTIONS

Fluid Management
Hypovolemia
  Management
	Bottle Feeding
	Diarrhea Management
	Electrolyte Management
	Electrolyte Monitoring
	Feeding
	Fever Treatment
	Fluid Monitoring
	Fluid/Electrolyte
	  Management
	Heat Exposure
	  Treatment
	Nutrition Management
	Nutritional Monitoring
	Urinary Elimination
	  Management
	Vital Signs Monitoring
		Bleeding Precautions
		Bleeding Reduction
		Bleeding Reduction:
		  Gastrointestinal
		Shock Management:
		  Volume
		Shock Prevention
		Temperature Regulation

Outcome: NUTRITIONAL STATUS: FOOD & FLUID INTAKE

MAJOR INTERVENTIONS	SUGGESTED INTERVENTIONS	OPTIONAL INTERVENTIONS

Fluid Monitoring
Nutritional Monitoring
	Enteral Tube Feeding
	Feeding
	Fluid Management
	Nutrition Management
	Self-Care Assistance:
	  Feeding
	Total Parenteral
	  Nutrition (TPN)
	  Administration
		Bottle Feeding
		Intravenous (IV)
		  Therapy
		Lactation Counseling
		Oral Health Restoration
		Swallowing Therapy
		Teaching:
		  Prescribed Diet

For interventions and outcomes related to specific risk factors refer to the following diagnoses: Diarrhea; Failure to Thrive, Adult; Hyperthermia; Infant Feeding Pattern, Ineffective; Knowledge, Deficit; Nausea; Nutrition, Altered: Less Than Body Requirements; Physical Mobility Impaired; Self-Care Deficit: Feeding; Swallowing, Impaired.

Nursing Diagnosis: FLUID VOLUME IMBALANCE, RISK FOR

DEFINITION: A risk of a decrease, increase, or rapid shift from one to the other of intravascular, interstitial, and/or intracellular fluid. This refers to the loss, excess, or both loss and excess of body fluids or replacement fluids.

Outcome: ELECTROLYTE & ACID/BASE BALANCE

MAJOR INTERVENTIONS	SUGGESTED INTERVENTIONS	OPTIONAL INTERVENTIONS
Electrolyte Management Fluid Management Fluid/Electrolyte Management	Acid-Base Management Acid-Base Monitoring Electrolyte Monitoring Fluid Monitoring Hemodialysis Therapy Hemodynamic Regulation Intravenous (IV) Therapy Laboratory Data Interpretation Neurologic Monitoring Vital Signs Monitoring	Electrolyte Management: Hypercalcemia Electrolyte Management: Hyperkalemia Electrolyte Management: Hypermagnesemia Electrolyte Management: Hypernatremia Electrolyte Management: Hyperphosphatemia Electrolyte Management: Hypocalcemia Electrolyte Management: Hypokalemia Electrolyte Management: Hypomagnesemia Electrolyte Management: Hyponatremia Electrolyte Management: Hypophosphatemia Respiratory Monitoring Specimen Management Total Parenteral Nutrition (TPN) Administration

Continued

Outcome: FLUID BALANCE

MAJOR INTERVENTIONS	SUGGESTED INTERVENTIONS	OPTIONAL INTERVENTIONS
Fluid Management Fluid Monitoring	Bedside Laboratory Testing Diarrhea Management Electrolyte Management Electrolyte Monitoring Fluid Resuscitation Fluid/Electrolyte Management Hypervolemia Management Hypovolemia Management Intravenous (IV) Insertion Intravenous (IV) Therapy Laboratory Data Interpretation Medication Administration Medication Management Medication Prescribing Nutrition Management Nutritional Monitoring Surveillance Total Parenteral Nutrition (TPN) Administration Urinary Elimination Management Vital Signs Monitoring	Bleeding Precautions Bleeding Reduction Bleeding Reduction: Gastrointestinal Blood Products Administration Hemodialysis Therapy Hemodynamic Regulation Hemorrhage Control Intracranial Pressure (ICP) Monitoring Invasive Hemodynamic Monitoring Peritoneal Dialysis Therapy Phlebotomy: Arterial Blood Sample Phlebotomy: Venous Blood Sample Respiratory Monitoring Shock Management Shock Management: Volume Shock Prevention Venous Access Devices (VAD) Maintenance

Outcome: HYDRATION

MAJOR INTERVENTIONS	SUGGESTED INTERVENTIONS	OPTIONAL INTERVENTIONS
Fluid Management Fluid Monitoring	Bottle Feeding Diarrhea Management Electrolyte Management Electrolyte Monitoring Feeding Fever Treatment Fluid Resuscitation Fluid/Electrolyte Management Heat Exposure Treatment Hypovolemia Management Intravenous (IV) Insertion Intravenous (IV) Therapy Nutrition Management Nutritional Monitoring Shock Management: Volume Urinary Elimination Management Vital Signs Monitoring	Bleeding Precautions Bleeding Reduction Hemorrhage Control Temperature Regulation

For interventions and outcomes related to specific risk factors refer to the following diagnoses: Diarrhea; Failure to Thrive, Adult; Fluid Volume Excess; Fluid Volume Deficit; Hyperthermia; Infant Feeding Pattern, Ineffective; Knowledge Deficit; Nausea; Nutrition, Altered: Less Than Body Requirements; Nutrition, Altered: More Than Body Requirements; Physical Mobility, Impaired; Self-Care Deficit: Feeding; Swallowing, Impaired; Urinary Elimination, Altered.

Nursing Diagnosis: GROWTH, RISK FOR ALTERED

DEFINITION: At risk for growth above the 97th percentile or below the 3rd percentile for age, crossing two percentile channels; disproportionate growth.

Outcome: CHILD DEVELOPMENT: 6 MONTHS

MAJOR INTERVENTIONS	SUGGESTED INTERVENTIONS	OPTIONAL INTERVENTIONS
Infant Care Teaching: Infant Nutrition	Attachment Promotion Bottle Feeding Health Screening Immunization/ Vaccination Management Kangaroo Care Lactation Counseling Parent Education: Infant Risk Identification Sleep Enhancement	Abuse Protection Support: Child Caregiver Support Health System Guidance Nutritional Monitoring Risk Identification: Genetic Sibling Support Surveillance Sustenance Support

Outcome: CHILD DEVELOPMENT: 12 MONTHS

MAJOR INTERVENTIONS	SUGGESTED INTERVENTIONS	OPTIONAL INTERVENTIONS
Infant Care Teaching: Infant Nutrition	Bottle Feeding Health Screening Immunization/ Vaccination Management Lactation Counseling Parent Education: Infant Risk Identification Sleep Enhancement	Abuse Protection Support: Child Attachment Promotion Caregiver Support Health System Guidance Nutrition Management Nutritional Monitoring Respite Care Sibling Support Surveillance Sustenance Support

Outcome: **CHILD DEVELOPMENT: 2 YEARS**		
MAJOR INTERVENTIONS	**SUGGESTED INTERVENTIONS**	**OPTIONAL INTERVENTIONS**

Health Screening
Teaching: Toddler
  Nutrition
	Nutrition Management
	Nutritional Monitoring
	Risk Identification
		Abuse Protection
		  Support: Child
		Family Therapy
		Health System Guidance
		Nutritional Counseling
		Support System
		  Enhancement
		Surveillance
		Sustenance Support

Outcome: **CHILD DEVELOPMENT: 3 YEARS**		
MAJOR INTERVENTIONS	**SUGGESTED INTERVENTIONS**	**OPTIONAL INTERVENTIONS**

Health Screening
Nutritional Monitoring
Teaching: Toddler
  Nutrition
	Nutrition Management
	Nutritional Counseling
	Risk Identification
	Support System
	  Enhancement
		Abuse Protection
		  Support: Child
		Energy Management
		Family Therapy
		Health System Guidance
		Sleep Enhancement
		Sustenance Support

Outcome: **CHILD DEVELOPMENT: 4 YEARS**		
MAJOR INTERVENTIONS	**SUGGESTED INTERVENTIONS**	**OPTIONAL INTERVENTIONS**

Health Screening
Nutritional Monitoring
Teaching: Toddler
  Nutrition
	Nutrition Management
	Risk Identification
	Support System
	  Enhancement
		Abuse Protection
		  Support: Child
		Behavior Management
		Behavior Modification
		Energy Management
		Health System Guidance
		Nutritional Counseling
		Sleep Enhancement
		Sustenance Support

Continued

Outcome: CHILD DEVELOPMENT: 5 YEARS

MAJOR INTERVENTIONS	SUGGESTED INTERVENTIONS	OPTIONAL INTERVENTIONS
Nutrition Management Nutritional Monitoring	Health Screening Nutritional Counseling Risk Identification	Abuse Protection Support: Child Behavior Management Behavior Modification Counseling Energy Management Health System Guidance Sleep Enhancement Sustenance Support

Outcome: CHILD DEVELOPMENT: MIDDLE CHILDHOOD (6-11 YEARS)

MAJOR INTERVENTIONS	SUGGESTED INTERVENTIONS	OPTIONAL INTERVENTIONS

Nutrition Management
Nutritional Monitoring
Weight Management
	Behavior Modification
	Counseling
	Eating Disorders
	  Management
	Exercise Promotion
	Health Screening
	Learning Facilitation
	Nutritional Counseling
	Patient Contracting
	Substance Use
	  Prevention
	Teaching:
	  Prescribed Diet
		Abuse Protection
		  Support: Child
		Behavior Management
		Coping Enhancement
		Family Support
		Family Therapy
		Health System Guidance
		Self-Modification
		  Assistance
		Self-Responsibility
		  Facilitation
		Weight Gain Assistance
		Weight Reduction
		  Assistance

Outcome: GROWTH

MAJOR INTERVENTIONS	SUGGESTED INTERVENTIONS	OPTIONAL INTERVENTIONS

Nutrition Management
Nutritional Monitoring
Weight Management
	Bottle Feeding
	Breastfeeding Assistance
	Counseling
	Developmental
	  Enhancement: Child
	Eating Disorders
	  Management
	Energy Management
	Health Education
	Health Screening
	Lactation Counseling
	Nutrition Therapy
	Nutritional Counseling
	Prenatal Care
	Teaching: Infant
	  Nutrition
	Teaching:
	  Prescribed Diet
	Teaching: Toddler
	  Nutrition
	Weight Gain Assistance
	Weight Reduction
	  Assistance
		Abuse Protection
		  Support: Child
		Enteral Tube Feeding
		Family Therapy
		High Risk Pregnancy
		  Care
		Parent Education:
		  Adolescent
		Parent Education:
		  Childrearing Family
		Preconception
		  Counseling
		Referral
		Substance Use
		  Prevention
		Substance Use Treatment
		Support System
		  Enhancement
		Sustenance Support
		Swallowing Therapy
		Total Parenteral
		  Nutrition (TPN)
		  Administration

For interventions and outcomes related to specific risk factors refer to the following diagnoses: Breastfeeding, Ineffective; Diarrhea; Health Maintenance, Altered; Infant Feeding Pattern, Ineffective; Infection, Risk for; Nutrition, Altered: Less than Body Requirements; Oral Mucous Membrane, Altered; Swallowing, Impaired; Violence, Risk for: Directed at Others.

Nursing Diagnosis: Infant Behavior, Disorganized, Risk for

Definition: Risk for alteration in integrating and modulation of the physiological and behavioral systems of functioning (i.e., autonomic, motor, state, organizational, self-regulatory, and attentional-interactional systems).

Outcome: Child Development: 2 months

MAJOR INTERVENTIONS	SUGGESTED INTERVENTIONS	OPTIONAL INTERVENTIONS
Infant Care	Attachment Promotion	Abuse Protection
Parent Education: Infant	Bottle Feeding	Support: Child
	Breastfeeding Assistance	Caregiver Support
	Family Integrity	Environmental
	Promotion:	Management
	Childbearing Family	Family Mobilization
	Family Process	Health System Guidance
	Maintenance	Nutritional Monitoring
	Family Support	Respite Care
	Lactation Counseling	Sibling Support
	Nonnutritive Sucking	Support System
	Sleep Enhancement	Enhancement
		Surveillance

Outcome: Child Development: 4 months

MAJOR INTERVENTIONS	SUGGESTED INTERVENTIONS	OPTIONAL INTERVENTIONS
Health Screening	Bottle Feeding	Abuse Protection
Infant Care	Family Integrity	Support: Child
Parent Education: Infant	Promotion:	Attachment Promotion
Risk Identification	Childbearing Family	Caregiver Support
	Family Process	Environmental
	Maintenance	Management
	Family Support	Family Mobilization
	Lactation Counseling	Health System Guidance
	Security Enhancement	Nonnutritive Sucking
	Sleep Enhancement	Nutrition Management
		Nutritional Monitoring
		Respite Care
		Sibling Support
		Support System
		Enhancement
		Surveillance

Outcome: PRETERM INFANT ORGANIZATION

MAJOR INTERVENTIONS	SUGGESTED INTERVENTIONS	OPTIONAL INTERVENTIONS
Environmental Management Newborn Monitoring Positioning	Developmental Care Environmental Management: Comfort Infant Care Kangaroo Care Lactation Counseling Neurologic Monitoring Nonnutritive Sucking Pain Management Respiratory Monitoring Surveillance Vital Signs Monitoring	Bottle Feeding Nutritional Monitoring Temperature Regulation

For interventions and outcomes related to specific risk factors refer to the following diagnoses: Growth and Development, Altered; Pain; Protection, Altered; Sensory, Perceptual Alterations.

Nursing Diagnosis: INFECTION, RISK FOR

DEFINITION: A state in which an individual is at increased risk for being invaded by pathogenic organisms.

Outcome: IMMUNE STATUS

MAJOR INTERVENTIONS	SUGGESTED INTERVENTIONS	OPTIONAL INTERVENTIONS
Health Screening Immunization/ Vaccination Management	Allergy Management Health Education Health System Guidance Infection Protection Laboratory Data Interpretation Medication Administration Parent Education: Infant Risk Identification Surveillance Teaching: Disease Process Teaching: Prescribed Medication	Newborn Care

Outcome: INFECTION STATUS

MAJOR INTERVENTIONS	SUGGESTED INTERVENTIONS	OPTIONAL INTERVENTIONS
Immunization/ Vaccination Management Infection Control Infection Protection	Bedside Laboratory Testing Communicable Disease Management Environmental Management Health Screening High-Risk Pregnancy Care Incision Site Care Infection Control: Intraoperative Labor Induction Laboratory Data Interpretation Medication Administration Medication Management Medication Prescribing Respiratory Monitoring Skin Surveillance Specimen Management Urinary Catheterization Vital Signs Monitoring Wound Care	Airway Management Allergy Management Amputation Care Artificial Airway Management Aspiration Precautions Bathing Birthing Cesarean Section Care Chest Physiotherapy Cough Enhancement Electronic Fetal Monitoring: Intrapartum Fever Treatment Health Education Intrapartal Care Intrapartal Care: High-Risk Delivery Nutrition Management Oral Health Maintenance Perineal Care Postpartal Care Pregnancy Termination Care Pressure Ulcer Care Tube Care Tube Care: Chest Tube Care: Gastrointestinal Tube Care: Umbilical Line Tube Care: Urinary Tube Care: Ventriculostomy/ Lumbar Drain Urinary Retention Care Venous Access Devices (VAD) Maintenance Wound Care

Continued

Outcome: Risk Control: Sexually Transmitted Diseases (STD)

MAJOR INTERVENTIONS	SUGGESTED INTERVENTIONS	OPTIONAL INTERVENTIONS
Infection Protection Teaching: Safe Sex Teaching: Sexuality	Active Listening Anticipatory Guidance Behavior Management: Sexual Behavior Modification Environmental Management: Community Health Education Health Screening Health System Guidance Patient Contracting Risk Identification Self-Responsibility Facilitation Sexual Counseling	Fertility Preservation Impulse Control Training Support Group

Outcome: Wound Healing: Primary Intention

MAJOR INTERVENTIONS	SUGGESTED INTERVENTIONS	OPTIONAL INTERVENTIONS
Incision Site Care Wound Care	Circulatory Precautions Fluid/Electrolyte Management Infection Control: Intraoperative Infection Protection Medication Administration Medication Administration: Skin Nutrition Management Skin Care: Topical Treatments Skin Surveillance Splinting Suturing Teaching: Prescribed Medication Teaching: Procedure/Treatment Wound Care: Closed Drainage	Bathing Bed Rest Care Cesarean Section Care Hyperglycemia Management Perineal Care

Outcome: WOUND HEALING: SECONDARY INTENTION

MAJOR INTERVENTIONS	SUGGESTED INTERVENTIONS	OPTIONAL INTERVENTIONS
Circulatory Care: Arterial Insufficiency Infection Control Wound Care	Circulatory Precautions Fluid/Electrolyte Management Infection Protection Medication Administration Medication Administration: Skin Nutrition Therapy Skin Care: Topical Treatments Skin Surveillance Splinting Teaching: Disease Process Teaching: Prescribed Medication Teaching: Procedure/ Treatment Transcutaneous Electrical Nerve Stimulation (TENS) Wound Care: Closed Drainage Wound Irrigation	Bathing Cutaneous Stimulation Hyperglycemia Management Leech Therapy Nutrition Management Positioning Pressure Ulcer Care Total Parenteral Nutrition (TPN) Administration

For interventions and outcomes related to specific risk factors refer to the following diagnoses: Dentition, Altered; Failure to Thrive, Adult; Health Maintenance, Altered; Individual Management of Therapeutic Regimen, Ineffective; Knowledge Deficit; Oral Mucous Membrane, Altered; Protection, Altered; Surgical Recovery, Delayed; Tissue Integrity, Impaired.

Nursing Diagnosis: INJURY, RISK FOR

DEFINITION: A state in which an individual is at risk of injury as a result of environmental conditions interacting with the individual's adaptive and defensive resources.

Outcome: FETAL STATUS: INTRAPARTUM

MAJOR INTERVENTIONS	SUGGESTED INTERVENTIONS	OPTIONAL INTERVENTIONS
Electronic Fetal Monitoring: Intrapartum	Labor Induction Intrapartal Care Intrapartal Care: High-Risk Delivery Newborn Monitoring Resuscitation: Neonate	Birthing High-Risk Pregnancy Care Newborn Care

Outcome: IMMUNE STATUS

MAJOR INTERVENTIONS	SUGGESTED INTERVENTIONS	OPTIONAL INTERVENTIONS
Allergy Management Health Screening Immunization/ Vaccination Management	Health Education Health System Guidance Infection Protection Latex Precautions Medication Administration Risk Identification Surveillance Teaching: Individual	Infection Control Surveillance

Outcome: MATERNAL STATUS: INTRAPARTUM

MAJOR INTERVENTIONS	SUGGESTED INTERVENTIONS	OPTIONAL INTERVENTIONS
Labor Induction Intrapartal Care: High-Risk Delivery	Bleeding Precautions Bleeding Reduction Environmental Management Infection Protection Intrapartal Care Labor Suppression Medication Administration Medication Management	High-Risk Pregnancy Care Neurologic Monitoring Seizure Management Surgical Precautions Ultrasonography: Limited Obstetric

Outcome: PARENTING: SOCIAL SAFETY

MAJOR INTERVENTIONS	SUGGESTED INTERVENTIONS	OPTIONAL INTERVENTIONS
Parent Education: Adolescent Parent Education: Childrearing Family Risk Identification Risk Identification: Childbearing Family	Abuse Protection Support: Child Anticipatory Guidance Developmental Enhancement: Child Family Integrity Promotion Family Integrity Promotion: Childbearing Family Family Mobilization Health Screening Socialization Enhancement Surveillance: Safety	Counseling Emotional Support Family Support Family Therapy Mutual Goal Setting Parent Education: Infant Self-Esteem Enhancement Self-Modification Assistance Self-Responsibility Facilitation Substance Use Prevention Support Group Teaching: Individual

Outcome: RISK CONTROL

MAJOR INTERVENTIONS	SUGGESTED INTERVENTIONS	OPTIONAL INTERVENTIONS
Behavior Modification Health Education Patient Contracting Self-Modification Assistance	Family Mobilization Health Screening Health System Guidance Learning Facilitation Learning Readiness Enhancement Mutual Goal Setting Risk Identification Self-Responsibility Facilitation Support System Enhancement	Allergy Management Bleeding Precautions Environmental Management: Safety Environmental Management: Violence Prevention Environmental Management: Worker Safety Family Involvement Promotion Immunization/ Vaccination Management Infection Control Laser Precautions Latex Precautions Suicide Prevention Surgical Precautions

Continued

Outcome: Safety Behavior: Home Physical Environment

MAJOR INTERVENTIONS	SUGGESTED INTERVENTIONS	OPTIONAL INTERVENTIONS
Environmental Management: Safety Surveillance: Safety	Area Restriction Environmental Management: Violence Prevention Environmental Management: Worker Safety Fire-Setting Precautions Home Maintenance Assistance Risk Identification	Dementia Management Hallucination Management Incident Reporting Parent Education: Childrearing Family Parent Education: Infant Seizure Precautions

Outcome: Safety Behavior: Personal

MAJOR INTERVENTIONS	SUGGESTED INTERVENTIONS	OPTIONAL INTERVENTIONS
Environmental Management: Safety Health Education	Anger Control Assistance Behavior Modification Environmental Management: Violence Prevention Home Maintenance Assistance Impulse Control Training Risk Identification Substance Use Prevention Surveillance: Safety Teaching: Safe Sex	Abuse Protection Support Allergy Management Area Restriction Behavior Management: Overactivity/ Inattention Behavior Management: Self-Harm Behavior Management: Sexual Environmental Management: Worker Safety Physical Restraint Security Enhancement

Outcome: SAFETY STATUS: FALLS OCCURRENCE

MAJOR INTERVENTIONS	SUGGESTED INTERVENTIONS	OPTIONAL INTERVENTIONS

Fall Prevention
Surveillance: Safety
	Environmental
	    Management: Safety
	Home Maintenance
	    Assistance
	Incident Reporting
	Risk Identification
	Security Enhancement
		Area Restriction
		Dementia Management
		Hallucination
		    Management
		Physical Restraint
		Seizure Precautions
		Teaching: Prescribed
		    Activity/Exercise

Outcome: SAFETY STATUS: PHYSICAL INJURY

MAJOR INTERVENTIONS	SUGGESTED INTERVENTIONS	OPTIONAL INTERVENTIONS

Fall Prevention
Surveillance: Safety
	Emergency Care
	Environmental
	    Management
	Environmental
	    Management: Safety
	Environmental
	    Management: Violence
	    Prevention
	Environmental
	    Management: Worker
	    Safety
	Home Maintenance
	    Assistance
	Incident Reporting
	Risk Identification
	Security Enhancement
		Area Restriction
		Delusion Management
		Dementia Management
		Elopement Precautions
		Hallucination
		    Management
		Physical Restraint
		Reality Orientation
		Seizure Management
		Seizure Precautions
		Sports-Injury Prevention:
		    Youth

For interventions and outcomes related to specific risk factors refer to the following diagnoses: Breathing Pattern, Ineffective; Community Coping, Ineffective; Individual Coping, Ineffective; Latex Allergy Response; Nutrition, Altered: Less Than Body Requirements; Post-Trauma Syndrome; Protection, Altered; Thermoregulation, Ineffective; Tissue Perfusion, Altered; Tissue Integrity, Impaired.

Nursing Diagnosis: LATEX ALLERGY RESPONSE, RISK FOR

DEFINITION: At risk for allergic response to natural latex rubber products.

Outcome: IMMUNE HYPERSENSITIVITY CONTROL

MAJOR INTERVENTIONS	SUGGESTED INTERVENTIONS	OPTIONAL INTERVENTIONS
Latex Precautions	Allergy Management Environmental Management Environmental Risk Protection Risk Identification Surveillance Teaching: Individual	Environmental Management: Worker Safety Health Care Information Exchange Health System Guidance Skin Surveillance Surveillance

For interventions and outcomes related to specific risk factors refer to the following diagnoses: Protection, Altered; Skin Integrity, Impaired; Tissue Integrity, Impaired.

Nursing Diagnosis: LONELINESS, RISK FOR

DEFINITION: A subjective state in which an individual is at risk of experiencing vague dysphoria.

Outcome: LONELINESS

MAJOR INTERVENTIONS	SUGGESTED INTERVENTIONS	OPTIONAL INTERVENTIONS
Socialization Enhancement	Activity Therapy	Art Therapy
Spiritual Support	Animal-Assisted Therapy	Bibliotherapy
Visitation Facilitation	Behavior Modification: Social Skills	Communication Enhancement: Hearing Deficit
	Complex Relationship Building	Communication Enhancement: Speech Deficit
	Coping Enhancement	Communication Enhancement: Visual Deficit
	Counseling	Family Therapy
	Emotional Support	Grief Work Facilitation
	Environmental Management	Reminiscence Therapy
	Family Integrity Promotion	Suicide Prevention
	Family Involvement Promotion	
	Family Mobilization	
	Hope Instillation	
	Mood Management	
	Presence	
	Recreation Therapy	
	Role Enhancement	
	Self-Awareness Enhancement	
	Self-Esteem Enhancement	
	Support Group	
	Support System Enhancement	
	Therapeutic Play	
	Therapy Group	
	Touch	

Continued

Outcome: SOCIAL INVOLVEMENT

MAJOR INTERVENTIONS	SUGGESTED INTERVENTIONS	OPTIONAL INTERVENTIONS
Socialization Enhancement	Activity Therapy Animal-Assisted Therapy Anxiety Reduction Art Therapy Recreation Therapy Reminiscence Therapy Role Enhancement Self-Awareness Enhancement Self-Esteem Enhancement Self-Responsibility Facilitation Therapeutic Play Visitation Facilitation	Active Listening Assertiveness Training Behavior Management Body Image Enhancement Complex Relationship Building Counseling Culture Brokerage Developmental Enhancement: Child Family Mobilization Family Therapy Milieu Therapy Mood Management Normalization Promotion Presence Support Group Support System Enhancement

For interventions and outcomes related to specific risk factors refer to the following diagnoses: Social Interaction, Impaired; Social Isolation; Sorrow, Chronic; Spiritual Distress.

Nursing Diagnosis: NUTRITION, ALTERED: RISK FOR MORE THAN BODY REQUIREMENTS

DEFINITION: The state in which an individual is at risk of experiencing an intake of nutrients that exceeds metabolic needs.

Outcome: NUTRITIONAL STATUS: FOOD & FLUID INTAKE

MAJOR INTERVENTIONS	SUGGESTED INTERVENTIONS	OPTIONAL INTERVENTIONS

Nutrition Management
Nutritional Monitoring
	Behavior Modification
	Fluid Management
	Fluid Monitoring
	Teaching:
	  Prescribed Diet
	Weight Management
	Weight Reduction
	  Assistance
		Behavior Management
		Mutual Goal Setting
		Patient Contracting
		Self-Responsibility
		  Facilitation

Outcome: WEIGHT CONTROL

MAJOR INTERVENTIONS	SUGGESTED INTERVENTIONS	OPTIONAL INTERVENTIONS

Nutrition Management
Weight Management
	Behavior Modification
	Exercise Promotion
	Nutritional Counseling
	Nutritional Monitoring
	Patient Contracting
	Self-Responsibility
	  Facilitation
		Behavior Management
		Mutual Goal Setting
		Teaching: Individual
		Teaching:
		  Prescribed Diet

For interventions and outcomes related to specific risk factors refer to the following diagnoses: Anxiety; Body Image Disturbance; Diversional Activity Deficit; Health Maintenance, Altered; Individual Coping, Ineffective; Physical Mobility, Impaired; Self-Esteem, Chronic Low; Sorrow, Chronic; Walking, Impaired.

Nursing Diagnosis: **PARENT/INFANT/CHILD ATTACHMENT, RISK FOR ALTERED**

DEFINITION: Disruption of the interactive process between parent/significant other and infant that fosters the development of a protective and nurturing reciprocal relationship.

Outcome: **PARENT-INFANT ATTACHMENT**

MAJOR INTERVENTIONS	SUGGESTED INTERVENTIONS	OPTIONAL INTERVENTIONS
Attachment Promotion	Anticipatory Guidance	Emotional Support
Environmental Management: Attachment Process	Anxiety Reduction	Family Integrity Promotion
Parent Education: Infant	Breastfeeding Assistance	Family Involvement Promotion
	Coping Enhancement	Family Process Maintenance
	Infant Care	
	Intrapartal Care	
	Kangaroo Care	
	Lactation Counseling	
	Normalization Promotion	
	Prenatal Care	
	Risk Identification: Childbearing Family	
	Role Enhancement	

Outcome: PARENTING

MAJOR INTERVENTIONS	SUGGESTED INTERVENTIONS	OPTIONAL INTERVENTIONS
Developmental Enhancement: Child Parenting Promotion	Abuse Protection Support: Child Anticipatory Guidance Coping Enhancement Counseling Environmental Management Family Integrity Promotion: Childbearing Family Family Involvement Promotion Family Mobilization Family Process Maintenance Family Support Normalization Promotion Parent Education: Adolescent Parent Education: Childrearing Family Respite Care Role Enhancement Self-Awareness Enhancement Self-Esteem Enhancement Self-Responsibility Facilitation Socialization Enhancement Support System Enhancement	Behavior Management: Overactivity/ Inattention Behavior Modification Breastfeeding Assistance Emotional Support Family Integrity Promotion Family Therapy Sibling Support Substance Use Prevention Substance Use Treatment Support Group Therapy Group

Continued

Outcome: ROLE PERFORMANCE

MAJOR INTERVENTIONS	SUGGESTED INTERVENTIONS	OPTIONAL INTERVENTIONS

Parenting Promotion
Role Enhancement
	Anticipatory Guidance
	Attachment Promotion
	Behavior Modification
	Caregiver Support
	Coping Enhancement
	Counseling
	Emotional Support
	Self-Awareness
	  Enhancement
	Self-Responsibility
	  Facilitation
	Values Clarification
		Childbirth Preparation
		Family Integrity
		  Promotion
		Family Therapy
		Kangaroo Care
		Parent Education:
		  Adolescent
		Parent Education:
		  Childrearing Family
		Parent Education: Infant
		Self-Esteem
		  Enhancement
		Support Group
		Support System
		  Enhancement

For interventions and outcomes related to specific risk factors refer to the following diagnoses: Breastfeeding, Ineffective; Breastfeeding, Interrupted; Caregiver Role Strain; Family Coping: Compromised, Ineffective; Family Processes, Altered; Individual Coping, Ineffective; Infant Behavior, Disorganized; Knowledge Deficit; Parental Role Conflict; Parenting, Altered; Role Performance, Altered; Self-Esteem, Situational Low.

Nursing Diagnosis: PARENTING, RISK FOR ALTERED

DEFINITION: Risk for inability of the primary caretaker to create, maintain, or regain an environment that promotes the optimum growth and development of the child.

Outcome: PARENT-INFANT ATTACHMENT

MAJOR INTERVENTIONS	SUGGESTED INTERVENTIONS	OPTIONAL INTERVENTIONS
Attachment Promotion Environmental Management: Attachment Process	Breastfeeding Assistance Family Integrity Promotion Infant Care Intrapartal Care Kangaroo Care Lactation Counseling Parent Education: Infant Prenatal Care Risk Identification: Childbearing Family	Anticipatory Guidance Coping Enhancement Emotional Support Role Enhancement Surveillance

Continued

Outcome: PARENTING

MAJOR INTERVENTIONS	SUGGESTED INTERVENTIONS	OPTIONAL INTERVENTIONS
Developmental Enhancement: Adolescent Developmental Enhancement: Child Family Integrity Promotion Parenting Promotion	Abuse Protection Support: Child Anticipatory Guidance Attachment Promotion Caregiver Support Coping Enhancement Counseling Normalization Promotion Parent Education: Adolescent Parent Education: Childrearing Family Parent Education: Infant Resiliency Promotion Role Enhancement Self-Esteem Enhancement Sibling Support Support System Enhancement	Breastfeeding Assistance Childbirth Preparation Emotional Support Family Integrity Promotion: Childbearing Family Family Involvement Promotion Family Process Maintenance Family Support Family Therapy Financial Resource Assistance Health Education Health System Guidance High-Risk Pregnancy Care Home Maintenance Assistance Infant Care Newborn Care Postpartal Care Prenatal Care Respite Care Security Enhancement Support Group

Outcome: PARENTING: SOCIAL SAFETY

MAJOR INTERVENTIONS	SUGGESTED INTERVENTIONS	OPTIONAL INTERVENTIONS
Abuse Protection Support: Child Family Integrity Promotion	Anticipatory Guidance Developmental Enhancement: Adolescent Developmental Enhancement: Child Family Integrity Promotion: Childbearing Family Health Screening Parent Education: Adolescent Parent Education: Childrearing Family Risk Identification Risk Identification: Childbearing Family Socialization Enhancement Surveillance: Safety	Counseling Emotional Support Family Support Family Therapy Self-Esteem Enhancement Self-Modification Assistance Self-Responsibility Facilitation Substance Use Prevention Support Group Teaching: Individual

Continued

Outcome: ROLE PERFORMANCE

MAJOR INTERVENTIONS	SUGGESTED INTERVENTIONS	OPTIONAL INTERVENTIONS

Parenting Promotion
Role Enhancement
	Anticipatory Guidance
	Behavior Modification
	Caregiver Support
	Coping Enhancement
	Counseling
	Emotional Support
	Resiliency Promotion
	Self-Awareness
	  Enhancement
	Support System
	  Enhancement
	Values Clarification
		Attachment Promotion
		Childbirth Preparation
		Decision-Making
		  Support
		Energy Management
		Family Integrity
		  Promotion
		Family Therapy
		Health Education
		Parent Education:
		  Adolescent
		Parent Education:
		  Childrearing Family
		Parent Education: Infant
		Self-Esteem
		  Enhancement
		Support Group
		Teaching: Sexuality

For interventions and outcomes related to specific risk factors refer to the following diagnoses: Breastfeeding, Ineffective; Breastfeeding, Interrupted; Caregiver Role Strain; Family Coping: Compromised, Ineffective; Family Processes, Altered; Individual Coping, Ineffective; Infant Behavior, Disorganized; Knowledge Deficit; Parental Role Conflict; Parenting, Altered; Role Performance, Altered; Self-Esteem, Situational Low.

Nursing Diagnosis: PERIOPERATIVE POSITIONING INJURY, RISK FOR

DEFINITION: A state in which the client is at risk for injury as a result of the environmental conditions found in the perioperative setting.

Outcome: CIRCULATION STATUS

MAJOR INTERVENTIONS	SUGGESTED INTERVENTIONS	OPTIONAL INTERVENTIONS
Circulatory Care: Arterial Insufficiency Circulatory Care: Venous Insufficiency Positioning: Intraoperative	Bleeding Reduction: Wound Circulatory Care: Mechanical Assist Device Circulatory Precautions Embolus Care: Peripheral Embolus Care: Pulmonary Embolus Precautions Hemodynamic Regulation Hemorrhage Control Hypovolemia Management Shock Prevention	Blood Products Administration Cerebral Perfusion Promotion Fluid Resuscitation Intravenous (IV) Insertion Intravenous (IV) Therapy Invasive Hemodynamic Monitoring Pneumatic Tourniquet Precautions

Outcome: NEUROLOGICAL STATUS

MAJOR INTERVENTIONS	SUGGESTED INTERVENTIONS	OPTIONAL INTERVENTIONS
Cerebral Profusion Promotion	Code Management Emergency Care Fluid Management Fluid Monitoring Neurologic Monitoring Peripheral Sensation Management Positioning: Intraoperative Respiratory Monitoring Seizure Management Seizure Precautions Surgical Precautions Surveillance Temperature Regulation: Intraoperative Vital Signs Monitoring	Invasive Hemodynamic Monitoring Medication Administration Medication Management

Continued

Outcome: RESPIRATORY STATUS: VENTILATION

MAJOR INTERVENTIONS	SUGGESTED INTERVENTIONS	OPTIONAL INTERVENTIONS
Airway Insertion and Stabilization Airway Management	Airway Suctioning Artificial Airway Management Aspiration Precautions Positioning: Intraoperative Respiratory Monitoring	Mechanical Ventilation Oxygen Therapy Ventilation Assistance

Outcome: TISSUE PERFUSION: PERIPHERAL

MAJOR INTERVENTIONS	SUGGESTED INTERVENTIONS	OPTIONAL INTERVENTIONS
Circulatory Precautions Embolus Care: Peripheral	Bleeding Reduction Cerebral Perfusion Promotion Circulatory Care: Arterial Insufficiency Circulatory Care: Mechanical Assist Device Circulatory Care: Venous Insufficiency Fluid Management Hemodynamic Regulation Hypovolemia Management Pressure Management Shock Prevention Skin Surveillance	Blood Products Administration Incision Site Care Pneumatic Tourniquet Precautions Positioning: Intraoperative Resuscitation

For interventions and outcomes related to specific risk factors refer to the following diagnoses: Environmental Interpretation Syndrome, Impaired; Failure to Thrive, Adult; Fluid Volume Excess; Mobility, Impaired Bed; Sensory/Perceptual Alterations; Thought Processes, Altered; Unilateral Neglect.

Nursing Diagnosis: PERIPHERAL NEUROVASCULAR DYSFUNCTION, RISK FOR

DEFINITION: A state in which an individual is at risk of experiencing a disruption in circulation, sensation, or motion of an extremity.

Outcome: JOINT MOVEMENT: ACTIVE

MAJOR INTERVENTIONS	SUGGESTED INTERVENTIONS	OPTIONAL INTERVENTIONS
Exercise Therapy: Joint Mobility	Energy Management Exercise Promotion: Stretching Exercise Therapy: Muscle Control	Body Mechanics Promotion Exercise Promotion Exercise Therapy: Ambulation Heat/Cold Application Pain Management Progressive Muscle Relaxation Splinting Teaching: Prescribed Activity/Exercise

Outcome: MUSCLE FUNCTION

MAJOR INTERVENTIONS	SUGGESTED INTERVENTIONS	OPTIONAL INTERVENTIONS
Exercise Promotion: Strength Training Exercise Therapy: Muscle Control	Body Mechanics Promotion Cutaneous Stimulation Energy Management Exercise Promotion: Stretching Exercise Therapy: Joint Mobility Heat/Cold Application Progressive Muscle Relaxation Simple Massage Simple Relaxation Therapy	Bed Rest Care Exercise Promotion Pain Management Teaching: Prescribed Activity/Exercise

Continued

Outcome: NEUROLOGICAL STATUS: SPINAL SENSORY/MOTOR FUNCTION

MAJOR INTERVENTIONS	SUGGESTED INTERVENTIONS	OPTIONAL INTERVENTIONS
Peripheral Sensation Management Positioning: Neurologic	Embolus Precautions Environmental Management: Safety Neurologic Monitoring Postanesthesia Care Pressure Ulcer Prevention Skin Surveillance Surveillance Traction/Immobilization Care Vital Signs Monitoring	Exercise Promotion: Stretching Exercise Therapy: Balance Exercise Therapy: Joint Mobility Exercise Therapy: Muscle Control Hope Instillation Risk Identification Seizure Precautions Sexual Counseling Skin Care: Topical Treatments Splinting

Outcome: TISSUE PERFUSION: PERIPHERAL

MAJOR INTERVENTIONS	SUGGESTED INTERVENTIONS	OPTIONAL INTERVENTIONS
Circulatory Care: Arterial Insufficiency Circulatory Care: Venous Insufficiency Circulatory Precautions	Bleeding Reduction Cardiac Care Cardiac Precautions Circulatory Care: Mechanical Assist Device Embolus Care: Peripheral Fluid Management Hemodynamic Regulation Pneumatic Tourniquet Precautions Pressure Management	Cutaneous Stimulation Heat/Cold Application Positioning Positioning: Wheelchair Prosthesis Care Skin Surveillance

For interventions and outcomes related to specific risk factors refer to the following diagnoses: Mobility, Impaired Bed; Perioperative Positioning Injury, Risk for; Physical Mobility, Impaired; Protection, Altered; Surgical Recovery, Delayed; Tissue Perfusion, Altered; Trauma, Risk for.

Nursing Diagnosis: POISONING, RISK FOR

DEFINITION: Accentuated risk of accidental exposure to or ingestion of drugs or dangerous products in doses sufficient to cause poisoning.

Outcome: SAFETY BEHAVIOR: HOME PHYSICAL ENVIRONMENT

MAJOR INTERVENTIONS	SUGGESTED INTERVENTIONS	OPTIONAL INTERVENTIONS
Environmental Management: Safety Surveillance: Safety	Environmental Management: Worker Safety Home Maintenance Assistance Risk Identification	Dementia Management Environmental Risk Protection Hallucination Management Parent Education: Childrearing Family Parent Education: Infant

Outcome: SAFETY BEHAVIOR: PERSONAL

MAJOR INTERVENTIONS	SUGGESTED INTERVENTIONS	OPTIONAL INTERVENTIONS
Environmental Management: Safety Health Education	Home Maintenance Assistance Medication Management Risk Identification Substance Use Prevention Surveillance: Safety	Environmental Management: Worker Safety Security Enhancement Surveillance

Outcome: SAFETY STATUS: PHYSICAL INJURY

MAJOR INTERVENTIONS	SUGGESTED INTERVENTIONS	OPTIONAL INTERVENTIONS
Environmental Management: Safety	Emergency Care Environmental Management: Worker Safety First Aid Home Maintenance Assistance Risk Identification Security Enhancement Surveillance: Safety	Dementia Management Hallucination Management

For interventions and outcomes related to specific risk factors refer to the following diagnoses: Confusion, Acute; Confusion, Chronic; Home Maintenance Management, Impaired; Memory, Impaired; Parenting, Altered.

Nursing Diagnosis: **POST-TRAUMA SYNDROME, RISK FOR**

DEFINITION: A risk for sustained maladaptive response to a traumatic, overwhelming event.

Outcome: **ABUSE RECOVERY: EMOTIONAL**

MAJOR INTERVENTIONS	SUGGESTED INTERVENTIONS	OPTIONAL INTERVENTIONS
Abuse Protection Support	Assertiveness Training	Anger Control Assistance
Coping Enhancement	Emotional Support	Anxiety Reduction
Counseling	Forgiveness Facilitation	Behavior Management: Self-Harm
	Mood Management	Behavior Modification: Social Skills
	Self-Esteem Enhancement	Complex Relationship Building
	Socialization Enhancement	Crisis Intervention
	Suicide Prevention	Family Involvement Promotion
	Support Group	Family Mobilization
		Mutual Goal Setting
		Self-Awareness Enhancement
		Spiritual Support
		Support System Enhancement

Outcome: ABUSE RECOVERY: SEXUAL

MAJOR INTERVENTIONS	SUGGESTED INTERVENTIONS	OPTIONAL INTERVENTIONS
Coping Enhancement Crisis Intervention Rape-Trauma Treatment	Abuse Protection Support Abuse Protection Support: Child Abuse Protection Support: Elder Active Listening Counseling Emotional Support Health System Guidance Presence Sexual Counseling	Activity Therapy Anger Control Assistance Animal-Assisted Therapy Anxiety Reduction Assertiveness Training Behavior Management: Self-Harm Behavior Management: Sexual Body Image Enhancement Cognitive Restructuring Complex Relationship Building Coping Enhancement Decision-Making Support Eating Disorders Management Guilt Work Facilitation Hope Instillation Hypnosis Meditation Facilitation Mood Management Self-Awareness Enhancement Self-Esteem Enhancement Simple Relaxation Therapy Socialization Enhancement Spiritual Support Substance Use Prevention Suicide Prevention Support Group Support System Enhancement Therapy Group

Continued

Outcome: COPING

MAJOR INTERVENTIONS	SUGGESTED INTERVENTIONS	OPTIONAL INTERVENTIONS

Coping Enhancement
Counseling
Crisis Intervention
	Active Listening
	Animal-Assisted
	  Therapy
	Anxiety Reduction
	Decision-Making
	  Support
	Emotional Support
	Exercise Promotion
	Guilt Work Facilitation
	Hope Instillation
	Hypnosis
	Meditation Facilitation
	Presence
	Progressive Muscle
	  Relaxation
	Simple Relaxation
	  Therapy
	Spiritual Support
	Support Group
	Support System
	  Enhancement
		Behavior Management:
		  Self-Harm
		Behavior Modification
		Cognitive Restructuring
		Environmental
		  Management
		Family Therapy
		Mood Management
		Normalization
		  Promotion
		Rape-Trauma Treatment
		Reminiscence Therapy
		Sibling Support
		Therapy Group
		Truth Telling

Outcome: DEPRESSION CONTROL

MAJOR INTERVENTIONS	SUGGESTED INTERVENTIONS	OPTIONAL INTERVENTIONS

Mood Management	Activity Therapy
	Behavior Management
	Behavior Management:
	  Self-Harm
	Exercise Promotion
	Medication Management
	Nutrition Management
	Self-Modification
	  Assistance
	Sleep Enhancement
		Grief Work Facilitation
		Guilt Work Facilitation
		Substance Use
		  Prevention

Outcome: DEPRESSION LEVEL

MAJOR INTERVENTIONS	SUGGESTED INTERVENTIONS	OPTIONAL INTERVENTIONS

Hope Instillation
Mood Management
	Behavior Modification:
	  Self-Harm
	Bibliotherapy
	Cognitive Restructuring
	Counseling
	Emotional Support
	Exercise Promotion
	Grief Work Facilitation
	Guilt Work Facilitation
	Medication Management
	Milieu Therapy
	Patient Contracting
	Self-Awareness
	  Enhancement
	Self-Esteem
	  Enhancement
	Self-Modification
	  Assistance
	Sleep Enhancement
	Support Group
	Therapy Group
		Activity Therapy
		Animal-Assisted
		  Therapy
		Crisis Intervention
		Nutrition Management
		Spiritual Support
		Substance Use
		  Prevention
		Support System
		  Enhancement
		Therapeutic Play

For interventions and outcomes related to specific risk factors refer to the following diagnoses: Grieving, Dysfunctional; Hopelessness; Powerlessness; Relocation Stress Syndrome; Self-Esteem Disturbance; Social Interaction, Impaired; Social Isolation; Sorrow, Chronic; Spiritual Distress.

Nursing Diagnosis: SELF-MUTILATION, RISK FOR

DEFINITION: A state in which an individual is at high risk to perform an act upon the self to injure, not kill, which produces tissue damage and tension relief.

Outcome: AGGRESSION CONTROL

MAJOR INTERVENTIONS	SUGGESTED INTERVENTIONS	OPTIONAL INTERVENTIONS
Anger Control Assistance Environmental Management: Violence Prevention Impulse Control Training	Area Restriction Assertiveness Training Behavior Management: Self-Harm Calming Technique Coping Enhancement Counseling Crisis Intervention Fire-Setting Precautions Limit Setting Patient Contracting Physical Restraint Seclusion Suicide Prevention Surveillance: Safety	Art Therapy Behavior Management Behavior Modification Delusion Management Environmental Management: Safety Hallucination Management Self-Awareness Enhancement Self-Modification Assistance Self-Responsibility Facilitation Socialization Enhancement

Outcome: IMPULSE CONTROL

MAJOR INTERVENTIONS	SUGGESTED INTERVENTIONS	OPTIONAL INTERVENTIONS
Behavior Management: Self-Harm Impulse Control Training	Anger Control Assistance Anxiety Reduction Area Restriction Behavior Management Behavior Modification Elopement Precautions Environmental Management: Safety Environmental Management: Violence Prevention Fire-Setting Precautions Limit Setting Milieu Therapy Patient Contracting Physical Restraint Seclusion Self-Modification Assistance Self-Responsibility Facilitation	Coping Enhancement Developmental Enhancement: Child Emotional Support Mood Management Risk Identification Security Enhancement Support Group Support System Enhancement Surveillance: Safety Therapy Group

Continued

Outcome: SELF-MUTILATION RESTRAINT

MAJOR INTERVENTIONS	SUGGESTED INTERVENTIONS	OPTIONAL INTERVENTIONS
Anger Control Assistance Behavior Management: Self-Harm Environmental Management: Safety	Anxiety Reduction Area Restriction Behavior Management Behavior Modification Calming Technique Cognitive Restructuring Coping Enhancement Counseling Crisis Intervention Emotional Support Environmental Management: Violence Prevention Impulse Control Training Limit Setting Milieu Therapy Mood Management Patient Contracting Physical Restraint Seclusion Security Enhancement Self-Esteem Enhancement Suicide Prevention Surveillance: Safety	Active Listening Animal-Assisted Therapy Family Therapy Fire-Setting Precautions Hallucination Management Mutual Goal Setting Presence Therapy Group

For interventions and outcomes related to specific risk factors refer to the following diagnoses: Anxiety; Body Image Disturbance; Individual, Coping, Ineffective; Family Processes, Altered; Hopelessness; Personal Identity Disturbance; Post-Trauma Syndrome; Rape-Trauma Syndrome; Self-Esteem Disturbance; Sorrow, Chronic; Spiritual Distress.

Nursing Diagnosis: SKIN INTEGRITY, RISK FOR IMPAIRED

DEFINITION: A state in which an individual's skin is at risk of being adversely altered.

Outcome: IMMOBILITY CONSEQUENCES: PHYSIOLOGICAL

MAJOR INTERVENTIONS	SUGGESTED INTERVENTIONS	OPTIONAL INTERVENTIONS

Bed Rest Care
Pressure Management
	Circulatory Precautions
	Embolus Care:
	  Peripheral
	Embolus Precautions
	Exercise Promotion:
	  Strength Training
	Exercise Promotion:
	  Stretching
	Exercise Therapy: Joint
	  Mobility
	Exercise Therapy:
	  Muscle Control
	Positioning
	Positioning:
	  Intraoperative
	Positioning: Wheelchair
	Pressure Ulcer
	  Prevention
	Simple Massage
	Skin Surveillance
	Traction/Immobilization
	  Care
		Skin Care: Topical
		  Treatments
		Surveillance
		Vital Signs Monitoring

Continued

Outcome: Tissue Integrity: Skin & Mucous Membranes

MAJOR INTERVENTIONS	SUGGESTED INTERVENTIONS	OPTIONAL INTERVENTIONS
Pressure Management	Amputation Care	Allergy Management
Pressure Ulcer Prevention	Bathing	Diarrhea Management
Skin Surveillance	Bed Rest Care	Fluid Management
	Bowel Incontinence Care	Lactation Counseling
	Cast Care: Maintenance	Nail Care
	Chemotherapy Management	Nutrition Therapy
	Circulatory Precautions	Perineal Care
	Cutaneous Stimulation	Positioning: Intraoperative
	Foot Care	Positioning: Wheelchair
	Health Screening	Prosthesis Care
	Incision Site Care	Self-Care Assistance: Bathing/Hygiene
	Infection Control	Self-Care Assistance: Toileting
	Infection Protection	Urinary Incontinence Care
	Latex Precautions	Urinary Incontinence Care: Enuresis
	Medication Administration: Skin	Wound Care
	Medication Management	
	Nutrition Management	
	Ostomy Care	
	Positioning	
	Radiation Therapy Management	
	Skin Care: Topical Treatments	
	Traction/Immobilization Care	

Outcome: WOUND HEALING: PRIMARY INTENTION

MAJOR INTERVENTIONS	SUGGESTED INTERVENTIONS	OPTIONAL INTERVENTIONS

Incision Site Care
Wound Care
	Circulatory Precautions
	Fluid Management
	Infection Control:
	    Intraoperative
	Infection Protection
	Medication
	    Administration
	Medication
	    Administration: Skin
	Nutrition Management
	Skin Care: Topical
	    Treatments
	Skin Surveillance
	Splinting
	Teaching: Prescribed
	    Medication
	Teaching: Procedure/
	    Treatment
	Wound Care: Closed
	    Drainage
		Bathing
		Bed Rest Care
		Cesarean Section Care
		Hyperglycemia
		    Management
		Perineal Care

Continued

Outcome: WOUND HEALING: SECONDARY INTENTION

MAJOR INTERVENTIONS	SUGGESTED INTERVENTIONS	OPTIONAL INTERVENTIONS
Wound Care	Circulatory Care: Arterial Insufficiency Circulatory Precautions Fluid/Electrolyte Management Infection Control Infection Protection Medication Administration Medication Administration: Skin Nutrition Therapy Skin Care: Topical Treatments Skin Surveillance Splinting Transcutaneous Electrical Nerve Stimulation (TENS) Wound Care: Closed Drainage Wound Irrigation	Bathing Cutaneous Stimulation Hyperglycemia Management Leech Therapy Nutrition Management Positioning Total Parenteral Nutrition (TPN) Administration

For interventions and outcomes related to specific risk factors refer to the following diagnoses: Diarrhea; Hyperthermia; Incontinence: Bowel; Latex Allergy Response; Nutrition, Altered: Less Than Body Requirements; Physical Mobility, Impaired; Sensory/Perceptual Alterations; Urinary Incontinence, Total.

Nursing Diagnosis: SPIRITUAL DISTRESS, RISK FOR

DEFINITION: At risk for an altered sense of harmonious connectedness with all of life and the universe in which dimensions that transcend and empower the self may be disrupted.

Outcome: HOPE

MAJOR INTERVENTIONS	SUGGESTED INTERVENTIONS	OPTIONAL INTERVENTIONS

Hope Installation
Spiritual Support
	Coping Enhancement
	Emotional Support
	Self-Awareness
	  Enhancement
	Self-Esteem
	  Enhancement
	Support Group
	Support System
	  Enhancement
	Values Clarification
		Animal-Assisted
		  Therapy
		Counseling
		Family Mobilization
		Milieu Therapy
		Mutual Goal Setting
		Presence
		Truth Telling

Outcome: SPIRITUAL WELL-BEING

MAJOR INTERVENTIONS	SUGGESTED INTERVENTIONS	OPTIONAL INTERVENTIONS

Spiritual Growth
  Facilitation
Spiritual Support
	Emotional Support
	Forgiveness Facilitation
	Grief Work Facilitation
	Hope Installation
	Meditation Facilitation
	Mood Management
	Resiliency Promotion
	Self-Awareness
	  Enhancement
	Support Group
	Values Clarification
		Abuse Protection
		  Support: Religious
		Bibliotherapy
		Caregiver Support
		Counseling
		Family Support
		Music Therapy
		Patient Rights Protection
		Referral
		Religious Addiction
		  Prevention
		Religious Ritual
		  Enhancement
		Reminiscence Therapy
		Self-Esteem
		  Enhancement
		Socialization
		  Enhancement
		Support System
		  Enhancement

For interventions and outcomes related to specific risk factors refer to the following diagnoses: Anxiety; Death Anxiety; Grieving, Dysfunctional; Hopelessness; Loneliness, Risk for; Self-Esteem, Chronic Low; Social Interaction, Impaired; Sorrow, Chronic.

Nursing Diagnosis: SUFFOCATION, RISK FOR

DEFINITION: Accentuated risk of accidental suffocation (inadequate air available for inhalation).

Outcome: ASPIRATION CONTROL

MAJOR INTERVENTIONS	SUGGESTED INTERVENTIONS	OPTIONAL INTERVENTIONS

Aspiration Precautions
Respiratory Monitoring
	Airway Management
	Airway Suctioning
	Artificial Airway
	   Management
	Environmental
	   Management: Safety
	Positioning
	Teaching: Infant Safety
	Ventilation Assistance
		Cough Enhancement
		Infant Care
		Parent Education: Infant
		Surveillance: Safety
		Swallowing Therapy
		Vital Signs Monitoring

Outcome: RESPIRATORY STATUS: VENTILATION

MAJOR INTERVENTIONS	SUGGESTED INTERVENTIONS	OPTIONAL INTERVENTIONS

Airway Management
Respiratory Monitoring
	Airway Insertion and
	   Stabilization
	Airway Suctioning
	Artificial Airway
	   Management
	Aspiration Precautions
	Energy Management
	Positioning
	Surveillance
	Ventilation Assistance
	Vital Signs Monitoring
		Chest Physiotherapy
		Cough Enhancement
		Infant Care
		Parent Education: Infant
		Teaching: Infant Safety

For interventions and outcomes related to specific risk factors refer to the following diagnoses: Airway Clearance, Ineffective; Confusion, Chronic; Home Maintenance Management, Impaired; Infant Feeding Pattern, Ineffective; Knowledge Deficit; Swallowing, Impaired.

Nursing Diagnosis: TRAUMA, RISK FOR

DEFINITION: Accentuated risk of accidental tissue injury (e.g., wound, burn, fracture).

Outcome: SAFETY BEHAVIOR: PERSONAL

MAJOR INTERVENTIONS	SUGGESTED INTERVENTIONS	OPTIONAL INTERVENTIONS
Environmental Management: Safety	Behavior Modification Health Education Home Maintenance Assistance Risk Identification Surveillance: Safety Teaching: Individual Teaching: Infant Safety Teaching: Toddler Safety Vehicle Safety Promotion	Area Restriction Behavior Management: Overactivity/ Inattention Environmental Management: Worker Safety Parent Education: Adolescent Parent Education: Childrearing Family Parent Education: Infant Physical Restraint Security Enhancement

Outcome: SAFETY STATUS: PHYSICAL INJURY

MAJOR INTERVENTIONS	SUGGESTED INTERVENTIONS	OPTIONAL INTERVENTIONS
Environmental Management: Safety	Environmental Management: Worker Safety Environmental Risk Protection Fall Prevention Home Maintenance Assistance Risk Identification Security Enhancement Surveillance: Safety Vital Signs Monitoring	Area Restriction Dementia Management Hallucination Management Seizure Precautions Sports-Injury Prevention: Youth

Continued

Outcome: Tissue Integrity: Skin & Mucous Membranes

MAJOR INTERVENTIONS	SUGGESTED INTERVENTIONS	OPTIONAL INTERVENTIONS
Pressure Management Skin Surveillance	Bathing Bed Rest Care Chemotherapy Management Circulatory Precautions Foot Care Health Screening Infection Protection Medication Administration: Skin Nutrition Management Oral Health Maintenance Oral Health Promotion Positioning Pressure Ulcer Prevention Radiation Therapy Management Self-Care Assistance: Bathing/Hygiene Self-Care Assistance: Toileting Simple Massage Skin Care: Topical Treatments	Eye Care Laser Precautions Nail Care Perineal Care Peripheral Sensation Management Positioning: Wheelchair

For interventions and outcomes related to specific risk factors refer to the following diagnoses:
Community Coping, Ineffective; Fatigue; Home Maintenance Management, Impaired; Parenting, Altered; Physical Mobility, Impaired; Protection, Altered; Sleep Deprivation.

Nursing Diagnosis: URINARY URGE INCONTINENCE, RISK FOR

DEFINITION: Risk for involuntary loss of urine associated with a sudden, strong sensation or urinary urgency.

Outcome: URINARY CONTINENCE

MAJOR INTERVENTIONS	SUGGESTED INTERVENTIONS	OPTIONAL INTERVENTIONS
Urinary Bladder Training Urinary Habit Training	Biofeedback Fluid Management Fluid Monitoring Medication Administration Medication Management Pelvic Muscle Exercise Self-Care Assistance: Toileting Urinary Elimination Management	Behavior Modification Environmental Management Exercise Promotion Health Screening Pessary Management Prompted Voiding Weight Management

Outcome: URINARY ELIMINATION

MAJOR INTERVENTIONS	SUGGESTED INTERVENTIONS	OPTIONAL INTERVENTIONS
Urinary Elimination Management	Fluid Management Fluid Monitoring Medication Administration Self-Care Assistance: Toileting Urinary Catheterization	Pelvic Muscle Exercise Tube Care: Urinary Urinary Bladder Training Urinary Habit Training

For interventions and outcomes related to specific risk factors refer to the following diagnoses: Growth and Development, Altered; Individual Management of Therapeutic Regimen, Ineffective; Self-Care Deficit: Toileting.

Nursing Diagnosis: VIOLENCE, RISK FOR: DIRECTED AT OTHERS

DEFINITION: Behaviors in which an individual demonstrates that he/she can be physically, emotionally, and/or sexually harmful to others.

Outcome: ABUSE CESSATION

MAJOR INTERVENTIONS	SUGGESTED INTERVENTIONS	OPTIONAL INTERVENTIONS
Abuse Protection Support	Abuse Protection Support: Child Abuse Protection Support: Domestic Partner Abuse Protection Support: Elder Anger Control Assistance Assertiveness Training Coping Enhancement Counseling Crisis Intervention Environmental Management: Violence Prevention Risk Identification Self-Esteem Enhancement	Calming Technique Caregiver Support Emotional Support Family Integrity Promotion Family Support Mood Management Parent Education: Childrearing Family Parent Education: Infant Role Enhancement Self-Awareness Enhancement Sexual Counseling Spiritual Support

Outcome: **Abusive Behavior Self-Control**

MAJOR INTERVENTIONS	SUGGESTED INTERVENTIONS	OPTIONAL INTERVENTIONS
Anger Control Assistance Environmental Management: Violence Prevention	Abuse Protection Support Abuse Protection Support: Child Abuse Protection Support: Domestic Partner Abuse Protection Support: Elder Behavior Management Behavior Management: Sexual Behavior Modification: Social Skills Coping Enhancement Counseling Emotional Support Environmental Management: Safety Impulse Control Training Referral Risk Identification Self-Modification Assistance Self-Responsibility Facilitation Substance Use Treatment Substance Use Treatment: Alcohol Withdrawal Substance Use Treatment: Drug Withdrawal	Assertiveness Training Medication Management Medication Prescribing Parent Education: Childrearing Family Self-Awareness Enhancement Self-Esteem Enhancement Support Group Support System Enhancement Teaching: Individual Values Clarification

Continued

Outcome: AGGRESSION CONTROL

MAJOR INTERVENTIONS	SUGGESTED INTERVENTIONS	OPTIONAL INTERVENTIONS
Anger Control Assistance Environmental Management: Violence Prevention	Abuse Protection Support Abuse Protection Support: Child Abuse Protection Support: Domestic Partner Abuse Protection Support: Elder Area Restriction Assertiveness Training Behavior Management: Self-Harm Behavior Management: Sexual Behavior Modification: Social Skills Calming Technique Coping Enhancement Counseling Crisis Intervention Fire-Setting Precautions Impulse Control Training Limit Setting Patient Contracting Physical Restraint Seclusion Suicide Prevention Surveillance: Safety	Animal-Assisted Therapy Art Therapy Behavior Management: Overactivity/ Inattention Behavior Modification Delusion Management Dementia Management Environmental Management Environmental Management: Safety Hallucination Management Self-Awareness Enhancement Self-Modification Assistance Self-Responsibility Facilitation Socialization Enhancement Therapeutic Play

Outcome: IMPULSE CONTROL

MAJOR INTERVENTIONS	SUGGESTED INTERVENTIONS	OPTIONAL INTERVENTIONS
Anger Control Assistance Impulse Control Training	Anxiety Reduction Area Restriction Behavior Management Behavior Management: Sexual Behavior Modification Behavior Modification: Social Skills Elopement Precautions Environmental Management: Safety Environmental Management: Violence Prevention Fire-Setting Precautions Limit Setting Milieu Therapy Patient Contracting Physical Restraint Seclusion Self-Modification Assistance Self-Responsibility Facilitation	Coping Enhancement Emotional Support Mood Management Risk Identification Security Enhancement Substance Use Prevention Substance Use Treatment Support Group Support System Enhancement Surveillance: Safety Therapy Group

For interventions and outcomes related to specific risk factors refer to the following diagnoses: Caregiver Role Strain; Family Coping: Disabling, Ineffective; Family Processes, Altered; Individual Coping, Ineffective; Parenteral Role Conflict; Personal Identity Disturbance; Thought Processes, Altered.

Nursing Diagnosis: VIOLENCE, RISK FOR: SELF-DIRECTED

DEFINITION: Behaviors in which an individual demonstrates that he/she can be physically, emotionally, and/or sexually harmful to self.

Outcome: IMPULSE CONTROL

MAJOR INTERVENTIONS	SUGGESTED INTERVENTIONS	OPTIONAL INTERVENTIONS
Impulse Control Training	Anger Control Assistance	Coping Enhancement
	Anxiety Reduction	Developmental Enhancement: Adolescent
	Area Restriction	Emotional Support
	Behavior Management	Mood Management
	Behavior Management: Overactivity/ Inattention	Risk Identification
		Security Enhancement
	Behavior Management: Self-Harm	Substance Use Prevention
	Behavior Management: Sexual	Substance Use Treatment
	Behavior Modification	Support Group
	Behavior Modification: Social Skills	Support System Enhancement
	Elopement Precautions	Surveillance: Safety
	Environmental Management: Safety	Therapy Group
	Environmental Management: Violence Prevention	
	Fire-Setting Precautions	
	Limit Setting	
	Milieu Therapy	
	Patient Contracting	
	Physical Restraint	
	Seclusion	
	Self-Modification Assistance	
	Self-Responsibility Facilitation	

Outcome: SELF-MUTILATION RESTRAINT

MAJOR INTERVENTIONS	SUGGESTED INTERVENTIONS	OPTIONAL INTERVENTIONS
Behavior Management: Self-Harm Environmental Management: Violence Prevention	Anger Control Assistance Anxiety Reduction Area Restriction Behavior Modification Cognitive Restructuring Coping Enhancement Counseling Crisis Intervention Emotional Support Environmental Management: Safety Impulse Control Training Limit Setting Mood Management Patient Contracting Physical Restraint Seclusion Security Enhancement Suicide Prevention Surveillance: Safety	Active Listening Delusion Management Family Involvement Promotion Fire-Setting Precautions Hallucination Management Mutual Goal Setting Presence

Continued

Outcome: Suicide Self-Restraint

MAJOR INTERVENTIONS	SUGGESTED INTERVENTIONS	OPTIONAL INTERVENTIONS
Environmental Management: Violence Prevention Hope Instillation Suicide Prevention	Area Restriction Behavior Management: Self-Harm Cognitive Restructuring Coping Enhancement Counseling Crisis Intervention Delusion Management Elopement Precautions Emotional Support Environmental Management: Safety Hallucination Management Impulse Control Training Milieu Therapy Mood Management Patient Contracting Physical Restraint Seclusion Substance Use Prevention Support Group Surveillance: Safety	Anger Control Assistance Anxiety Reduction Assertiveness Training Behavior Modification Body Image Enhancement Family Involvement Promotion Family Support Grief Work Facilitation Guilt Work Facilitation Limit Setting Self-Esteem Enhancement Substance Use Treatment Substance Use Treatment: Overdose

For interventions and outcomes related to specific risk factors refer to the following diagnoses: Anxiety; Body Image Disturbance; Family Processes, Altered; Hopelessness; Individual Coping, Ineffective; Personal Identity Disturbance; Post-Trauma Syndrome; Rape-Trauma Syndrome; Self-Esteem Disturbance; Sexual Dysfunction; Social Isolation; Sorrow, Chronic; Spiritual Distress.

PART III

Appendixes

NOC Outcome Labels and Definitions
(260 Outcomes)

2500	**Abuse Cessation** Evidence that the victim is no longer abused
2501	**Abuse Protection** Protection of self or dependent others from abuse
2502	**Abuse Recovery: Emotional** Healing of psychological injuries due to abuse
2503	**Abuse Recovery: Financial** Regaining monetary and legal control or benefits following financial exploitation
2504	**Abuse Recovery: Physical** Healing of physical injuries due to abuse
2505	**Abuse Recovery: Sexual** Healing following sexual abuse or exploitation
1400	**Abusive Behavior Self-Control** Self-restraint of own behaviors to avoid abuse and neglect of dependents or significant others
1300	**Acceptance: Health Status** Reconciliation to health circumstances
0005	**Activity Tolerance** Responses to energy-consuming body movements involved in required or desired daily activities
1600	**Adherence Behavior** Self-initiated action taken to promote wellness, recovery, and rehabilitation
1401	**Aggression Control** Self-restraint of assaultive, combative, or destructive behavior toward others
0200	**Ambulation: Walking** Ability to walk from place to place
0201	**Ambulation: Wheelchair** Ability to move from place to place in a wheelchair
1402	**Anxiety Control** Personal actions to eliminate or reduce feelings of apprehension and tension from an unidentifiable source
1918	**Aspiration Control** Personal actions to prevent the passage of fluid and solid particles into the lung
0704	**Asthma Control** Personal actions to reverse inflammatory condition resulting in bronchial constriction of the airways
0202	**Balance** Ability to maintain body equilibrium
2300	**Blood Glucose Control** Extent to which plasma glucose levels are maintained in expected range

From Johnson, M., Maas, M., & Moorhead, S. (Eds.). (2000). *Nursing outcomes classification (NOC)* (2nd ed.). St. Louis: Mosby.

0700   **Blood Transfusion Reaction Control**   Extent to which complications of blood transfusions are minimized

1200   **Body Image**   Positive perception of own appearance and body functions

0203   **Body Positioning: Self-Initiated**   Ability to change own body positions

1104   **Bone Healing**   The extent to which cellsand tissues have regenerated following bone injury

0500   **Bowel Continence**   Control of passage of stool from the bowel

0501   **Bowel Elimination**   Ability of the gastrointestinal tract to form and evacuate stool effectively

1000   **Breastfeeding Establishment: Infant**   Proper attachment of an infant to and sucking from the mother's breast for nourishment during the first 2 to 3 weeks

1001   **Breastfeeding Establishment: Maternal**   Maternal establishment of proper attachment of an infant to and sucking from the breast for nourishment during the first 2 to 3 weeks

1002   **Breastfeeding Maintenance**   Continued nourishment of an infant through breastfeeding

1003   **Breastfeeding Weaning**   Process leading to the eventual discontinuation of breastfeeding

0400   **Cardiac Pump Effectiveness**   Extent to which blood is ejected from the left ventricle per minute to support systemic perfusion pressure

2200   **Caregiver Adaptation to Patient Institutionalization**   Family caregiver adaptation of role when the care recipient is transferred outside the home

2506   **Caregiver Emotional Health**   Feelings, attitudes, and emotions of a family care provider while caring for a family member or significant other over an extended period of time

2202   **Caregiver Home Care Readiness**   Preparedness to assume responsibility for the health care of a family member or significant other in the home

2203   **Caregiver Lifestyle Disruption**   Disturbances in the lifestyle of a family member due to caregiving

2204   **Caregiver-Patient Relationship**   Positive interactions and connections between the caregiver and care recipient

2205   **Caregiver Performance: Direct Care**   Provision by family care provider of appropriate personal and health care for a family member or significant other

2206   **Caregiver Performance: Indirect Care**   Arrangement and oversight of appropriate care for a family member or significant other by family care provider

2507   **Caregiver Physical Health**   Physical well-being of a family care provider while caring for a family member or significant other over an extended period of time

2208   **Caregiver Stressors**   The extent of biopsychosocial pressure on a family care provider caring for a family member or significant other over an extended period of time

2508   **Caregiver Well-Being**   Primary care provider's satisfaction with health and life circumstances

2210   **Caregiving Endurance Potential**   Factors that promote family care provider continuance over an extended period of time

1301	**Child Adaptation to Hospitalization** Child's adaptive response to hospitalization
0100	**Child Development: 2 months** Milestones of physical, cognitive, and psychosocial progression by 2 months of age
0101	**Child Development: 4 months** Milestones of physical, cognitive, and psychosocial progression by 4 months of age
0102	**Child Development: 6 months** Milestones of physical, cognitive, and psychosocial progression by 6 months of age
0103	**Child Development: 12 months** Milestones of physical, cognitive, and psychosocial progression by 12 months of age
0104	**Child Development: 2 years** Milestones of physical, cognitive, and psychosocial progression by 2 years of age
0105	**Child Development: 3 years** Milestones of physical, cognitive, and psychosocial progression by 3 years of age
0106	**Child Development: 4 years** Milestones of physical, cognitive, and psychosocial progression by 4 years of age
0107	**Child Development: 5 years** Milestones of physical, cognitive, and psychosocial progression by 5 years of age
0108	**Child Development: Middle Childhood (6-11 years)** Milestones of physical, cognitive, and psychosocial progression between 6 and 11 years of age
0109	**Child Development: Adolescence (12-17 years)** Milestones of physical, cognitive, and psychosocial progression between 12 and 17 years of age
0401	**Circulation Status** Extent to which blood flows unobstructed, unidirectionally, and at an appropriate pressure through large vessels of the systemic and pulmonary circuits
0409	**Coagulation Status** Extent to which blood clots within expected period of time
0900	**Cognitive Ability** Ability to execute complex mental processes
0901	**Cognitive Orientation** Ability to identify person, place, and time
2100	**Comfort Level** Feelings of physical and psychological ease
0902	**Communication Ability** Ability to receive, interpret, and express spoken, written, and non-verbal messages
0903	**Communication: Expressive Ability** Ability to express and interpret verbal and/or non-verbal messages
0904	**Communication: Receptive Ability** Ability to receive and interpret verbal and/or non-verbal messages
2700	**Community Competence** The ability of a community to collectively problem solve to achieve goals
2701	**Community Health Status** The general state of well-being of a community or population
2800	**Community Health: Immunity** Resistance of a group to the invasion and spread of an infectious agent
2801	**Community Risk Control: Chronic Disease** Community actions to reduce the risk of chronic diseases and related complications
2802	**Community Risk Control: Communicable Disease** Community actions to eliminate or reduce the spread of infectious agents (bacteria, fungi, parasites, and viruses) that threaten public health
2803	**Community Risk Control: Lead Exposure** Community actions to reduce lead exposure and poisoning

1601   **Compliance Behavior**   Actions taken on the basis of professional advice to promote wellness, recovery, and rehabilitation

0905   **Concentration**   Ability to focus on a specific stimulus

1302   **Coping**   Actions to manage stressors that tax an individual's resources

0906   **Decision Making**   Ability to choose between two or more alternatives

1409   **Depression Control**   Personal actions to minimize melancholy and maintain interest in life events

1208   **Depression Level**   Severity of melancholic mood and loss of interest in life events

1105   **Dialysis Access Integrity**   The extent to which a dialysis access site is functional and free of inflammation

1303   **Dignified Dying**   Maintaining personal control and comfort with the approaching end of life

1403   **Distorted Thought Control**   Self-restraint of disruption in perception, thought processes, and thought content

0600   **Electrolyte & Acid/Base Balance**   Balance of the electrolytes and non-electrolytes in the intracellular and extracellular compartments of the body

0001   **Endurance**   Extent that energy enables a person to sustain activity

0002   **Energy Conservation**   Extent of active management of energy to initiate and sustain activity

2600   **Family Coping**   Family actions to manage stressors that tax family resources

2601   **Family Environment: Internal**   Social climate as characterized by family member relationships and goals

2602   **Family Functioning**   Ability of the family to meet the needs of its members through developmental transitions

2606   **Family Health Status**   Overall health status and social competence of family unit

2603   **Family Integrity**   Extent that family members' behaviors collectively demonstrate cohesion, strength, and emotional bonding

2604   **Family Normalization**   Ability of the family to develop and maintain routines and management strategies that contribute to optimal functioning when a member has a chronic illness or disability

2605   **Family Participation in Professional Care**   Family involvement in decision-making, delivery, and evaluation of care provided by health care personnel

1404   **Fear Control**   Personal actions to eliminate or reduce disabling feelings of alarm aroused by an identifiable source

0111   **Fetal Status: Antepartum**   Conditions indicative of fetal physical well-being from conception to the onset of labor

0112   **Fetal Status: Intrapartum**   Conditions and behaviors indicative of fetal well-being from onset of labor to delivery

0601   **Fluid Balance**   Balance of water in the intracellular and extracellular compartments of the body

1304   **Grief Resolution**   Adjustment to actual or impending loss

0110   **Growth**   A normal increase in body size and weight

1700   **Health Beliefs**   Personal convictions that influence health behaviors

1701   **Health Beliefs: Perceived Ability to Perform**   Personal conviction that one can carry out a given health behavior

1702   **Health Beliefs: Perceived Control**   Personal conviction that one can influence a health outcome

1703   **Health Beliefs: Perceived Resources**   Personal conviction that one has adequate means to carry out a health behavior

1704   **Health Beliefs: Perceived Threat**   Personal conviction that a health problem is serious and has potential negative consequences for lifestyle

1705   **Health Orientation**   Personal view of health and health behaviors as priorities

1602   **Health Promoting Behavior**   Actions to sustain or increase wellness

1603   **Health Seeking Behavior**   Actions to promote optimal wellness, recovery, and rehabilitation

1610   **Hearing Compensation Behavior**   Actions to identify, monitor, and compensate for hearing loss

1201   **Hope**   Presence of internal state of optimism that is personally satisfying and life-supporting

0602   **Hydration**   Amount of water in the intracellular and extracellular compartments of the body

1202   **Identity**   Ability to distinguish between self and non-self and to characterize one's essence

0204   **Immobility Consequences: Physiological**   Extent of compromise in physiological functioning due to impaired physical mobility

0205   **Immobility Consequences: Psycho-Cognitive**   Extent of compromise in psycho-cognitive functioning due to impaired physical mobility

0701   **Immune Hypersensitivity Control**   Extent to which inappropriate immune responses are suppressed

0702   **Immune Status**   Adequacy of natural and acquired appropriately targeted resistance to internal and external antigens

1900   **Immunization Behavior**   Actions to obtain immunization to prevent a communicable disease

1405   **Impulse Control**   Self-restraint of compulsive or impulsive behaviors

0703   **Infection Status**   Presence and extent of infection

0907   **Information Processing**   Ability to acquire, organize, and use information

0206   **Joint Movement: Active**   Range of motion of joints with self-initiated movement

0207   **Joint Movement: Passive**   Range of motion of joints with assisted movement

1800   **Knowledge: Breastfeeding**   Extent of understanding conveyed about lactation and nourishment of infant through breastfeeding

1801   **Knowledge: Child Safety**   Extent of understanding conveyed about safely caring for a child

1821   **Knowledge: Conception Prevention**   Extent of understanding conveyed about pregnancy prevention

1820   **Knowledge: Diabetes Management**   Extent of understanding conveyed about diabetes mellitus and its control

1802   **Knowledge: Diet**   Extent of understanding conveyed about diet

1803   **Knowledge: Disease Process**   Extent of understanding conveyed about a specific disease process

1804   **Knowledge: Energy Conservation**   Extent of understanding conveyed about energy conservation techniques

1816   **Knowledge: Fertility Promotion**   Extent of understanding conveyed about fertility testing and the conditions that affect conception

1805   **Knowledge: Health Behaviors**   Extent of understanding conveyed about the promotion and protection of health

1823   **Knowledge: Health Promotion**   Extent of understanding of information needed to obtain and maintain optimal health

1806   **Knowledge: Health Resources**   Extent of understanding conveyed about health care resources

1824   **Knowledge: Illness Care**   Extent of understanding of illness-related information needed to achieve and maintain optimal health

1819   **Knowledge: Infant Care**   Extent of understanding conveyed about caring for a baby up to 12 months

1807   **Knowledge: Infection Control**   Extent of understanding conveyed about prevention and control of infection

1817   **Knowledge: Labor and Delivery**   Extent of understanding conveyed about labor and delivery

1825   **Knowledge: Maternal-Child Health**   Extent of understanding of information needed to achieve and maintain optimal health of a mother and child

1808   **Knowledge: Medication**   Extent of understanding conveyed about the safe use of medication

1809   **Knowledge: Personal Safety**   Extent of understanding conveyed about preventing unintentional injuries

1818   **Knowledge: Postpartum**   Extent of understanding conveyed about maternal health following delivery

1822   **Knowledge: Preconception**   Extent of understanding conveyed about maternal health prior to conception to insure a healthy pregnancy

1810   **Knowledge: Pregnancy**   Extent of understanding conveyed about maintenance of a healthy pregnancy and prevention of complications

1811   **Knowledge: Prescribed Activity**   Extent of understanding conveyed about prescribed activity and exercise

1815   **Knowledge: Sexual Functioning**   Extent of understanding conveyed about sexual development and responsible sexual practices

1812   **Knowledge: Substance Use Control**   Extent of understanding conveyed about managing substance use safely

1814   **Knowledge: Treatment Procedure(s)**   Extent of understanding conveyed about procedure(s) required as part of a treatment regimen

1813   **Knowledge: Treatment Regimen**   Extent of understanding conveyed about a specific treatment regimen

1604   **Leisure Participation**   Use of restful or relaxing activities as needed to promote well-being

1203   **Loneliness**   The extent of emotional, social, or existential isolation response

2509   **Maternal Status: Antepartum**   Conditions and behaviors indicative of maternal well-being from conception to the onset of labor

2510   **Maternal Status: Intrapartum**   Conditions and behaviors indicative of maternal well-being from onset of labor to delivery

2511   **Maternal Status: Postpartum**   Conditions and behaviors indicative of maternal well-being from delivery of placenta to completion of involution

2301   **Medication Response**   Therapeutic and adverse effects of prescribed medication

0908   **Memory**   Ability to cognitively retrieve and report previously stored information

0208   **Mobility Level**   Ability to move purposefully

1204   **Mood Equilibrium**   Appropriate adjustment of prevailing emotional tone in response to circumstances

0209   **Muscle Function**   Adequacy of muscle contraction needed for movement

2512   **Neglect Recovery**   Healing following the cessation of substandard care

0909   **Neurological Status**   Extent to which the peripheral and central nervous systems receive, process, and respond to internal and external stimuli

0910   **Neurological Status: Autonomic**   Extent to which the autonomic nervous system coordinates visceral function

0911   **Neurological Status: Central Motor Control**   Extent to which skeletal muscle activity (body movement) is coordinated by the central nervous system

0912   **Neurological Status: Consciousness**   Extent to which an individual arouses, orients, and attends to the environment

0913   **Neurological Status: Cranial Sensory/Motor Function**   Extent to which cranial nerves convey sensory and motor information

0914   **Neurological Status: Spinal Sensory/Motor Function**   Extent to which spinal nerves convey sensory and motor information

0118   **Newborn Adaptation**   Adaptation to the extrauterine environment by a physiologically mature newborn during the first 28 days

1004   **Nutritional Status**   Extent to which nutrients are available to meet metabolic needs

1005   **Nutritional Status: Biochemical Measures**   Body fluid components and chemical indices of nutritional status

1006   **Nutritional Status: Body Mass**   Congruence of body weight, muscle, and fat to height, frame, and gender

1007   **Nutritional Status: Energy**   Extent to which nutrients provide cellular energy

1008   **Nutritional Status: Food & Fluid Intake**   Amount of food and fluid taken into the body over a 24-hour period

1009   **Nutritional Status: Nutrient Intake**   Adequacy of nutrients taken into the body

1100   **Oral Health**   Condition of the mouth, teeth, gums, and tongue

1605   **Pain Control**   Personal actions to control pain

2101   **Pain: Disruptive Effects**   Observed or reported disruptive effects of pain on emotions and behavior

2102   **Pain Level**   Severity of reported or demonstrated pain

1306   **Pain: Psychological Response**   Cognitive and emotional responses to physical pain

1500   **Parent-Infant Attachment**   Behaviors which demonstrate an enduring affectionate bond between a parent and infant

2211   **Parenting**   Provision of an environment that promotes optimum growth and development of dependent children

1901   **Parenting: Social Safety**   Parental actions to avoid social relationships that might cause harm or injury

1606   **Participation: Health Care Decisions**   Personal involvement in selecting and evaluating health care options

0113   **Physical Aging Status**   Physical changes that commonly occur with adult aging

2004   **Physical Fitness**   Ability to perform physical activities with vigor

0114   **Physical Maturation: Female**   Normal physical changes in the female that occur with the transition from childhood to adulthood

0115   **Physical Maturation: Male**   Normal physical changes in the male that occur with the transition from childhood to adulthood

0116   **Play Participation**   Use of activities as needed for enjoyment, entertainment, and development by children

1607   **Prenatal Health Behavior**   Personal actions to promote a healthy pregnancy

0117   **Preterm Infant Organization**   Extrauterine integration of physiological and behavioral function by the infant born 24 to 37 (term) weeks gestation

0006   **Psychomotor Energy**   Ability to maintain activities of daily living (ADLs), nutrition, personal safety

1305   **Psychosocial Adjustment: Life Change**   Psychosocial adaptation of an individual to a life change

2000   **Quality of Life**   An individual's expressed satisfaction with current life circumstances

0410   **Respiratory Status: Airway Patency**   Extent to which the tracheobronchial passages remain open

0402   **Respiratory Status: Gas Exchange**   Alveolar exchange of CO_2 or O_2 to maintain arterial blood gas concentrations

0403   **Respiratory Status: Ventilation**   Movement of air in and out of the lungs

0003   **Rest**   Extent and pattern of diminished activity for mental and physical rejuvenation

1902   **Risk Control**   Actions to eliminate or reduce actual, personal, and modifiable health threats

1903   **Risk Control: Alcohol Use**   Actions to eliminate or reduce alcohol use that poses a threat to health

1917   **Risk Control: Cancer**   Actions to reduce or detect the possibility of cancer

1914   **Risk Control: Cardiovascular Health**   Actions to eliminate or reduce threats to cardiovascular health

1904   **Risk Control: Drug Use**   Actions to eliminate or reduce drug use that poses a threat to health

1915   **Risk Control: Hearing Impairment**   Actions to eliminate or reduce the possibility of altered hearing function

1905   **Risk Control: Sexually Transmitted Diseases (STD)**   Actions to eliminate or reduce behaviors associated with sexually transmitted disease

1906   **Risk Control: Tobacco Use**   Actions to eliminate or reduce tobacco use

1907   **Risk Control: Unintended Pregnancy**   Actions to reduce the possibility of unintended pregnancy

1916   **Risk Control: Visual Impairment**   Actions to eliminate or reduce the possibility of altered visual function

1908   **Risk Detection**   Actions taken to identify personal health threats

1501   **Role Performance**   Congruence of an individual's role behavior with role expectations

1909   **Safety Behavior: Fall Prevention**   Individual or caregiver actions to minimize risk factors that might precipitate falls

1910   **Safety Behavior: Home Physical Environment**   Individual or caregiver actions to minimize environmental factors that might cause physical harm or injury in the home

1911   **Safety Behavior: Personal**   Individual or caregiver efforts to control behaviors that might cause physical injury

1912   **Safety Status: Falls Occurrence**   Number of falls in the past week

1913   **Safety Status: Physical Injury**   Severity of injuries from accidents and trauma

0300   **Self-Care: Activities of Daily Living (ADL)**   Ability to perform the most basic physical tasks and personal care activities

0301   **Self-Care: Bathing**   Ability to cleanse own body

0302   **Self-Care: Dressing**   Ability to dress self

0303   **Self-Care: Eating**   Ability to prepare and ingest food

0304   **Self-Care: Grooming**   Ability to maintain kempt appearance

0305   **Self-Care: Hygiene**   Ability to maintain own hygiene

0306   **Self-Care: Instrumental Activities of Daily Living (IADL)**   Ability to perform activities needed to function in the home or community

0307   **Self-Care: Non-Parenteral Medication**   Ability to administer oral and topical medications to meet therapeutic goals

0308   **Self-Care: Oral Hygiene**   Ability to care for own mouth and teeth

0309   **Self-Care: Parenteral Medication**   Ability to administer parenteral medications to meet therapeutic goals

0310   **Self-Care: Toileting**   Ability to toilet self

1613   **Self-Direction of Care**   Directing others to assist with or perform physical tasks, personal care, and activities needed to function in the home or the community

1205   **Self-Esteem**   Personal judgement of self-worth

1406   **Self-Mutilation Restraint**   Ability to refrain from intentional self-inflicted injury (non-lethal)

2400   **Sensory Function: Cutaneous**   Extent to which stimulation of the skin is sensed in an impaired area

2401   **Sensory Function: Hearing**   Extent to which sounds are sensed, with or without assistive devices

2402   **Sensory Function: Proprioception**   Extent to which the position and movement of the head and body are sensed

2403   **Sensory Function: Taste & Smell**   Extent to which chemicals inhaled or dissolved in saliva are sensed

2404   **Sensory Function: Vision**   Extent to which visual images are sensed, with or without assistive devices

0119   **Sexual Functioning**   Integration of physical, socioemotional, and intellectual aspects of sexual expression

1207   **Sexual Identity: Acceptance**   Acknowledgment and acceptance of own sexual identity

0211   **Skeletal Function**   The functional ability of the bones to support the body and facilitate movement

0004   **Sleep**   Extent and pattern of natural periodic suspension of consciousness during which the body is restored

1502   **Social Interaction Skills**   An individual's use of effective interaction behaviors

1503   **Social Involvement**   Frequency of an individual's social interactions with persons, groups, or organizations

1504 **Social Support** Perceived availability and actual provision of reliable assistance from other persons

2001 **Spiritual Well-Being** Personal expressions of connectedness with self, others, higher power, all life, nature, and the universe that transcend and empower the self

1407 **Substance Addiction Consequences** Compromise in health status and social functioning due to substance addiction

2003 **Suffering Level** Severity of anguish associated with a distressing symptom, injury, or loss with potential long-term effects

1408 **Suicide Self-Restraint** Ability to refrain from gestures and attempts at killing self

1010 **Swallowing Status** Extent of safe passage of fluids and/or solids from the mouth to the stomach

1011 **Swallowing Status: Esophageal Phase** Adequacy of the passage of fluids and/or solids from the pharynx to the stomach

1012 **Swallowing Status: Oral Phase** Adequacy of preparation, containment, and posterior movement of fluids and/or solids in the mouth for swallowing

1013 **Swallowing Status: Pharyngeal Phase** Adequacy of the passage of fluids and/or solids from the mouth to the esophagus

1608 **Symptom Control** Personal actions to minimize perceived adverse changes in physical and emotional functioning

2103 **Symptom Severity** Extent of perceived adverse changes in physical, emotional, and social functioning

2104 **Symptom Severity: Perimenopause** Extent of symptoms caused by declining hormonal levels

2105 **Symptom Severity: Premenstrual Syndrome (PMS)** Extent of symptoms caused by cyclic hormonal fluctuations

2302 **Systemic Toxin Clearance: Dialysis** Extent to which toxins are cleared from the body with peritoneal or hemodialysis

0800 **Thermoregulation** Balance among heat production, heat gain, and heat loss

0801 **Thermoregulation: Neonate** Balance among heat production, heat gain, and heat loss during the neonatal period

1101 **Tissue Integrity: Skin & Mucous Membranes** Structural intactness and normal physiological function of skin and mucous membranes

0404 **Tissue Perfusion: Abdominal Organs** Extent to which blood flows through the small vessels of the abdominal viscera and maintains organ function

0405 **Tissue Perfusion: Cardiac** Extent to which blood flows through the coronary vasculature and maintains heart function

0406 **Tissue Perfusion: Cerebral** Extent to which blood flows through the cerebral vasculature and maintains brain function

0407 **Tissue Perfusion: Peripheral** Extent to which blood flows through the small vessels of the extremities and maintains tissue function

0408 **Tissue Perfusion: Pulmonary** Extent to which blood flows through intact pulmonary vasculature with appropriate pressure and volume, perfusing alveoli/capillary unit

0210 **Transfer Performance** Ability to change body locations

1609 **Treatment Behavior: Illness or Injury** Personal actions to palliate or eliminate pathology

0502   **Urinary Continence**   Control of the elimination of urine

0503   **Urinary Elimination**   Ability of the urinary system to filter wastes,
conserve solutes, and to collect and discharge urine in a healthy pattern

1611   **Vision Compensation Behavior**   Actions to compensate for visual
impairment

0802   **Vital Signs Status**   Temperature, pulse, respiration, and blood pressure
within expected range for the individual

1612   **Weight Control**   Personal actions resulting in achievement and
maintenance of optimum body weight for health

2002   **Well-Being**   An individual's expressed satisfaction with health status

1206   **Will to Live**   Desire, determination, and effort to survive

1102   **Wound Healing: Primary Intention**   The extent to which cells and
tissues have regenerated following intentional closure

1103   **Wound Healing: Secondary Intention**   The extent to which cells and
tissues in an open wound have regenerated

NIC Intervention Labels and Definitions (486 Interventions)

6400   **Abuse Protection Support**   Identification of high-risk, dependent relationships and actions to prevent further infliction of physical or emotional harm

6402   **Abuse Protection Support: Child**   Identification of high-risk, dependent child relationships and actions to prevent possible or further infliction of physical, sexual, or emotional harm or neglect of basic necessities of life

6403   **Abuse Protection Support: Domestic Partner**   Identification of high-risk, dependent domestic relationships and actions to prevent possible or further infliction of physical, sexual, or emotional harm, or exploitation of a domestic partner

6404   **Abuse Protection Support: Elder**   Identification of high-risk dependent elder relationships and actions to prevent possible or further infliction of physical, sexual, or emotional harm; neglect of basic necessities of life; or exploitation

6408   **Abuse Protection Support: Religious**   Identification of high-risk, controlling, religious relationships and actions to prevent infliction of physical, sexual, or emotional harm and/or exploitation

1910   **Acid-Base Management**   Promotion of acid-base balance and prevention of complications resulting from acid-base imbalance

1911   **Acid-Base Management: Metabolic Acidosis**   Promotion of acid-base balance and prevention of complications resulting from serum HCO_3 levels lower than desired

1912   **Acid-Base Management: Metabolic Alkalosis**   Promotion of acid-base balance and prevention of complications resulting from serum HCO_3 levels higher than desired

1913   **Acid-Base Management: Respiratory Acidosis**   Promotion of acid-base balance and prevention of complications resulting from serum pCO_2 levels higher than desired

From McCloskey, J.C., & Bulechek, G.M. (Eds.). (2000). *Nursing interventions classification (NIC)* (3rd ed.). St. Louis: Mosby.

1914   **Acid-Base Management: Respiratory Alkalosis** Promotion of acid-base balance and prevention of complications resulting from serum pCO_2 levels lower than desired

1920   **Acid-Base Monitoring** Collection and analysis of patient data to regulate acid-base balance

4920   **Active Listening** Attending closely to and attaching significance to a patient's verbal and nonverbal messages

4310   **Activity Therapy** Prescription of and assistance with specific physical, cognitive, social, and spiritual activities to increase the range, frequency, or duration of an individual's (or group's) activity

1320   **Acupressure** Application of firm, sustained pressure to special points on the body to decrease pain, produce relaxation, and prevent or reduce nausea

7310   **Admission Care** Facilitating entry of a patient into a health care facility

3120   **Airway Insertion and Stabilization** Insertion or assisting with insertion and stabilization of an artificial airway

3140   **Airway Management** Facilitation of patency of air passages

3160   **Airway Suctioning** Removal of airway secretions by inserting a suction catheter into the patient's oral airway and/or trachea

6410   **Allergy Management** Identification, treatment, and prevention of allergic responses to food, medications, insect bites, contrast material, blood, or other substances

6700   **Amnioinfusion** Infusion of fluid into the uterus during labor to relieve umbilical cord compression or to dilute meconium-stained fluid

3420   **Amputation Care** Promotion of physical and psychological healing after amputation of a body part

2210   **Analgesic Administration** Use of pharmacologic agents to reduce or eliminate pain

2214   **Analgesic Administration: Intraspinal** Administration of pharmacologic agents into the epidural or intrathecal space to reduce or eliminate pain

6412   **Anaphylaxis Management** Promotion of adequate ventilation and tissue perfusion for a patient with a severe allergic (antigen-antibody) reaction

2840   **Anesthesia Administration** Preparation for and administration of anesthetic agents and monitoring of patient responsiveness during administration

4640   **Anger Control Assistance** Facilitation of the expression of anger in an adaptive nonviolent manner

4320   **Animal-Assisted Therapy** Purposeful use of animals to provide affection, attention, diversion, and relaxation

5210   **Anticipatory Guidance** Preparation of patient for an anticipated developmental and/or situational crisis

5820   **Anxiety Reduction** Minimizing apprehension, dread, foreboding, or uneasiness related to an unidentified source of anticipated danger

6420   **Area Restriction** Limitation of patient mobility to a specified area for purposes of safety or behavior management

4330   **Art Therapy** Facilitation of communication through drawings or other art forms

3180   **Artificial Airway Management** Maintenance of endotracheal and tracheostomy tubes and preventing complications associated with their use

3200   **Aspiration Precautions**   Prevention or minimization of risk factors in the patient at risk for aspiration

4340   **Assertiveness Training**   Assistance with the effective expression of feelings, needs, and ideas while respecting the rights of others

6710   **Attachment Promotion**   Facilitation of the development of the parent-infant relationship

5840   **Autogenic Training**   Assisting with self-suggestions about feelings of heaviness and warmth for the purpose of inducing relaxation

2860   **Autotransfusion**   Collecting and reinfusing blood that has been lost intraoperatively or postoperatively from clean wounds

1610   **Bathing**   Cleaning of the body for the purposes of relaxation, cleanliness, and healing

0740   **Bed Rest Care**   Promotion of comfort and safety and prevention of complications for a patient unable to get out of bed

7610   **Bedside Laboratory Testing**   Performance of laboratory tests at the bedside or point of care

4350   **Behavior Management**   Helping a patient to manage negative behavior

4352   **Behavior Management: Overactivity/Inattention**   Provision of a therapeutic milieu that safely accommodates the patient's attention deficit and/or overactivity while promoting optimal function

4354   **Behavior Management: Self-Harm**   Assisting the patient to decrease or eliminate self-mutilating or self-abusive behaviors

4356   **Behavior Management: Sexual**   Delineation and prevention of socially unacceptable sexual behaviors

4360   **Behavior Modification**   Promotion of a behavior change

4362   **Behavior Modification: Social Skills**   Assisting the patient to develop or improve interpersonal social skills

4680   **Bibliotherapy**   Use of literature to enhance the expression of feelings and the gaining of insight

5860   **Biofeedback**   Assisting the patient to modify a body function using feedback from instrumentation

6720   **Birthing**   Delivery of a baby

0550   **Bladder Irrigation**   Instillation of a solution into the bladder to provide cleansing or medication

4010   **Bleeding Precautions**   Reduction of stimuli that may induce bleeding or hemorrhage in at-risk patients

4020   **Bleeding Reduction**   Limitation of the loss of blood volume during an episode of bleeding

4021   **Bleeding Reduction: Antepartum Uterus**   Limitation of the amount of blood loss from the pregnant uterus during third trimester of pregnancy

4022   **Bleeding Reduction: Gastrointestinal**   Limitation of the amount of blood loss from the upper and lower gastrointestinal tract and related complications

4024   **Bleeding Reduction: Nasal**   Limitation of the amount of blood loss from the nasal cavity

4026   **Bleeding Reduction: Postpartum Uterus**   Limitation of the amount of blood loss from the postpartum uterus

4028   **Bleeding Reduction: Wound**   Limitation of the blood loss from a wound that may be a result of trauma, incisions, or placement of a tube or catheter

4030   **Blood Products Administration**   Administration of blood or blood products and monitoring of patient's response

5220   **Body Image Enhancement**   Improving a patient's conscious and unconscious perceptions and attitudes toward his/her body

0140   **Body Mechanics Promotion**   Facilitating the use of posture and movement in daily activities to prevent fatigue and musculoskeletal strain or injury

1052   **Bottle Feeding**   Preparation and administration of fluids to an infant via a bottle

0410   **Bowel Incontinence Care**   Promotion of bowel continence and maintenance of perianal skin integrity

0412   **Bowel Incontinence Care: Encopresis**   Promotion of bowel continence in children

0420   **Bowel Irrigation**   Instillation of a substance into the lower gastrointestinal tract

0430   **Bowel Management**   Establishment and maintenance of a regular pattern of bowel elimination

0440   **Bowel Training**   Assisting the patient to train the bowel to evacuate at specific intervals

6522   **Breast Examination**   Inspection and palpation of the breasts and related areas

1054   **Breastfeeding Assistance**   Preparing a new mother to breastfeed her infant

5880   **Calming Technique**   Reducing anxiety in patient experiencing acute distress

4040   **Cardiac Care**   Limitation of complications resulting from an imbalance between myocardial oxygen supply and demand for a patient with symptoms of impaired cardiac function

4044   **Cardiac Care: Acute**   Limitation of complications for a patient recently experiencing an episode of an imbalance between myocardial oxygen supply and demand resulting in impaired cardiac function

4046   **Cardiac Care: Rehabilitative**   Promotion of maximum functional activity level for a patient who has suffered an episode of impaired cardiac function that resulted from an imbalance between myocardial oxygen supply and demand

4050   **Cardiac Precautions**   Prevention of an acute episode of impaired cardiac function by minimizing myocardial oxygen consumption or increasing myocardial oxygen supply

7040   **Caregiver Support**   Provision of the necessary information, advocacy, and support to facilitate primary patient care by someone other than a health care professional

7320   **Case Management**   Coordinating care and advocating for specified individuals and patient populations across settings to reduce cost, reduce resource use, improve quality of health care, and achieve desired outcomes

0762   **Cast Care: Maintenance**   Care of a cast after the drying period

0764   **Cast Care: Wet**   Care of a new cast during the drying period

2540   **Cerebral Edema Management**   Limitation of secondary cerebral injury resulting from swelling of brain tissue

2550   **Cerebral Perfusion Promotion**   Promotion of adequate perfusion and limitation of complications for a patient experiencing, or at risk for, inadequate cerebral perfusion

6750 **Cesarean Section Care** Preparation and support of patient delivering a baby by cesarean section

2240 **Chemotherapy Management** Assisting the patient and family to understand the action and minimize side effects of antineoplastic agents

3230 **Chest Physiotherapy** Assisting the patient to move airway secretions from peripheral airways to more central airways for expectoration and/or suctioning

6760 **Childbirth Preparation** Providing information and support to facilitate childbirth and to enhance the ability of an individual to develop and perform the role of parent

4062 **Circulatory Care: Arterial Insufficiency** Promotion of arterial circulation

4064 **Circulatory Care: Mechanical Assist Device** Temporary support of the circulation through the use of mechanical devices or pumps

4066 **Circulatory Care: Venous Insufficiency** Promotion of venous circulation

4070 **Circulatory Precautions** Protection of a localized area with limited perfusion

6140 **Code Management** Coordination of emergency measures to sustain life

4700 **Cognitive Restructuring** Challenging a patient to alter distorted thought patterns and view self and the world more realistically

4720 **Cognitive Stimulation** Promotion of awareness and comprehension of surroundings by utilization of planned stimuli

8820 **Communicable Disease Management** Working with a community to decrease and manage the incidence and prevalence of contagious diseases in a specific population

4974 **Communication Enhancement: Hearing Deficit** Assistance in accepting and learning alternate methods for living with diminished hearing

4976 **Communication Enhancement: Speech Deficit** Assistance in accepting and learning alternate methods for living with impaired speech

4978 **Communication Enhancement: Visual Deficit** Assistance in accepting and learning alternate methods for living with diminished vision

8840 **Community Disaster Preparedness** Preparing for an effective response to a large-scale disaster

8500 **Community Health Development** Facilitating members of a community to identify a community's health concerns, mobilize resources, and implement solutions

5000 **Complex Relationship Building** Establishing a therapeutic relationship with a patient who has difficulty interacting with others

5020 **Conflict Mediation** Facilitation of constructive dialogue between opposing parties with a goal of resolving disputes in a mutually acceptable manner

2260 **Conscious Sedation** Administration of sedatives, monitoring of the patient's response, and provision of necessary physiological support during a diagnostic or therapeutic procedure

0450 **Constipation/Impaction Management** Prevention and alleviation of constipation/impaction

7910   **Consultation**   Using expert knowledge to work with those who seek help in problem-solving to enable individuals, families, groups or agencies to achieve identified goals

1620   **Contact Lens Care**   Prevention of eye injury and lens damage by proper use of contact lenses

7620   **Controlled Substance Checking**   Promoting appropriate use and maintaining security of controlled substances

5230   **Coping Enhancement**   Assisting a patient to adapt to perceived stressors, changes, or threats which interfere with meeting life demands and roles

7630   **Cost Containment**   Management and facilitation of efficient and effective use of resources

3250   **Cough Enhancement**   Promotion of deep inhalation by the patient with subsequent generation of high intrathoracic pressures and compression of underlying lung parenchyma for the forceful expulsion of air

5240   **Counseling**   Use of an interactive helping process focusing on the needs, problems, or feelings of the patient and significant others to enhance or support coping, problem-solving, and interpersonal relationships

6160   **Crisis Intervention**   Use of short-term counseling to help the patient cope with a crisis and resume a state of functioning comparable to or better than the pre-crisis state

7640   **Critical Path Development**   Constructing and using a timed sequence of patient care activities to enhance desired patient outcomes in a cost-efficient manner

7330   **Culture Brokerage**   The deliberate use of culturally competent strategies to bridge or mediate between the patient's culture and the biomedical health care system

1340   **Cutaneous Stimulation**   Stimulation of the skin and underlying tissues for the purpose of decreasing undesirable signs and symptoms such as pain, muscle spasm, or inflammation

5250   **Decision-Making Support**   Providing information and support for a patient who is making a decision regarding health care

7650   **Delegation**   Transfer of responsibility for the performance of patient care while retaining accountability for the outcome

6440   **Delirium Management**   Provision of a safe and therapeutic environment for the patient who is experiencing an acute confusional state

6450   **Delusion Management**   Promoting the comfort, safety, and reality orientation of a patient experiencing false, fixed beliefs that have little or no basis in reality

6460   **Dementia Management**   Provision of a modified environment for the patient who is experiencing a chronic confusional state

8250   **Developmental Care**   Structuring the environment and providing care in response to the behavioral cues and states of the preterm infant

8272   **Developmental Enhancement: Adolescent**   Facilitating optimal physical, cognitive, social, and emotional growth of individuals during the transition from childhood to adulthood

8274   **Developmental Enhancement: Child**   Facilitating or teaching parents/caregivers to facilitate the optimal gross motor, fine motor, language, cognitive, social and emotional growth of preschool and school-aged children

0460   **Diarrhea Management**   Prevention and alleviation of diarrhea

1020   **Diet Staging**   Instituting required diet restrictions with subsequent progression of diet as tolerated

7370   **Discharge Planning**   Preparation for moving a patient from one level of care to another within or outside the current health care agency

5900   **Distraction**   Purposeful focusing of attention away from undesirable sensations

7920   **Documentation**   Recording of pertinent patient data in a clinical record

1630   **Dressing**   Choosing, putting on, and removing clothes for a person who cannot do this for self

5260   **Dying Care**   Promotion of physical comfort and psychological peace in the final phase of life

2560   **Dysreflexia Management**   Prevention and elimination of stimuli that cause hyperactive reflexes and inappropriate autonomic responses in a patient with a cervical or high thoracic cord lesion

4090   **Dysrhythmia Management**   Preventing, recognizing, and facilitating treatment of abnormal cardiac rhythms

1640   **Ear Care**   Prevention or minimization of threats to ear or hearing

1030   **Eating Disorders Management**   Prevention and treatment of severe diet restriction and overexercising or binging and purging of food and fluids

2000   **Electrolyte Management**   Promotion of electrolyte balance and prevention of complications resulting from abnormal or undesired serum electrolyte levels

2001   **Electrolyte Management: Hypercalcemia**   Promotion of calcium balance and prevention of complications resulting from serum calcium levels higher than desired

2002   **Electrolyte Management: Hyperkalemia**   Promotion of potassium balance and prevention of complications resulting from serum potassium levels higher than desired

2003   **Electrolyte Management: Hypermagnesemia**   Promotion of magnesium balance and prevention of complications resulting from serum magnesium levels higher than desired

2004   **Electrolyte Management: Hypernatremia**   Promotion of sodium balance and prevention of complications resulting from serum sodium levels higher than desired

2005   **Electrolyte Management: Hyperphosphatemia**   Promotion of phosphate balance and prevention of complications resulting from serum phosphate levels higher than desired

2006   **Electrolyte Management: Hypocalcemia**   Promotion of calcium balance and prevention of complications resulting from serum calcium levels lower than desired

2007   **Electrolyte Management: Hypokalemia**   Promotion of potassium balance and prevention of complications resulting from serum potassium levels lower than desired

2008   **Electrolyte Management: Hypomagnesemia**   Promotion of magnesium balance and prevention of complications resulting from serum magnesium levels lower than desired

2009   **Electrolyte Management: Hyponatremia**   Promotion of sodium balance and prevention of complications resulting from serum sodium levels lower than desired

2010 **Electrolyte Management: Hypophosphatemia** Promotion of phosphate balance and prevention of complications resulting from serum phosphate levels lower than desired

2020 **Electrolyte Monitoring** Collection and analysis of patient data to regulate electrolyte balance

6771 **Electronic Fetal Monitoring: Antepartum** Electronic evaluation of fetal heart rate response to movement, external stimuli, or uterine contractions during antepartal testing

6772 **Electronic Fetal Monitoring: Intrapartum** Electronic evaluation of fetal heart rate response to uterine contractions during intrapartal care

6470 **Elopement Precautions** Minimizing the risk of a patient leaving a treatment setting without authorization when departure presents a threat to the safety of patient or others

4104 **Embolus Care: Peripheral** Limitation of complications for a patient experiencing, or at risk for, occlusion of peripheral circulation

4106 **Embolus Care: Pulmonary** Limitation of complications for a patient experiencing, or at risk for, occlusion of pulmonary circulation

4110 **Embolus Precautions** Reduction of the risk of an embolus in a patient with thrombi or at risk for developing thrombus formation

6200 **Emergency Care** Providing life-saving measures in life-threatening situations

7660 **Emergency Cart Checking** Systematic review of the contents of an emergency cart at established time intervals

5270 **Emotional Support** Provision of reassurance, acceptance, and encouragement during times of stress

3270 **Endotracheal Extubation** Purposeful removal of the endotracheal tube from the nasopharyngeal or oropharyngeal airway

0180 **Energy Management** Regulating energy use to treat or prevent fatigue and optimize function

1056 **Enteral Tube Feeding** Delivering nutrients and water through a gastrointestinal tube

6480 **Environmental Management** Manipulation of the patient's surroundings for therapeutic benefit

6481 **Environmental Management: Attachment Process** Manipulation of the patient's surroundings to facilitate the development of the parent-infant relationship

6482 **Environmental Management: Comfort** Manipulation of the patient's surroundings for promotion of optimal comfort

6484 **Environmental Management: Community** Monitoring and influencing of the physical, social, cultural, economic, and political conditions that affect the health of groups and communities

6485 **Environmental Management: Home Preparation** Preparing the home for safe and effective delivery of care

6486 **Environmental Management: Safety** Monitoring and manipulation of the physical environment to promote safety

6487 **Environmental Management: Violence Prevention** Monitoring and manipulation of the physical environment to decrease the potential for violent behavior directed toward self, others, or environment

6489 **Environmental Management: Worker Safety** Monitoring and manipulating of the work-site environment to promote safety and health of workers

8880   **Environmental Risk Protection** Preventing and detecting disease and injury in populations at risk from environmental hazards

7680   **Examination Assistance** Providing assistance to the patient and another health care provider during a procedure or exam

0200   **Exercise Promotion** Facilitation of regular physical exercise to maintain or advance to a higher level of fitness and health

0201   **Exercise Promotion: Strength Training** Facilitating regular resistive muscle training to maintain or increase muscle strength

0202   **Exercise Promotion: Stretching** Facilitation of systematic slow-stretch-hold muscle exercises to induce relaxation, to prepare muscles/joints for more vigorous exercise, or to increase or maintain body flexibility

0221   **Exercise Therapy: Ambulation** Promotion and assistance with walking to maintain or restore autonomic and voluntary body functions during treatment and recovery from illness or injury

0222   **Exercise Therapy: Balance** Use of specific activities, postures, and movements to maintain, enhance, or restore balance

0224   **Exercise Therapy: Joint Mobility** Use of active or passive body movement to maintain or restore joint flexibility

0226   **Exercise Therapy: Muscle Control** Use of specific activity or exercise protocols to enhance or restore controlled body movement

1650   **Eye Care** Prevention or minimization of threats to eye or visual integrity

6490   **Fall Prevention** Instituting special precautions with patient at risk for injury from falling

7100   **Family Integrity Promotion** Promotion of family cohesion and unity

7104   **Family Integrity Promotion: Childbearing Family** Facilitation of the growth of individuals or families who are adding an infant to the family unit

7110   **Family Involvement Promotion** Facilitating family participation in the emotional and physical care of the patient

7120   **Family Mobilization** Utilization of family strengths to influence patient's health in a positive direction

6784   **Family Planning: Contraception** Facilitation of pregnancy prevention by providing information about the physiology of reproduction and methods to control conception

6786   **Family Planning: Infertility** Management, education, and support of the patient and significant other undergoing evaluation and treatment for infertility

6788   **Family Planning: Unplanned Pregnancy** Facilitation of decision-making regarding pregnancy outcome

7130   **Family Process Maintenance** Minimization of family process disruption effects

7140   **Family Support** Promotion of family values, interests, and goals

7150   **Family Therapy** Assisting family members to move their family toward a more productive way of living

1050   **Feeding** Providing nutritional intake for patient who is unable to feed self

7160   **Fertility Preservation** Providing information, counseling, and treatment that facilitate reproductive health and the ability to conceive

3740   **Fever Treatment** Management of a patient with hyperpyrexia caused by nonenvironmental factors

7380   **Financial Resource Assistance**   Assisting an individual/family to secure and manage finances to meet health care needs

6500   **Fire-Setting Precautions**   Prevention of fire-setting behaviors

6240   **First Aid**   Providing initial care of a minor injury

8550   **Fiscal Resource Management**   Procuring and directing the use of financial resources to assure to development and continuation of programs and services

0470   **Flatulence Reduction**   Prevention of flatus formation and facilitation of passage of excessive gas

4120   **Fluid Management**   Promotion of fluid balance and prevention of complications resulting from abnormal or undesired fluid levels

4130   **Fluid Monitoring**   Collection and analysis of patient data to regulate fluid balance

4140   **Fluid Resuscitation**   Administering prescribed intravenous fluids rapidly

2080   **Fluid/Electrolyte Management**   Regulation and prevention of complications from altered fluid and/or electrolyte levels

1660   **Foot Care**   Cleansing and inspecting the feet for the purposes of relaxation, cleanliness, and healthy skin

5280   **Forgiveness Facilitation**   Assisting an individual to forgive and/or experience forgiveness in relationship with self, others, and higher power

1080   **Gastrointestinal Intubation**   Insertion of a tube into the gastrointestinal tract

5242   **Genetic Counseling**   Use of an interactive helping process focusing on assisting an individual, family, or group, manifesting or at risk for developing or transmitting a birth defect or genetic condition, to cope

5290   **Grief Work Facilitation**   Assistance with the resolution of a significant loss

5294   **Grief Work Facilitation: Perinatal Death**   Assistance with the resolution of a perinatal loss

5300   **Guilt Work Facilitation**   Helping another to cope with painful feelings of responsibility, actual or perceived

1670   **Hair Care**   Promotion of neat, clean, attractive hair

6510   **Hallucination Management**   Promoting the safety, comfort, and reality orientation of a patient experiencing hallucinations

7960   **Health Care Information Exchange**   Providing patient care information to health professionals in other agencies

5510   **Health Education**   Developing and providing instruction and learning experiences to facilitate voluntary adaptation of behavior conducive to health in individuals, families, groups, or communities

7970   **Health Policy Monitoring**   Surveillance and influence of government and organization regulations, rules, and standards that affect nursing systems and practices to ensure quality care of patients

6520   **Health Screening**   Detecting health risks or problems by means of history, examination, and other procedures

7400   **Health System Guidance**   Facilitating a patient's location and use of appropriate health services

3780   **Heat Exposure Treatment**   Management of patient overcome by heat due to excessive environmental heat exposure

1380   **Heat/Cold Application**   Stimulation of the skin and underlying tissues with heat or cold for the purpose of decreasing pain, muscle spasms, or inflammation

2100	**Hemodialysis Therapy** Management of extracorporeal passage of the patient's blood through a dialyzer
4150	**Hemodynamic Regulation** Optimization of heart rate, preload, afterload, and contractility
2110	**Hemofiltration Therapy** Cleansing of acutely ill patient's blood via a hemofilter controlled by the patient's hydrostatic pressure
4160	**Hemorrhage Control** Reduction or elimination of rapid and excessive blood loss
6800	**High-Risk Pregnancy Care** Identification and management of a high-risk pregnancy to promote healthy outcomes for mother and baby
7180	**Home Maintenance Assistance** Helping the patient/family to maintain the home as a clean, safe, and pleasant place to live
5310	**Hope Instillation** Facilitation of the development of a positive outlook in a given situation
5320	**Humor** Facilitating the patient to perceive, appreciate, and express what is funny, amusing, or ludicrous in order to establish relationships, relieve tension, release anger, facilitate learning, or cope with painful feelings
2120	**Hyperglycemia Management** Preventing and treating above-normal blood glucose levels
4170	**Hypervolemia Management** Reduction in extracellular and/or intracellular fluid volume and prevention of complications in a patient who is fluid overloaded
5920	**Hypnosis** Assisting a patient to induce an altered state of consciousness to create an acute awareness and a directed focus experience
2130	**Hypoglycemia Management** Preventing and treating low blood glucose levels
3800	**Hypothermia Treatment** Rewarming and surveillance of a patient whose core body temperature is below 35° C
4180	**Hypovolemia Management** Expansion of intravascular fluid volume in a patient who is volume depleted
6530	**Immunization/Vaccination Management** Monitoring immunization status, facilitating access to immunizations, and provision of immunizations to prevent communicable disease
4370	**Impulse Control Training** Assisting the patient to mediate impulsive behavior through application of problem-solving strategies to social and interpersonal situations
7980	**Incident Reporting** Written and verbal reporting of any event in the process of patient care that is inconsistent with desired patient outcomes or routine operations of the health care facility
3440	**Incision Site Care** Cleansing, monitoring, and promotion of healing in a wound that is closed with sutures, clips, or staples
6820	**Infant Care** Provision of developmentally appropriate family-centered care to the child under 1 year of age
6540	**Infection Control** Minimizing the acquisition and transmission of infectious agents
6545	**Infection Control: Intraoperative** Preventing nosocomial infection in the operating room
6550	**Infection Protection** Prevention and early detection of infection in a patient at risk

7410   **Insurance Authorization**   Assisting the patient and provider to secure payment for health services or equipment from a third party

2590   **Intracranial Pressure (ICP) Monitoring**   Measurement and interpretation of patient data to regulate intracranial pressure

6830   **Intrapartal Care**   Monitoring and management of stages one and two of the birth process

6834   **Intrapartal Care: High-Risk Delivery**   Assisting vaginal birth of multiple or malpositioned fetuses

4190   **Intravenous (IV) Insertion**   Insertion of a needle into a peripheral vein for the purpose of administering fluids, blood, or medications

4200   **Intravenous (IV) Therapy**   Administration and monitoring of intravenous fluids and medications

4210   **Invasive Hemodynamic Monitoring**   Measurement and interpretation of invasive hemodynamic parameters to determine cardiovascular function and regulate therapy as appropriate

6840   **Kangaroo Care**   Promoting closeness between parent and physiologically stable preterm infant by preparing the parent and providing the environment for skin-to-skin contact

6850   **Labor Induction**   Initiation or augmentation of labor by mechanical or pharmacological methods

6860   **Labor Suppression**   Controlling uterine contractions prior to 37 weeks of gestation to prevent preterm birth

7690   **Laboratory Data Interpretation**   Critical analysis of patient laboratory data in order to assist with clinical decision-making

5244   **Lactation Counseling**   Use of an interactive helping process to assist in maintenance of successful breastfeeding

6870   **Lactation Suppression**   Facilitating the cessation of milk production and minimizing breast engorgement after giving birth

6560   **Laser Precautions**   Limiting the risk of injury to the patient related to use of a laser

6570   **Latex Precautions**   Reducing the risk of systemic reaction to latex

5520   **Learning Facilitation**   Promoting the ability to process and comprehend information

5540   **Learning Readiness Enhancement**   Improving the ability and willingness to receive information

3460   **Leech Therapy**   Application of medicinal leeches to help drain replanted or transplanted tissue engorged with venous blood

4380   **Limit Setting**   Establishing the parameters of desirable and acceptable patient behavior

3840   **Malignant Hyperthermia Precautions**   Prevention or reduction of hypermetabolic response to pharmacological agents used during surgery

3300   **Mechanical Ventilation**   Use of an artificial device to assist a patient to breathe

3310   **Mechanical Ventilatory Weaning**   Assisting the patient to breathe without the aid of a mechanical ventilator

2300   **Medication Administration**   Preparing, giving, and evaluating the effectiveness of prescription and nonprescription drugs

2308   **Medication Administration: Ear**   Preparing and instilling otic medications

2301   **Medication Administration: Enteral**   Delivering medications through an intestinal tube

2309   **Medication Administration: Epidural** Preparing and administering medications via the epidural route

2310   **Medication Administration: Eye** Preparing and instilling opthalmic medications

2311   **Medication Administration: Inhalation** Preparing and administering inhaled medications

2302   **Medication Administration: Interpleural** Administration of medication through an interpleural catheter for reduction of pain

2312   **Medication Administration: Intradermal** Preparing and giving medications via the intradermal route

2313   **Medication Administration: Intramuscular (IM)** Preparing and giving medications via the intramuscular route

2303   **Medication Administration: Intraosseous** Insertion of a needle through the bone cortex into the medullary cavity for the purpose of short-term, emergency administration of fluid, blood, or medication

2314   **Medication Administration: Intravenous (IV)** Preparing and giving medications via the intravenous route

2304   **Medication Administration: Oral** Preparing and giving medications by mouth and monitoring patient responsiveness

2315   **Medication Administration: Rectal** Preparing and inserting rectal suppositories

2316   **Medication Administration: Skin** Preparing and applying medications to the skin

2317   **Medication Administration: Subcutaneous** Preparing and giving medications via the subcutaneous route

2318   **Medication Administration: Vaginal** Preparing and inserting vaginal medications

2307   **Medication Administration: Ventricular Reservoir** Administration and monitoring of medication through an indwelling catheter into the lateral ventricle

2380   **Medication Management** Facilitation of safe and effective use of prescription and over-the-counter drugs

2390   **Medication Prescribing** Prescribing medication for a health problem

5960   **Meditation Facilitation** Facilitating a person to alter his/her level of awareness by focusing specifically on an image or thought

4760   **Memory Training** Facilitation of memory

4390   **Milieu Therapy** Use of people, resources, and events in the patient's immediate environment to promote optimal psychosocial functioning

5330   **Mood Management** Providing for safety, stabilization, recovery, and maintenance of a patient who is experiencing dysfunctionally depressed mood or elevated mood

8020   **Multidisciplinary Care Conference** Planning and evaluating patient care with health professionals from other disciplines

4400   **Music Therapy** Using music to help achieve a specific change in behavior, feeling, or physiology

4410   **Mutual Goal Setting** Collaborating with patient to identify and prioritize care goals, then developing a plan for achieving those goals

1680   **Nail Care** Promotion of clean, neat, attractive nails and prevention of skin lesions related to improper care of nails

1450   **Nausea Management** Prevention and alleviation of nausea

2620   **Neurologic Monitoring**   Collection and analysis of patient data to prevent or minimize neurological complications

6880   **Newborn Care**   Management of neonate during the transition to extrauterine life and subsequent period of stabilization

6890   **Newborn Monitoring**   Measurement and interpretation of physiologic status of the neonate the first 24 hours after delivery

6900   **Nonnutritive Sucking**   Provision of sucking opportunities for the infant

7200   **Normalization Promotion**   Assisting parents and other family members of children with chronic illnesses or disabilities in providing normal life experiences for their children and families

1100   **Nutrition Management**   Assisting with or providing a balanced dietary intake of foods and fluids

1120   **Nutrition Therapy**   Administration of food and fluids to support metabolic processes of a patient who is malnourished or at high risk for becoming malnourished

5246   **Nutritional Counseling**   Use of an interactive helping process focusing on the need for diet modification

1160   **Nutritional Monitoring**   Collection and analysis of patient data to prevent or minimize malnourishment

1710   **Oral Health Maintenance**   Maintenance and promotion of oral hygiene and dental health for the patient at risk for developing oral or dental lesions

1720   **Oral Health Promotion**   Promotion of oral hygiene and dental care for a patient with normal oral and dental health

1730   **Oral Health Restoration**   Promotion of healing for a patient who has an oral mucosa or dental lesion

8060   **Order Transcription**   Transferring information from order sheets to the nursing patient care planning and documentation system

6260   **Organ Procurement**   Guiding families through the donation process to ensure timely retrieval of vital organs and tissue for transplant

0480   **Ostomy Care**   Maintenance of elimination through a stoma and care of surrounding tissue

3320   **Oxygen Therapy**   Administration of oxygen and monitoring of its effectiveness

1400   **Pain Management**   Alleviation of pain or a reduction in pain to a level of comfort that is acceptable to the patient

5562   **Parent Education: Adolescent**   Assisting parents to understand and help their adolescent children

5566   **Parent Education: Childrearing Family**   Assisting parents to understand and promote the physical, psychological, and social growth and development of their toddler, preschool, or school-aged child/children

5568   **Parent Education: Infant**   Instruction on nurturing and physical care needed during the first year of life

8300   **Parenting Promotion**   Providing parenting information, support and coordination of comprehensive services to high-risk families

7440   **Pass Facilitation**   Arranging a leave for a patient from a health care facility

4420   **Patient Contracting**   Negotiating an agreement with a patient that reinforces a specific behavior change

2400 **Patient-Controlled Analgesia (PCA) Assistance**   Facilitating patient control of analgesic administration and regulation

7460 **Patient Rights Protection**   Protection of health care rights of a patient, especially a minor, incapacitated, or incompetent patient unable to make decisions

7700 **Peer Review**   Systematic evaluation of a peer's performance compared with professional standards of practice

0560 **Pelvic Muscle Exercise**   Strengthening and training the levator ani and urogenital muscles through voluntary, repetitive contraction to decrease stress, urge, or mixed types of urinary incontinence

1750 **Perineal Care**   Maintenance of perineal skin integrity and relief of perineal discomfort

2660 **Peripheral Sensation Management**   Prevention or minimization of injury or discomfort in the patient with altered sensation

4220 **Peripherally Inserted Central (PIC) Catheter Care**   Insertion and maintenance of a peripherally inserted central catheter

2150 **Peritoneal Dialysis Therapy**   Administration and monitoring of dialysis solution into and out of the peritoneal cavity

0630 **Pessary Management**   Placement and monitoring of a vaginal device for treating stress urinary incontinence, uterine retroversion, genital prolapse, or incompetent cervix

4232 **Phlebotomy: Arterial Blood Sample**   Obtaining a blood sample from an uncannulated artery to assess oxygen and carbon dioxide levels and acid-base balance

4234 **Phlebotomy: Blood Unit Acquisition**   Procuring blood and blood products from donors

4238 **Phlebotomy: Venous Blood Sample**   Removal of a sample of venous blood from an uncannulated vein

6924 **Phototherapy: Neonate**   Use of light therapy to reduce bilirubin levels in newborn infants

6580 **Physical Restraint**   Application, monitoring, and removal of mechanical restraining devices or manual restraints, which are used to limit physical mobility of a patient

7710 **Physician Support**   Collaborating with physicians to provide quality patient care

6590 **Pneumatic Tourniquet Precautions**   Applying a pneumatic tourniquet, while minimizing the potential for patient injury from use of the device

0840 **Positioning**   Deliberative placement of the patient or a body part to promote physiological and/or psychological well-being

0842 **Positioning: Intraoperative**   Moving the patient or body part to promote surgical exposure while reducing the risk of discomfort and complications

0844 **Positioning: Neurologic**   Achievement of optimal, appropriate body alignment for the patient experiencing or at risk for spinal cord injury or vertebrae irritability

0846 **Positioning: Wheelchair**   Placement of a patient in a properly selected wheelchair to enhance comfort, promote skin integrity, and foster independence

2870 **Postanesthesia Care**   Monitoring and management of the patient who has recently undergone general or regional anesthesia

1770   **Postmortem Care** Providing physical care of the body of an expired patient and support for the family viewing the body

6930   **Postpartal Care** Monitoring and management of the patient who has recently given birth

7722   **Preceptor: Employee** Assisting and supporting a new or transferred employee through a planned orientation to a specific clinical area

7726   **Preceptor: Student** Assisting and supporting learning experiences for a student

5247   **Preconception Counseling** Screening and providing information and support to individuals of childbearing age before pregnancy to promote health and reduce risks

6950   **Pregnancy Termination Care** Management of the physical and psychological needs of the woman undergoing a spontaneous or elective abortion

6960   **Prenatal Care** Monitoring and management of patient during pregnancy to prevent complications of pregnancy and promote a healthy outcome for both mother and infant

2880   **Preoperative Coordination** Facilitating preadmission diagnostic testing and preparation of the surgical patient

5580   **Preparatory Sensory Information** Describing in concrete and objective terms the typical sensory experiences and events associated with an upcoming stressful health care procedure/treatment

5340   **Presence** Being with another, both physically and psychologically, during times of need

3500   **Pressure Management** Minimizing pressure to body parts

3520   **Pressure Ulcer Care** Facilitation of healing in pressure ulcers

3540   **Pressure Ulcer Prevention** Prevention of pressure ulcers for a patient at high risk for developing them

7760   **Product Evaluation** Determining the effectiveness of new products or equipment

8700   **Program Development** Planning, implementing, and evaluating a coordinated set of activities designed to enhance wellness, or to prevent, reduce, or eliminate one or more health problems of a group or community

1460   **Progressive Muscle Relaxation** Facilitating the tensing and releasing of successive muscle groups while attending to the resulting differences in sensation

0640   **Prompted Voiding** Promotion of urinary continence through the use of timed verbal toileting reminders and positive social feedback for successful toileting

1780   **Prosthesis Care** Care of a removable appliance worn by a patient and the prevention of complications associated with its use

3550   **Pruritus Management** Preventing and treating itching

7800   **Quality Monitoring** Systematic collection and analysis of an organization's quality indicators for the purpose of improving patient care

6600   **Radiation Therapy Management** Assisting the patient to understand and minimize the side effects of radiation treatments

6300   **Rape-Trauma Treatment** Provision of emotional and physical support immediately following a reported rape

4820	**Reality Orientation** Promotion of patient's awareness of personal identity, time, and environment
5360	**Recreation Therapy** Purposeful use of recreation to promote relaxation and enhancement of social skills
0490	**Rectal Prolapse Management** Prevention and/or manual reduction of rectal prolapse
8100	**Referral** Arrangement for services by another care provider or agency
5422	**Religious Addiction Prevention** Prevention of a self-imposed controlling religious life-style
5424	**Religious Ritual Enhancement** Facilitating participation in religious practices
4860	**Reminiscence Therapy** Using the recall of past events, feelings, and thoughts to facilitate pleasure, quality of life, or adaptation to present circumstances
7886	**Reproductive Technology Management** Assisting a patient through the steps of complex infertility treatment
8120	**Research Data Collection** Collecting research data
8340	**Resiliency Promotion** Assisting individuals, families, and communities in development, use, and strengthening of protective factors to be used in coping with environmental and societal stressors
3350	**Respiratory Monitoring** Collection and analysis of patient data to ensure airway patency and adequate gas exchange
7260	**Respite Care** Provision of short-term care to provide relief for family caregiver
6320	**Resuscitation** Administering emergency measures to sustain life
6972	**Resuscitation: Fetus** Administering emergency measures to improve placental perfusion or correct fetal acid-base status
6974	**Resuscitation: Neonate** Administering emergency measures to support newborn adaptation to extrauterine life
6610	**Risk Identification** Analysis of potential risk factors, determination of health risks, and prioritization of risk reduction strategies for an individual or group
6612	**Risk Identification: Childbearing Family** Identification of an individual or family likely to experience difficulties in parenting and prioritization of strategies to prevent parenting problems
6614	**Risk Identification: Genetic** Identification and analysis of potential genetic risk factors in an individual, family, or group
5370	**Role Enhancement** Assisting a patient, significant other, and/or family to improve relationships by clarifying and supplementing specific role behaviors
6630	**Seclusion** Solitary containment in a fully protective environment with close surveillance by nursing staff for purposes of safety or behavior management
5380	**Security Enhancement** Intensifying a patient's sense of physical and psychological safety
2680	**Seizure Management** Care of a patient during a seizure and the postictal state
2690	**Seizure Precautions** Prevention or minimization of potential injuries sustained by a patient with a known seizure disorder
5390	**Self-Awareness Enhancement** Assisting a patient to explore and understand his/her thoughts, feelings, motivations, and behaviors

1800   **Self-Care Assistance**   Assisting another to perform activities of daily living

1801   **Self-Care Assistance: Bathing/Hygiene**   Assisting patient to perform personal hygiene

1802   **Self-Care Assistance: Dressing/Grooming**   Assisting patient with clothes and makeup

1803   **Self-Care Assistance: Feeding**   Assisting a person to eat

1804   **Self-Care Assistance: Toileting**   Assisting another with elimination

5400   **Self-Esteem Enhancement**   Assisting a patient to increase his/her personal judgment of self worth

4470   **Self-Modification Assistance**   Reinforcement of self-directed change initiated by the patient to achieve personally important goals

4480   **Self-Responsibility Facilitation**   Encouraging a patient to assume more responsibility for own behavior

5248   **Sexual Counseling**   Use of an interactive helping process focusing on the need to make adjustments in sexual practice or to enhance coping with a sexual event/disorder

8140   **Shift Report**   Exchanging essential patient care information with other nursing staff at change of shift

4250   **Shock Management**   Facilitation of the delivery of oxygen and nutrients to systemic tissue with removal of cellular waste products in a patient with severely altered tissue perfusion

4254   **Shock Management: Cardiac**   Promotion of adequate tissue perfusion for a patient with severely compromised pumping function of the heart

4256   **Shock Management: Vasogenic**   Promotion of adequate tissue perfusion for a patient with severe loss of vascular tone

4258   **Shock Management: Volume**   Promotion of adequate tissue perfusion for a patient with severely compromised intravascular volume

4260   **Shock Prevention**   Detecting and treating a patient at risk for impending shock

7280   **Sibling Support**   Assisting a sibling to cope with a brother's or sister's illness/chronic condition/disability

6000   **Simple Guided Imagery**   Purposeful use of imagination to achieve relaxation and/or direct attention away from undesirable sensations

1480   **Simple Massage**   Stimulation of the skin and underlying tissues with varying degrees of hand pressure to decrease pain, produce relaxation, and/or improve circulation

6040   **Simple Relaxation Therapy**   Use of techniques to encourage and elicit relaxation for the purpose of decreasing undesirable signs and symptoms such as pain, muscle tension, or anxiety

3584   **Skin Care: Topical Treatments**   Application of topical substances or manipulation of devices to promote skin integrity and minimize skin breakdown

3590   **Skin Surveillance**   Collection and analysis of patient data to maintain skin and mucous membrane integrity

1850   **Sleep Enhancement**   Facilitation of regular sleep/wake cycles

4490   **Smoking Cessation Assistance**   Helping another to stop smoking

5100   **Socialization Enhancement**   Facilitation of another person's ability to interact with others

7820   **Specimen Management**   Obtaining, preparing, and preserving a specimen for a laboratory test

5426   **Spiritual Growth Facilitation** Facilitation of growth in patient's capacity to identify, connect with, and call upon the source of meaning, purpose, comfort, strength, and hope in his/her life

5420   **Spiritual Support** Assisting the patient to feel balance and connection with a greater power

0910   **Splinting** Stabilization, immobilization, and/or protection of an injured body part with a supportive appliance

6648   **Sports-Injury Prevention: Youth** Reduce the risk of sport-related injury in young athletes

7850   **Staff Development** Developing, maintaining, and monitoring competence of staff

7830   **Staff Supervision** Facilitating the delivery of high-quality patient care by others

2720   **Subarachnoid Hemorrhage Precautions** Reduction of internal and external stimuli or stressors to minimize risk of rebleeding prior to aneurysm surgery

4500   **Substance Use Prevention** Prevention of an alcoholic or drug use life-style

4510   **Substance Use Treatment** Supportive care of patient/family members with physical and psychosocial problems associated with the use of alcohol or drugs

4512   **Substance Use Treatment: Alcohol Withdrawal** Care of the patient experiencing sudden cessation of alcohol consumption

4514   **Substance Use Treatment: Drug Withdrawal** Care of a patient experiencing drug detoxification

4516   **Substance Use Treatment: Overdose** Monitoring, treatment, and emotional support of a patient who has ingested prescription or over-the-counter drugs beyond the therapeutic range

6340   **Suicide Prevention** Reducing risk of self-inflicted harm with intent to end life

7840   **Supply Management** Ensuring acquisition and maintenance of appropriate items for providing patient care

5430   **Support Group** Use of a group environment to provide emotional support and health-related information for members

5440   **Support System Enhancement** Facilitation of support to patient by family, friends, and community

2900   **Surgical Assistance** Assisting the surgeon/dentist with operative procedures and care of the surgical patient

2920   **Surgical Precautions** Minimizing the potential for iatrogenic injury to the patient related to a surgical procedure

2930   **Surgical Preparation** Providing care to a patient immediately prior to surgery and verification of required procedures/tests and documentation in the clinical record

6650   **Surveillance** Purposeful and ongoing acquisition, interpretation, and synthesis of patient data for clinical decision-making

6652   **Surveillance: Community** Purposeful and on-going acquisition, interpretation, and synthesis of data for decision-making in the community

6656   **Surveillance: Late Pregnancy** Purposeful and ongoing acquisition, interpretation, and synthesis of maternal-fetal data for treatment, observation, or admission

6658   **Surveillance: Remote Electronic**   Purposeful and ongoing acquisition of patient data via electronic modalities (telephone, video, conferencing, e-mail) from distant locations as well as interpretation and synthesis of patient data for clinical decision-making with individuals or populations

6654   **Surveillance: Safety**   Purposeful and ongoing collection and analysis of information about the patient and the environment for use in promoting and maintaining patient safety

7500   **Sustenance Support**   Helping a needy individual/family to locate food, clothing, or shelter

3620   **Suturing**   Approximating edges of a wound using sterile suture material and a needle

1860   **Swallowing Therapy**   Facilitating swallowing and preventing complications of impaired swallowing

5602   **Teaching: Disease Process**   Assisting the patient to understand information related to a specific disease process

5604   **Teaching: Group**   Development, implementation, and evaluation of a patient teaching program for a group of individuals experiencing the same health condition

5606   **Teaching: Individual**   Planning, implementation, and evaluation of a teaching program designed to address a patient's particular needs

5626   **Teaching: Infant Nutrition**   Instruction on nutrition and feeding practices during the first year of life

5628   **Teaching: Infant Safety**   Instruction on safety during first year of life

5610   **Teaching: Preoperative**   Assisting a patient to understand and mentally prepare for surgery and the postoperative recovery period

5612   **Teaching: Prescribed Activity/Exercise**   Preparing a patient to achieve and/or maintain a prescribed level of activity

5614   **Teaching: Prescribed Diet**   Preparing a patient to correctly follow a prescribed diet

5616   **Teaching: Prescribed Medication**   Preparing a patient to safely take prescribed medications and monitor for their effects

5618   **Teaching: Procedure/Treatment**   Preparing a patient to understand and mentally prepare for a prescribed procedure or treatment

5620   **Teaching: Psychomotor Skill**   Preparing a patient to perform a psychomotor skill

5622   **Teaching: Safe Sex**   Providing instruction concerning sexual protection during sexual activity

5624   **Teaching: Sexuality**   Assisting individuals to understand physical and psychosocial dimensions of sexual growth and development

5630   **Teaching: Toddler Nutrition**   Instruction on nutrition and feeding practices during the second and third years of life

5632   **Teaching: Toddler Safety**   Instruction on safety during the second and third years of life

7880   **Technology Management**   Use of technical equipment and devices to monitor patient condition or sustain life

8180   **Telephone Consultation**   Eliciting patient's concerns, listening, and providing support, information, or teaching in response to patient's stated concerns, over the telephone

8190   **Telephone Follow-up**   Providing results of testing or evaluating patient's response and determining potential for problems as a result of previous treatment, examination, or testing, over the telephone

3900 **Temperature Regulation** Attaining and/or maintaining body temperature within a normal range

3902 **Temperature Regulation: Intraoperative** Attaining and/or maintaining desired intraoperative body temperature

4430 **Therapeutic Play** Purposeful and directive use of toys or other materials to assist a children in communicating their perception and knowledge of their world and to help in gaining mastery of their environment

5465 **Therapeutic Touch** Attuning to the universal healing field, seeking to act as an instrument for healing influence, and using the natural sensitivity of the hands to gently focus and direct the intervention process

5450 **Therapy Group** Application of psychotherapeutic techniques to a group, including the utilization of interactions between members of the group

1200 **Total Parenteral Nutrition (TPN) Administration** Preparation and delivery of nutrients intravenously and monitoring of patient responsiveness

5460 **Touch** Providing comfort and communication through purposeful tactile contact

0940 **Traction/Immobilization Care** Management of a patient who has traction and/or a stabilizing device to immobilize and stabilize a body part

1540 **Transcutaneous Electrical Nerve Stimulation (TENS)** Stimulation of skin and underlying tissues with controlled, low-voltage electrical vibration via electrodes

0960 **Transport** Moving a patient from one location to another

6362 **Triage: Disaster** Establishing priorities of patient care for urgent treatment while allocating scarce resources

6364 **Triage: Emergency Center** Establishing priorities and initiating treatment for patients in an emergency center

6366 **Triage: Telephone** Determining the nature and urgency of a problem(s) and providing directions for the level of care required, over the telephone

5470 **Truth Telling** Use of whole truth, partial truth, or decision delay to promote the patient's self-determination and well-being

1870 **Tube Care** Management of a patient with an external drainage device exiting the body

1872 **Tube Care: Chest** Management of a patient with an external water-seal drainage device exiting the chest cavity

1874 **Tube Care: Gastrointestinal** Management of a patient with a gastrointestinal tube

1875 **Tube Care: Umbilical Line** Management of a newborn with an umbilical catheter

1876 **Tube Care: Urinary** Management of a patient with urinary drainage equipment

1878 **Tube Care: Ventriculostomy/Lumbar Drain** Management of a patient with an external cerebrospinal fluid drainage system

6982 **Ultrasonography: Limited Obstetric** Performance of ultrasound exams to determine ovarian, uterine, or fetal status

2760   **Unilateral Neglect Management**   Protecting and safely reintegrating the affected part of the body while helping the patient adapt to disturbed perceptual abilities

0570   **Urinary Bladder Training**   Improving bladder function for those with urge incontinence by increasing the bladder's ability to hold urine and the patient's ability to suppress urination

0580   **Urinary Catheterization**   Insertion of a catheter into the bladder for temporary or permanent drainage of urine

0582   **Urinary Catheterization: Intermittent**   Regular periodic use of a catheter to empty the bladder

0590   **Urinary Elimination Management**   Maintenance of an optimum urinary elimination pattern

0600   **Urinary Habit Training**   Establishing a predictable pattern of bladder emptying to prevent incontinence for persons with limited cognitive ability who have urge, stress, or functional incontinence

0610   **Urinary Incontinence Care**   Assistance in promoting continence and maintaining perineal skin integrity

0612   **Urinary Incontinence Care: Enuresis**   Promotion of urinary continence in children

0620   **Urinary Retention Care**   Assistance in relieving bladder distention

5480   **Values Clarification**   Assisting another to clarify her/his own values in order to facilitate effective decision-making

9050   **Vehicle Safety Promotion**   Assisting individuals, families, and communities to increase awareness of measures to reduce unintentional injuries in motorized and nonmotorized vehicles

2440   **Venous Access Devices (VAD) Maintenance**   Management of the patient with prolonged venous access via tunneled and nontunneled (percutaneous) catheters, and implanted ports

3390   **Ventilation Assistance**   Promotion of an optimal spontaneous breathing pattern that maximizes oxygen and carbon dioxide exchange in the lungs

7560   **Visitation Facilitation**   Promoting beneficial visits by family and friends

6680   **Vital Signs Monitoring**   Collection and analysis of cardiovascular, respiratory, and body temperature data to determine and prevent complications

1570   **Vomiting Management**   Prevention and alleviation of vomiting

1240   **Weight Gain Assistance**   Facilitating gain of body weight

1260   **Weight Management**   Facilitating maintenance of optimal body weight and percent body fat

1280   **Weight Reduction Assistance**   Facilitating loss of weight and/or body fat

3660   **Wound Care**   Prevention of wound complications and promotion of wound healing

3662   **Wound Care: Closed Drainage**   Maintenance of a pressure drainage system at the wound site

3680   **Wound Irrigation**   Flushing of an open wound to cleanse and remove debris and excessive drainage

Index

Page numbers followed by *t* indicate
tables.